Fungal Infections

Editors

LUIS OSTROSKY-ZEICHNER
JACK D. SOBEL

INFECTIOUS DISEASE CLINICS OF NORTH AMERICA

www.id.theclinics.com

Consulting Editor
HELEN W. BOUCHER

March 2016 • Volume 30 • Number 1

ELSEVIER

1600 John F. Kennedy Boulevard • Suite 1800 • Philadelphia, Pennsylvania, 19103-2899.
http://www.theclinics.com

INFECTIOUS DISEASE CLINICS OF NORTH AMERICA Volume 30, Number 1
March 2016 ISSN 0891–5520, ISBN-13: 978-0-323-41649-8

Editor: Kerry Holland
Developmental Editor: Donald Mumford

Infectious Disease Clinics of North America (ISSN 0891–5520) is published in March, June, September, and December by Elsevier Inc., 360 Park Avenue South, New York, NY 10010-1710. Periodicals postage paid at New York, NY and additional mailing offices. Subscription prices are $295.00 per year for US individuals, $560.00 per year for US institutions, $100.00 per year for US students, $350.00 per year for Canadian individuals, $699.00 per year for Canadian institutions, $420.00 per year for international individuals, $699.00 per year for international institutions, and $200.00 per year for Canadian and international students. To receive student rate, orders must be accompanied by name of affiliated institution, date of term, and the *signature* of program/ residency coordinator on institution letterhead. Orders will be billed at individual rate until proof of status is received. Foreign air speed delivery is included in all *Clinics* subscription prices. All prices are subject to change without notice. **POSTMASTER**: Send address changes to *Infectious Disease Clinics of North America,* Elsevier Health Sciences Division, Subcription Customer Service, 3251 Riverport Lane, Maryland Heights, MO 63043. **Customer Service: 1-800-654-2452 (US). From outside of the US and Canada, call 1-314-447-8871. Fax: 1-314-447-8029. E-mail: JournalsCustomerService-usa@elsevier.com (print support) or JournalsOnlineSupport-usa@elsevier.com (online support).**

Infectious Disease Clinics of North America is also published in Spanish by Editorial Inter-Médica, Junin 917, 1er A 1113, Buenos Aires, Argentina.

Reprints. For copies of 100 or more, of articles in this publication, please contact the Commercial Reprints Department, Elsevier Inc., 360 Park Avenue South, New York, New York 10010-1710. Tel. 212-633-3874, Fax: 212-633-3820, E-mail: reprints@elsevier.com.

Infectious Disease Clinics of North America is covered in *MEDLINE/PubMed (Index Medicus), Current Contents/ Clinical Medicine, Science Citation Alert, SCISEARCH,* and *Research Alert.*

Contributors

CONSULTING EDITOR

HELEN W. BOUCHER, MD, FIDSA, FACP
Director, Infectious Diseases Fellowship Program, Division of Geographic Medicine and Infectious Diseases, Tufts Medical Center; Associate Professor of Medicine, Tufts University School of Medicine, Boston, Massachusetts

EDITORS

LUIS OSTROSKY-ZEICHNER, MD
Professor and Vice Chairman of Medicine, Division of Infectious Diseases, McGovern Medical School, Medical Director for Epidemiology, Memorial Hermann Texas Medical Center, Houston, Texas

JACK D. SOBEL, MD
Professor of Medicine, Division of Infectious Diseases, Wayne State University School of Medicine, Detroit, Michigan

AUTHORS

MOHAMMAD T. ALBATAINEH, MD, PhD
Fungus Testing Laboratory, Department of Pathology, University of Texas Health Science Center at San Antonio, San Antonio, Texas

DAVID R. ANDES, MD
Departments of Medicine and Medical Microbiology and Immunology, University of Wisconsin, Madison, Wisconsin

JUDITH A. ANESI, MD
Fellow, Division of Infectious Diseases, University of Pennsylvania, Philadelphia, Pennsylvania

MARWAN M. AZAR, MD
Section of Infectious Diseases, Infectious Disease Fellow, Yale School of Medicine, New Haven, Connecticut

JOHN W. BADDLEY, MD, MSPH
Professor, Department of Medicine, University of Alabama at Birmingham; Professor, Department of Medicine, Birmingham VA Medical Center, Birmingham, Alabama

NATHAN C. BAHR, MD
Division of Infectious Diseases, University of Kansas, Kansas City, Kansas

JOSE CADENA, MD
Assistant Professor of Medicine, Division of Infectious Diseases, Department of Medicine, The University of Texas Health Science Center and South Texas Veterans Health Care System, San Antonio, Texas

CAROLINE G. CASTILLO, MD
Division of Infectious Diseases, University of Michigan Health System, Ann Arbor, Michigan

TOM CHILLER, MD, MPHTM
Deputy Branch Chief, Medical Epidemiologist, Mycotic Diseases Branch, Centers for Disease Control and Prevention, Atlanta, Georgia

OLIVER A. CORNELY, MD
Department I of Internal Medicine, University Hospital of Cologne; Cologne Excellence Cluster on Cellular Stress Responses in Aging-Associated Diseases (CECAD), University of Cologne; Clinical Trials Centre Cologne, ZKS Köln; German Centre for Infection Research, Partner Site Bonn-Cologne, Cologne, Germany

DIMITRIOS FARMAKIOTIS, MD
Assistant Professor of Medicine, Division of Infectious Diseases, Rhode Island Hospital, Warren Alpert Medical School of Brown University, Providence, Rhode Island

ANNETTE W. FOTHERGILL, MA, MBA, MT
Fungus Testing Laboratory, Department of Pathology, University of Texas Health Science Center at San Antonio, San Antonio, Texas

CHADI HAGE, MD
Methodist Professional Center, Indianapolis, Indiana

KIMBERLY E. HANSON, MD, MHS
Associate Professor, Departments of Medicine and Pathology, University of Utah School of Medicine, Salt Lake City, Utah

CAROL A. KAUFFMAN, MD
Division of Infectious Diseases, University of Michigan Health System; Division of Infectious Diseases, Veterans Affairs Ann Arbor Healthcare System, Ann Arbor, Michigan

PHILIPP KOEHLER, MD
Department I of Internal Medicine, University Hospital of Cologne; Cologne Excellence Cluster on Cellular Stress Responses in Aging-Associated Diseases (CECAD), University of Cologne, Cologne, Germany

DIMITRIOS P. KONTOYIANNIS, MD, ScD, FACP, FIDSA
Frances King Black endowed Professor of Medicine, Department of Infectious Diseases, Infection Control and Employee Health, The University of Texas MD Anderson Cancer Center, Houston, Texas

EILEEN K. MAZIARZ, MD
Medical Instructor, Division of Infectious Diseases and International Health, Department of Medicine, Duke University Medical Center, Durham, North Carolina

TODD P. McCARTY, MD
Instructor in Medicine, Director of Antimicrobial Stewardship, Division of Infectious Diseases, Birmingham VA Medical Center, University of Alabama at Birmingham, Birmingham, Alabama

MARISA H. MICELI, MD
Division of Infectious Diseases, University of Michigan Health System, Ann Arbor, Michigan

RAJAL K. MODY, MD, MPH
Medical Epidemiologist, Mycotic Diseases Branch, Centers for Disease Control and Prevention, Atlanta, Georgia

MIHAI G. NETEA, MD, PhD
Department of Internal Medicine, Radboud University Medical Center; Radboud Center for Infectious Diseases (RCI), Nijmegen, The Netherlands

JENIEL E. NETT, MD, PhD
Departments of Medicine and Medical Microbiology and Immunology, University of Wisconsin, Madison, Wisconsin

PETER G. PAPPAS, MD, FACP
Professor of Medicine, Director, Division of Infectious Diseases, Mycoses Study Group Education and Research Consortium, University of Alabama at Birmingham, Birmingham, Alabama

THOMAS F. PATTERSON, MD
Professor of Medicine and Chief, Division of Infectious Diseases, Department of Medicine, The University of Texas Health Science Center and South Texas Veterans Health Care System, San Antonio, Texas

JOHN R. PERFECT, MD
James B. Duke Professor of Medicine, Chief, Division of Infectious Diseases and International Health, Department of Medicine, Duke University Medical Center, Durham, North Carolina

MARGARET V. POWERS-FLETCHER, PhD
Medical and Public Health Laboratory Microbiology Fellow, Department of Pathology, ARUP Laboratories, University of Utah School of Medicine, Salt Lake City, Utah

RYAN F. RELICH, MD, PhD, D(ABMM), MLS(ASCP)[CM]SM[CM]
Division of Clinical Microbiology, Department of Pathology and Laboratory Medicine, Indiana University Health Pathology Laboratory, Indiana University School of Medicine, Indianapolis, Indiana

SANJAY G. REVANKAR, MD
Professor of Medicine, Division of Infectious Diseases, Harper University Hospital, Wayne State University, Detroit, Michigan

ANDREJ SPEC, MD
Infectious Disease Fellow, Washington University School of Medicine, Saint Louis, Missouri

NATHAN W. STOCKAMP, MD
Division of Infectious Disease, Department of Internal Medicine, University of California, San Francisco, Fresno, San Francisco, California

DEANNA A. SUTTON, PhD
Fungus Testing Laboratory, Department of Pathology, University of Texas Health Science Center at San Antonio, San Antonio, Texas

GEORGE R. THOMPSON III, MD
Associate Professor of Internal Medicine, Division of Infectious Diseases, Department of Internal Medicine; Associate Professor of Medicine, Department of Medical Microbiology and Immunology; Division of Infectious Diseases, Department of Medicine, University of California, Davis, Davis, California

SNIGDHA VALLABHANENI, MD, MPH
Medical Epidemiologist, Mycotic Diseases Branch, Centers for Disease Control and Prevention, Atlanta, Georgia

FRANK L. VAN DE VEERDONK, MD, PhD
Department of Internal Medicine, Radboud University Medical Center; Radboud Center for Infectious Diseases (RCI), Nijmegen, The Netherlands

TIFFANY WALKER, MD
Epidemic Intelligence Service Officer, Mycotic Diseases Branch, Centers for Disease Control and Prevention, Atlanta, Georgia

XIAOWEN WANG, MD
Department of Internal Medicine, Radboud University Medical Center, Nijmegen, The Netherlands; Department of Dermatology, Peking University First Hospital, Beijing, China

LAWRENCE J. WHEAT, MD
MiraVista Diagnostics, Indianapolis, Indiana

NATHAN P. WIEDERHOLD, PharmD
Fungus Testing Laboratory, Department of Pathology, University of Texas Health Science Center at San Antonio, San Antonio, Texas

EUNICE H. WONG, MD
Fellow, Division of Infectious Diseases, Harper University Hospital, Wayne State University, Detroit, Michigan

Contents

Preface: Fungal Infections   xiii

Luis Ostrosky-Zeichner and Jack D. Sobel

The Global Burden of Fungal Diseases   1

Snigdha Vallabhaneni, Rajal K. Mody, Tiffany Walker, and Tom Chiller

Fungal diseases require greater attention today than ever before, given the expanding population of immunosuppressed patients who are at higher risk for these diseases. This article reports on distribution, incidence, and prevalence of various fungal diseases and points out gaps in knowledge where such data are not available. Fungal diseases that contribute substantially to global morbidity and mortality are highlighted. Long-term, sustainable surveillance programs for fungal diseases and better noninvasive and reliable diagnostic tools are needed to estimate the burden of these diseases more accurately.

Update from the Laboratory: Clinical Identification and Susceptibility Testing of Fungi and Trends in Antifungal Resistance   13

Mohammad T. Albataineh, Deanna A. Sutton, Annette W. Fothergill, and Nathan P. Wiederhold

Despite the availability of new diagnostic assays and broad-spectrum antifungal agents, invasive fungal infections remain a significant challenge to clinicians and are associated with marked morbidity and mortality. In addition, the number of etiologic agents of invasive mycoses has increased accompanied by an expansion in the immunocompromised patient populations, and the use of molecular tools for fungal identification and characterization has resulted in the discovery of several cryptic species. This article reviews various methods used to identify fungi and perform antifungal susceptibility testing in the clinical laboratory. Recent developments in antifungal resistance are also discussed.

Nonculture Diagnostics in Fungal Disease   37

Margaret V. Powers-Fletcher and Kimberly E. Hanson

Fungal diagnostics that utilize antibody, antigen or nucleic acid detection offer several advantages that supplement traditional culture-based methods. As a group, nonculture assays can help identify patients with invasive fungal infection (IFI) sooner than is possible with culture, are often more sensitive, and can be used to guide early interventions. Challenges associated with these techniques include the possibility for contamination or cross-reactivity as well as the potential for false negative tests. This review summarizes the test characteristics and clinical utility of nonculture-based laboratory methods.

Antifungal Agents: Spectrum of Activity, Pharmacology, and Clinical Indications   51

Jeniel E. Nett and David R. Andes

The currently available antifungal therapies vary significantly in terms of spectrum of activity, pharmacologic properties, toxicity, and potential for drug–drug interactions. This article provides a history of antifungal development and discusses the characteristics of individual drugs and drug classes, including the amphotericin B formulations, the triazoles, the echinocandins, and flucytosine. For each drug, the clinically relevant pharmacokinetics are reviewed, the spectrum of activity described, and the Food and Drug Administration–approved clinical indications examined. Antifungal side-effects, therapeutic drug monitoring, and drug–drug interactions are summarized. The variations among different formulations are highlighted.

Basic Genetics and Immunology of Candida Infections   85

Xiaowen Wang, Frank L. van de Veerdonk, and Mihai G. Netea

Candida infections can cause superficial and invasive disease. Several essential mechanisms underlying the pathogenesis of these infections were known for some time, such as neutropenia predisposing to invasive disease, and CD4 lymphopenia causing increased susceptibility to mucosal candidiasis. However, the development of novel genetic screening techniques has led to several new insights in the genetics and immunology of candida infections. This article highlights novel insights in the pathogenesis of mucocutaneous and invasive candidiasis that have been identified in recent years.

Invasive Candidiasis   103

Todd P. McCarty and Peter G. Pappas

Invasive candidiasis is a collective term that refers to a group of infectious syndromes caused by a variety of species of *Candida*, 5 of which cause most cases. Candidemia is the most commonly recognized syndrome associated with invasive candidiasis. Certain conditions may influence the likelihood for one species versus another in a specific clinical scenario, and this can have important implications for selection of antifungal therapy and the duration of treatment. Molecular diagnostic technology plays an ever-increasing role as an adjunct to traditional culture-based diagnostics, offering significant potential toward improvement in patient care.

Invasive Aspergillosis: Current Strategies for Diagnosis and Management   125

Jose Cadena, George R. Thompson III, and Thomas F. Patterson

Aspergillosis remains a significant cause of morbidity and mortality in the immunocompromised population. The spectrum of disease is broad, ranging from severe and rapidly fatal infection to noninvasive disease. The diversity of patients and risk factors complicates diagnostic and therapeutic decision-making. Invasive procedures are often precluded by host status; noninvasive diagnostic tests vary in their sensitivity and specificity. Advancements in understanding the pathophysiology of invasive aspergillosis and host genetics in differential risk have also occurred. Future work may assist in therapeutic decision-making and patient prognosis.

Voriconazole remains the preferred agent for treatment. Additional alternatives have emerged.

Mucormycoses 143

Dimitrios Farmakiotis and Dimitrios P. Kontoyiannis

Life-threatening infections from virulent, angioinvasive molds of the order Mucorales are being recognized with increasing frequency in immunosuppressed hosts. Advances in the understanding of pathogenesis, early diagnosis, and the recent availability of active, nontoxic drugs have improved the prospects for effective control and even cure of this devastating infection. However, rates of delayed diagnosis and mortality are still high, partially because of the low yield and complexity of culture-based and molecular diagnostic methods. Therefore, there is an urgent need for novel diagnostic modalities and effective therapeutic approaches.

Dematiaceous Molds 165

Eunice H. Wong and Sanjay G. Revankar

Dematiaceous fungi are the cause of phaeohyphomycosis, a term that encompasses many clinical syndromes, from local infections due to trauma to widely disseminated infection in immunocompromised patients. These fungi are unique owing to the presence of melanin in their cell walls, which imparts the characteristic dark color to their spores and hyphae. Melanin may also be a virulence factor. Local infection may be cured with excision alone, whereas systemic disease is often refractory to therapy. Azoles have the most consistent in vitro activity. Further studies are needed to better understand the pathogenesis and treatment of these uncommon infections.

Cryptococcosis 179

Eileen K. Maziarz and John R. Perfect

Cryptococcosis is an invasive mycosis caused by pathogenic encapsulated yeasts in the genus Cryptococcus. Cryptococcus gained prominence as a pathogen capable of widespread disease outbreaks in vulnerable populations. We have gained insight into the pathobiology of Cryptococcus, including the yeast's capacity to adapt to environmental pressures, exploit new geographic environments, and cause disease in both immunocompromised and apparently immunocompetent hosts. Inexpensive, point-of-care testing makes diagnosis more feasible than ever. The associated worldwide burden and mortality remains unacceptably high. Novel screening strategies and preemptive therapy offer promise at making a sustained and much needed impact on this sugar-coated opportunistic mycosis.

Histoplasmosis 207

Lawrence J. Wheat, Marwan M. Azar, Nathan C. Bahr, Andrej Spec, Ryan F. Relich, and Chadi Hage

Although histoplasmosis is highly endemic in certain regions of the Americas, disease may be seen globally and should not be overlooked in patients with unexplained pulmonary or systemic illnesses. Most patients exhibit pulmonary signs and symptoms, accompanied by radiographic abnormalities, which often are mistaken for community-acquired pneumonia caused by bacterial or viral agents. Once a diagnosis is considered, a panel of mycologic and non–culture-based assays is adequate to establish a diagnosis in a few days to a week in most patients. Once diagnosed, the treatment is highly effective even in immunocompromised patients.

Coccidioidomycosis   229

Nathan W. Stockamp and George R. Thompson III

Coccidioides immitis and *C posadasii* are pathogenic dimorphic fungi responsible for causing coccidioidomycosis in the Southwestern United States and Central and South America. Antifungal therapy is beneficial and entails careful periodic assessment with therapies ranging from none or short courses of therapy to prolonged antifungal therapy. Factors that influence the decision to treat are the duration or severity of infection, radiographic findings, anticomplementary titers, presence of underlying immunosuppression, and comorbidities. Cure for disseminated infection is infrequent with current treatment regimens. This review summarizes the management guidelines for various disease manifestations and reviews data on challenging cases with newer agents.

Blastomycosis   247

Caroline G. Castillo, Carol A. Kauffman, and Marisa H. Miceli

Blastomycosis is an endemic fungal infection due to *Blastomyces dermatitidis* that most commonly causes pneumonia; but the organism can disseminate to any organ system, most commonly the skin, bones/joints, and genitourinary tract. Both immunocompetent and immunocompromised persons can be infected, but more severe disease occurs in the immunocompromised. Blastomycosis can be diagnosed by culture, direct visualization of the yeast in affected tissue, and/or antigen testing. Treatment course and duration depend on severity of illness. For mild to moderate pulmonary disease the treatment is itraconazole. For severe blastomycosis, lipid formulation amphotericin B is given, followed by step-down therapy with itraconazole.

Contemporary Strategies in the Prevention and Management of Fungal Infections   265

Philipp Koehler and Oliver A. Cornely

Major patient groups at risk for invasive fungal infection are found in hematology, intensive care, and abdominal surgery units. The vast majority of invasive fungal infections are candidemia, pulmonary aspergillosis, and pulmonary or sinunasal mucormycosis, the latter typically in the context of diabetes. Clinical presentation is highly variable and depends on host, fungus, and organs involved. Symptoms are unspecific and, outside of fungemia, diagnosis is established by radiographic imaging combined with microbiological, serologic, and histopathological workup. Complex prevention and management strategies have been developed, and it is recommended to follow institutional pathways to standardize diagnostic and therapeutic strategies.

Approach to the Solid Organ Transplant Patient with Suspected Fungal Infection   277

Judith A. Anesi and John W. Baddley

In solid organ transplant (SOT) recipients, invasive fungal infections (IFIs) are associated with significant morbidity and mortality. Detection of IFIs can be difficult because the signs and symptoms are similar to those of viral or bacterial infections, and diagnostic techniques have limited sensitivity and specificity. Clinicians must rely on knowledge of the patient's risk factors for fungal infection to make a diagnosis. The authors describe their approach to the SOT recipient with suspected fungal infection. The epidemiology of IFIs in the SOT population is reviewed, and a syndromic approach to suspected IFI in SOT recipients is described.

Index   297

INFECTIOUS DISEASE CLINICS OF NORTH AMERICA

FORTHCOMING ISSUES

June 2016
Antibiotic Resistance
Robert A. Bonomo and
Richard R. Watkins, *Editors*

September 2016
**Infection Prevention and Control in
Healthcare, Part I: Facility Planning
and Management**
Keith S. Kaye and Sorabh Dhar, *Editors*

December 2016
**Infection Prevention and Control in
Healthcare, Part II: Clinical Management
of Infections**
Keith S. Kaye and Sorabh Dhar, *Editors*

RECENT ISSUES

December 2015
Pediatric Infectious Disease: Part II
Mary Anne Jackson and Angela L. Myers,
Editors

September 2015
Pediatric Infectious Disease: Part I
Mary Anne Jackson and Angela L. Myers,
Editors

June 2015
**Lyme Disease and Other Infections
Transmitted by *Ixodes scapularis***
Paul G. Auwaerter, *Editor*

RELATED INTEREST

Clinics in Laboratory Medicine, December 2015 (Volume 35, Issue 4)
Tickborne Borrelia Infections
Elitza S. Theel, *Editor*

THE CLINICS ARE AVAILABLE ONLINE!
Access your subscription at:
www.theclinics.com

Preface

Fungal Infections

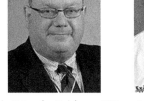 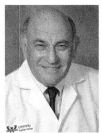

Luis Ostrosky-Zeichner, MD   Jack D. Sobel, MD
Editors

The *Infectious Disease Clinics of North America* had dedicated fungal infections issues in 2002 (Walsh and Rex, editors) and 2006 (Patterson, editor). It's been 10 years since the last thematic issue, and it is a pleasure to present an update on contemporary data and issues in medical mycology.

Fungal infections have gone from diseases caused by obscure pathogens often studied in the basement of medical schools, and rare patient events with only one or two therapeutic options, to highly complex diseases affecting the most vulnerable patients. An increase in frequency in fungal infections is also widely reported, this being mainly related to advances in medical science that allow patients to survive devastating diseases at the cost of a compromised immune system. In the diagnostic area, we have gone from relying on histopathology and culture for diagnosis, to an array of contemporary diagnostic techniques, including sophisticated culturing techniques, genetic detection/sequencing, serodiagnostics, and biomarkers. The one or two therapeutic options have expanded to an arsenal of antifungals, with new drug classes and an encouraging pipeline of new agents.

In this issue of the *Infectious Diseases Clinics of North America*, experts in the field address the global burden of fungal infections and recent epidemiologic trends and provide an in-depth review at current antifungal agents. Authors present the state of the art in culture, identification, and resistance testing; introduce an article of non-culture-based diagnostics; discuss new antifungal management strategies such as prophylaxis and pre-emptive therapy; and describe critical new information on the major fungal diseases, including invasive candidiasis, invasive aspergillosis, mucormycosis, infections by dematiaceous molds, cryptococcosis, and the endemic mycoses. Unique to this latest review is an article dealing with host determinants of the genetics and immunology of fungal infections. Finally, a systematic and timely approach to solid organ transplant patients with a suspected fungal infection is described.

Infect Dis Clin N Am 30 (2016) xiii–xiv
http://dx.doi.org/10.1016/j.idc.2015.12.001
0891-5520/16/$ – see front matter © 2016 Published by Elsevier Inc.

The past 10 years have been exciting with major developments in multiple areas of medical mycology, and we anticipate similar advances in the next 10 years.

Luis Ostrosky-Zeichner, MD
Division of Infectious Diseases
McGovern Medical School
Memorial Hermann Texas Medical Center
Houston, TX 77030, USA

Jack D. Sobel, MD
Infectious Diseases
Wayne State University School of Medicine
Detroit, MI 48322, USA

E-mail addresses:
Luis.Ostrosky-Zeichner@uth.tmc.edu (L. Ostrosky-Zeichner)
jsobel@med.wayne.edu (J.D. Sobel)

The Global Burden of Fungal Diseases

Snigdha Vallabhaneni, MD, MPH*, Rajal K. Mody, MD, MPH, Tiffany Walker, MD, Tom Chiller, MD, MPHTM

KEYWORDS

- Global burden • Epidemiology • Fungal diseases • *Candida* • *Cryptococcus*
- *Aspergillus* • Mold • Endemic mycoses

KEY POINTS

- Fungal pathogens are emerging as an even more important cause of disease as the number of people with severely immunocompromising conditions, such as HIV, cancer, and organ transplantation, who are at higher risk for fungal diseases, increases.
- *Candida* species are the most important cause of serious invasive fungal infections, but infections caused by *Cryptococcus*, *Pneumocystis*, invasive molds, and dimorphic molds also contribute to a substantial burden of disease.
- Systematic surveillance for fungal infections is scarce and is needed to make informed estimates of the global burden of fungal diseases.

INTRODUCTION

Assessment of the global burden and epidemiologic trends of fungal diseases is critical to prioritizing prevention strategies, diagnostic modalities, and therapeutic interventions. The global burden of fungal diseases is increasing, given the expanding number of patients at risk for these infections, including people living with human immunodeficiency virus (PLHIV), transplant recipients, patients with cancer, patients receiving immunomodulators (eg, tumor necrosis factor-α inhibitors), premature neonates, and the elderly. Recent increases in travel and changes in climate may also result in changes in geographic distribution of fungi.

Disclaimer: The findings and conclusions in this report are those of the authors and do not necessarily represent the official position of the Centers for Disease Control and Prevention.
Funding Source: No funding source to report.
Conflict of Interest: The authors have no relevant conflicts of interest to report.
Mycotic Diseases Branch, Centers for Disease Control and Prevention, Atlanta, GA, USA
* Corresponding author. Centers for Disease Control and Prevention, 1600 Clifton Road Northeast, Mailstop C-09, Atlanta, GA 30329.
E-mail address: fco6@cdc.gov

Infect Dis Clin N Am 30 (2016) 1–11
http://dx.doi.org/10.1016/j.idc.2015.10.004
0891-5520/16/$ – see front matter Published by Elsevier Inc.

id.theclinics.com

Quantifying the global burden of fungal diseases is challenging. Fungal diseases are often difficult to diagnose because they manifest with nonspecific symptoms and are not routinely suspected. Diagnosis frequently requires invasive tissue specimens, fungi do not always grow in culture, histopathologic identification is challenging, fungal antibody tests may cross-react, and skin testing for latent infection is generally not available. The most comprehensive estimates of any disease come from surveillance (formal systematic case counts within a specified population). In some parts of the world, limited single institution-based, population-based, or sentinel surveillance for some fungal diseases provides helpful information on trends in the burden of that infection. However, the lack of routine surveillance for most fungal diseases greatly limits the availability of data needed to inform burden estimates. In some cases, administrative health care data documenting hospital discharge diagnoses or registries of patients with fungal diseases have been used in lieu of surveillance.[1] Although helpful, these assessments do not capture the full burden of disease. Recent attempts to estimate fungal disease burden have been made using far-reaching extrapolations from limited available data on susceptible populations and prevalence of disease.[2] These estimates highlight important data gaps and should be interpreted cautiously.

This article reports on distribution, incidence, and prevalence of selected fungal disease, and points out the gaps in knowledge where such data were not available. The review is organized by pathogen and by global region, highlighting the fungal diseases that contribute the most to global morbidity and mortality.

YEASTS
Candida

Candida bloodstream infection (candidemia) is the most common form of invasive *Candida* infection and is associated with substantial morbidity and mortality. The incidence of candidemia in the general population and hospitalized and intensive care unit patients has been reported from multiple countries. These estimates vary widely within regions of the same country and over time.[3] Representative studies are listed in **Table 1**.[4–14] The reasons for these differences in candidemia incidence are likely multifactorial, including underlying ecology of *Candida* spp, differences in underlying patient populations, resources available for medical care and training programs, difficulties in implementing hospital infection control programs, and differences in surveillance methodologies.[3] Although a plethora of single-institution studies have been reported, only a few countries have conducted geographically widespread surveillance, and in still fewer countries has this been sustained over time to describe trends in candidemia.[5,12,15] To truly understand the global burden of candidemia, there is a need for within- and between-country collaborations to systematically study candidemia in different settings.

Species distribution of *Candida* infections in various parts of the world are listed in **Box 1**.[5,8,16–19] The differences in species distribution may relate to local ecology of *Candida* spp and is important because variation in antifungal susceptibility patterns by species has implications for treatment success. Furthermore, the predominance of some species, such as *Candida parapsilosis*, signals a need for examination of hospital infection control practices.

Invasive infection caused by antifungal-resistant *Candida* spp is an emerging problem. Fluconazole resistance among *Candida albicans* isolates is estimated between 0% and 5%, with the highest rate reported in South Africa.[20] Fluconazole resistance is a much bigger problem among non-*albicans* spp and ranges between 5% and

Table 1
Incidence of candidemia by year, country, and patient population, select studies

Year	Country	Candidemia Incidence			Ref
		Per 100,000 Population	Per 10,000 Patient Days	Per 1000 Discharges	
1992	USA	9	—	—	4
2008	USA	14	—	—	4
2013	USA	10	—	—	5
1999–2004	Canada	2.9	—	—	6
1995–1999	Finland	2	—	—	7
2004–2012	Norway	3.9	—	—	8
2002–2003	Spain	4.3	—	—	9
2003–2004	Brazil	—	3.7	—	10
1998–2000	USA	—	1.5	—	11
2004–2009	France	—	1.0–1.2	—	12
2010–2011	Asia (25 hospitals across Asia)	—	—	1.2	13
	India	—	—	6 (per 1000 ICU admission)	14

65%, with the highest rate reported in Denmark.[20] Fluconazole resistance is problematic because it is the only antifungal drug available for treatment of *Candida* infections in many parts of the world. Echinocandin resistance has also been reported in some settings; in the United States, approximately 6% of *Candida glabrata* isolates are resistant to echinocandins.[5]

Cryptococcus

Disseminated *Cryptococcus neoformans* disease is largely associated with HIV infection. A 2009 study estimated that nearly 1 million cases of cryptococcal meningitis occurred worldwide each year, with more than 600,000 deaths annually.[21] More than 700,000 cases were estimated to occur in sub-Saharan Africa annually, where the burden of HIV is also the highest. This study was based on limited published reports of the burden of cryptococcal meningitis at that time, and as such, the estimated range of total infections per year was very wide (371,700–1,544,000). Increased efforts aimed at earlier diagnosis of HIV, rapid antiretroviral treatment initiation, and improved

Box 1
Patterns of *Candida* species distribution

- *C albicans* was the leading cause of candidemia worldwide, but its predominance has decreased during the past two decades.[5,8]

- Currently, only about one-third of candidemia in the United States and Western Europe is caused by *C albicans*; the second leading cause of candidemia is *C glabrata* followed by *C parapsilosis*.[5]

- In many regions of the world, *C albicans* candidemia still predominates, but *C tropicalis* or *C parapsilosis* are the second leading cause rather than *C glabrata*.[16,17]

- In some countries in Asia and South America, *C tropicalis* is the most common agent and *C albicans* has dropped to third or fourth in frequency.[18,19]

retention in care, along with cryptococcal antigen screening efforts, should reduce the burden of cryptococcal disease in coming years.[22] Revised estimates of the burden of cryptococcosis are needed based on current epidemiology.

C neoformans infection can also affect patients with immunosuppression resulting from solid organ or bone marrow transplantation, and those receiving short- and long-term treatment with steroids or tumor necrosis factor-α inhibitors,[23] but the burden of disease in this population has not been well-reported.

Cryptococcus gattii infections are emerging in some areas of the world. *C gattii* is endemic in Papua New Guinea, Australia, and South America. Starting in the late 1990s, *C gattii* infections were recognized in British Columbia, Canada (218 cases reported during 1999–2007) and in the US Pacific Northwest since 2004 (approximately 100 cases reported in the United States).[24] Unlike *C neoformans*, which usually affects immunocompromised individuals, *C gattii* infections can also cause serious disease in immunocompetent hosts.

OTHER FUNGUS
Pneumocystis jirovecii

Pneumocystis pneumonia (PCP) was a rare disease until the AIDS epidemic began in the early 1980s. PCP became the leading AIDS-defining diagnosis among PLHIV in the United States and Europe. Since the advent of highly active antiretroviral therapy, combined with aggressive PCP prophylaxis with trimethoprim-sulfamethoxazole, the incidence of PCP decreased dramatically in North America and Europe; in one study, incidence decreased from 4.9 cases per 100 person-years to 0.3 cases per 100 person-years among PLHIV between 1995 and 1998.[25] Despite this decline, PCP is still an important opportunistic infection among PLHIV in the United States and Europe. Initial reports from developing countries suggested that PCP was a less important cause of morbidity and mortality than tuberculosis and enteric pathogens, but these rates may have been artificially low because of poor access to PCP diagnostic testing and competing risk of death from other opportunistic infections.

PCP is also a leading cause of opportunistic infections in HIV-negative persons with malignancies, inflammatory disease, organ transplant recipients, and those receiving prolonged courses of corticosteroids,[26] but the burden in this population is unclear.

MOLDS
Aspergillus

In a multicenter study of invasive fungal infections (IFI) among transplant recipients at 23 US transplant centers during 2001 to 2006, invasive aspergillosis accounted for nearly 20% of all IFIs, second only to invasive candidiasis. The annual incidence of invasive aspergillosis among transplant recipients was 0.65%[27,28] and incidence of invasive aspergillosis was highest (3.9%) among hematopoietic stem cell transplant (HSCT) recipients with a matched, unrelated donor.[28] A multicenter French study describing trends in IFIs based on hospital discharge data found a 4.4% increase in invasive aspergillosis each year during 2001 to 2010[29]; similar increases have been noted in other parts of the world.

Data describing invasive aspergillosis in other parts of the world are sparse. A multicenter Brazilian study of patients with HSCT and hematologic malignancy reported invasive aspergillosis to be the most common IFI, with 6.5% of patients developing the disease.[30] Published data on prevalence from most of Asia or Africa are lacking.[16] Although the current burden is not known, aspergillosis is likely to increase as resource-limited countries increase organ and bone marrow transplantation.

Mucormycetes

Although mucormycosis is less common than invasive aspergillosis, its incidence seems to be rising.[29] Several studies have shown a rise in the proportion of HSCT recipients developing mucormycosis (8% during 2001–2006 vs 1% in the 1990s) after widespread use of voriconazole prophylaxis to prevent invasive aspergillosis and other fungal infections.[31] Although data on mucormycosis are sparse, India contributes substantially to the global burden of this disease. Unlike the United States and Europe, mucormycosis is largely associated with diabetes in India.[16] This burden is likely to grow given the rising rates of obesity and diabetes in India and many other parts of the world.

Scedosporium

Scedosporium (Pseudallescheria) spp are rare mold pathogens of concern because of echinocandin resistance and variable susceptibility to azoles and high mortality.[32] The actual burden of this disease is largely unknown but a single-institution retrospective review from the United States revealed increasing incidence from 0.82 cases per 100,000 inpatient days during 1993 to 1998 to 1.33 cases during 1999 to 2005.[33]

Fusarium

Invasive infections with Fusarium spp occurs in the setting of severe immunosuppression and mortality ranges from 50% to 80%.[34] One prospective study of several transplant centers in the United States noted a cumulative incidence of rare molds, including Fusarium, of 0.25%,[27,28] which was significantly lower than the incidence of 2.5% among patients with HSCT and hematologic malignancy reported from eight centers in Brazil.[30] The global burden of fusariosis is unknown.

ENDEMIC MOLDS
Histoplasma capsulatum

The epidemiology of histoplasmosis in the United States has shifted from an HIV-related disease to one that affects individuals after organ transplantation or chronic immunosuppression from inflammatory conditions,[35] and now is the most common transplant-related endemic mycosis in the United States.[36] One study evaluating a random sample of US Medicare data reported an incidence of 6.1 cases per 100,000 person-years in the Midwest during 1999 to 2008.[37] The actual burden in the United States is unknown outside of a few states because histoplasmosis is not nationally notifiable.

In Latin America, histoplasmosis is the most clinically significant endemic mycosis,[38] and the most common opportunistic infection among PLHIV, with an incidence reported by one study of 0.15 per 100,000 person-years.[39] Histoplasmosis has also been described in China[40] and India.[41] More than 1200 Thai cases that have been reported to date have mostly occurred among PLHIV.[41] African histoplasmosis has been described in Central and Western Africa and Madagascar. More than 200 cases have been reported in the literature from Nigeria, Niger, Senegal, Congo, and Uganda.[42] There is no way to estimate the burden of this disease in this region because it has no systematic surveillance.

Coccidioides immitis and Coccidioides posadasii

The most reliable burden estimates of coccidioidomycosis are from the United States, where it is a nationally notifiable disease. During 1998 to 2011, the incidence of reported coccidioidomycosis increased substantially in the endemic area from 5.3 to

42.6 per 100,000.[43] Subsequent reports show a decline in incidence since 2011; the reasons for the initial increase and subsequent decline are not clear. These estimates are likely to be gross underestimations of the actual burden because an estimated 60% of those with disease do not seek medical care, and many symptomatic infections go undiagnosed.[44]

The incidence of disease in Central and South America has not been clearly defined. Skin testing surveys in Mexico found positivity rates between 40% and 90% in certain states,[45] indicating a high frequency of exposure to the fungus. Endemic regions have been defined in Mexico, Guatemala, Honduras, Nicaragua, northern Venezuela, northeastern Brazil, Argentina, Bolivia, and Paraguay.[38,46]

Paracoccidioides brasiliensis

Paracoccidioidomycosis has an endemic zone that extends south from Mexico to Argentina.[47] Based on skin testing studies in humans and animals, it is estimated that 50% to 75% of adults in endemic areas have been exposed to the fungus. Brazil, where the disease was first described, has the highest burden of disease, with more than 80% of all cases of paracoccidioidomycosis occurring in six Brazilian states.[38] Brazilian data also suggest that the reported incidence of paracoccidioidomycosis is between one and three cases per 100,000 persons living in the endemic areas; in Colombia, the reported incidence is lower at 0.05 to 0.22 per 100,000 persons.[48]

Blastomyces dermatitidis

The incidence of blastomycosis from certain areas in the United States and Canada, where the disease is reportable, ranges from 0.3 to 41.9 cases per 100,000, with north-central parts of Wisconsin showing the highest incidence rate.[49–51] There were approximately 1000 blastomycosis-related hospitalizations in the United States during 2007 to 2011.[1] Again, the true burden in the United States is unknown because of the lack of reporting beyond a few states. Data on the burden of blastomycosis in other parts of the world are not available.

Talaromyces (Penicillium) marneffei

Infections with *Talaromyces (Penicillium) marneffei* are primarily seen as HIV-associated opportunistic infections in Southeast Asia. Although the true incidence of *T marneffei* is unknown, it was the third most commonly reported opportunistic infection after tuberculosis and cryptococcosis in northern Thailand in the 1990s.[52] Eastern India[53] and Southern China[54] are also endemic for *T marneffei*. In a retrospective study of the 8000 stored serum samples from Chinese PLHIV during 2004 to 2011, nearly 10% had evidence of *T marneffei* antigen[55]; the prevalence of antigen positivity (28%) was higher among those with CD4 counts less than 50 cells/mm^3. It remains unclear how these results correlate with the actual burden of infection.

OTHER FUNGAL ORGANISMS
Organisms Causing Eumycetoma

Mycetoma has a worldwide distribution, but is endemic primarily in tropical and subtropical regions.[56] Based on a review of 8000 published cases, Mexico, India, and Sudan seem to carry the highest burden of mycetoma.[57,58] Mycetoma has been recognized by the World Health Organization as a neglected tropical disease. It affects many people in the prime of their lives, yet little is known about its incidence, prevalence, diagnosis, or treatment.

Table 2
Emerging fungal infections

Organism	Years First Detected	Global Region to Date	Notes	Ref
Emmonsia spp	2008–2011	South Africa	Finding of a new species of dimorphic fungus that is pathogenic to humans	59
Candida auris	2004–2006	Korea, India, Pakistan, South Africa, Kuwait	Intrinsically resistant to multiple antifungal agents	60
Sporothrix schenckii	1987–present	Brazil	Acquired from contact with cats (in addition to inoculation after contact with plants)	61
Azole-resistant *Aspergillus fumigatus*	—	Multiple regions including in Europe, Japan, India, Iran	Clinical and environmental *A fumigatus* found to be azole-resistant; possibly linked to fungicide use in agriculture	62

Emerging Pathogens

Newly emerging fungal pathogens are described each year, as fungal species not previously known to cause disease are recognized as agents of opportunistic infections in high-risk patients. Several recently described emerging fungal pathogens are listed in **Table 2**[59–62] along with their significance and implications. Many other established and emerging fungal organisms are not included in this review. Infections caused by yeast, such as *Trichosporon*, and rare molds, such as *Exserohilum*, *Bipolaris*, and *Sarocladium*, are conditions that are relevant in certain susceptible populations, but the burden of these conditions is not known.

SUMMARY

Fungal diseases cause considerable morbidity and mortality globally, but their burden is largely undetermined. The prevalence of invasive *Candida* infection has been the best-studied of all fungal diseases. Several population-based estimates describe rates of candidemia, especially in North America and Europe. Nevertheless, it is difficult to estimate the worldwide burden of this disease because of major data gaps from Africa and some parts of Asia. Estimates of the global burden of cryptococcal disease, which is probably the next best-studied fungal disease, have been attempted but relied on limited data from a few settings.[21] Regional burden estimates for other diseases, such as histoplasmosis and coccidioidomycosis, exist but lack of data from other endemic areas makes global burden estimation challenging.

In general, lack of surveillance data, especially in the developing world, makes calculating reliable burden estimates very challenging. Establishing the incidence and prevalence of infection through institution of surveillance systems is critical to understand disease burden and to describe emerging fungal threats and antimicrobial resistance. Developing much needed, long-term, sustainable, surveillance programs for fungal diseases should be a priority. To begin with, efforts to improve the diagnosis and recognition of fungal infections are paramount. Focusing surveillance activities on populations at risk (candidemia in intensive care unit patients, mold infections in transplant recipients, and so forth) may help narrow the scope of surveillance programs and reduce cost. Developing better noninvasive and reliable diagnostic tools for fungal diseases will facilitate laboratory diagnosis and thereby increase case detection and reporting to surveillance. Such information serves as a foundation for appropriate, targeted, and measurable prevention and control efforts.

REFERENCES

1. Seitz AE, Younes N, Steiner CA, et al. Incidence and trends of blastomycosis-associated hospitalizations in the United States. PLoS One 2014;9(8):e105466.
2. Brown GD, Denning DW, Gow NA, et al. Hidden killers: human fungal infections. Sci Transl Med 2012;4(165):165rv113.
3. Pfaller MA, Diekema DJ. Epidemiology of invasive candidiasis: a persistent public health problem. Clin Microbiol Rev 2007;20(1):133–63.
4. Cleveland AA, Farley MM, Harrison LH, et al. Changes in incidence and antifungal drug resistance in candidemia: results from population-based laboratory surveillance in Atlanta and Baltimore, 2008–2011. Clin Microbiol Rev 2012; 55(10):1352–61.
5. Cleveland AA, Harrison LH, Farley MM, et al. Declining incidence of candidemia and the shifting epidemiology of Candida resistance in two US metropolitan areas, 2008-2013: results from population-based surveillance. PLoS One 2015; 10(3):e0120452.
6. Laupland KB, Gregson DB, Church DL, et al. Invasive Candida species infections: a 5 year population-based assessment. J Antimicrob Chemother 2005;56(3):532–7.
7. Poikonen E, Lyytikainen O, Anttila VJ, et al. Candidemia in Finland, 1995-1999. Emerg Infect Dis 2003;9(8):985–90.
8. Hesstvedt L, Gaustad P, Andersen CT, et al. Twenty-two years of candidaemia surveillance: results from a Norwegian national study. Clin Microbiol Infect 2015;21(10):938–45.
9. Almirante B, Rodriguez D, Park BJ, et al. Epidemiology and predictors of mortality in cases of Candida bloodstream infection: results from population-based surveillance, Barcelona, Spain, from 2002 to 2003. J Clin Microbiol 2005;43(4):1829–35.
10. Colombo AL, Nucci M, Park BJ, et al. Epidemiology of candidemia in Brazil: a nationwide sentinel surveillance of candidemia in eleven medical centers. J Clin Microbiol 2006;44(8):2816–23.
11. Hajjeh RA, Sofair AN, Harrison LH, et al. Incidence of bloodstream infections due to Candida species and in vitro susceptibilities of isolates collected from 1998 to 2000 in a population-based active surveillance program. J Clin Microbiol 2004; 42(4):1519–27.
12. Lortholary O, Renaudat C, Sitbon K, et al. Worrisome trends in incidence and mortality of candidemia in intensive care units (Paris area, 2002-2010). Intensive Care Med 2014;40(9):1303–12.
13. Tan BH, Chakrabarti A, Li RY, et al. Incidence and species distribution of candidaemia in Asia: a laboratory-based surveillance study. Clin Microbiol Infect 2015; 21(10):946–53.
14. Chakrabarti A, Sood P, Rudramurthy SM, et al. Incidence, characteristics and outcome of ICU-acquired candidemia in India. Intensive Care Med 2015;41(2): 285–95.
15. Pfaller MA, Andes DR, Diekema DJ, et al. Epidemiology and outcomes of invasive candidiasis due to non-albicans species of Candida in 2,496 patients: data from the Prospective Antifungal Therapy (PATH) registry 2004-2008. PLoS One 2014; 9(7):e101510.

16. Chakrabarti A, Chatterjee SS, Shivaprakash MR. Overview of opportunistic fungal infections in India. Nihon Ishinkin Gakkai Zasshi 2008;49(3):165–72.
17. Tan TY, Tan AL, Tee NW, et al. A retrospective analysis of antifungal susceptibilities of *Candida* bloodstream isolates from Singapore hospitals. Ann Acad Med Singapore 2008;37(10):835–40.
18. Kumar S, Kalam K, Ali S, et al. Frequency, clinical presentation and microbiological spectrum of candidemia in a tertiary care center in Karachi, Pakistan. J Pak Med Assoc 2014;64(3):281–5.
19. Tang JL, Kung HC, Lei WC, et al. High incidences of invasive fungal infections in acute myeloid leukemia patients receiving induction chemotherapy without systemic antifungal prophylaxis: a prospective observational study in Taiwan. PLoS One 2015;10(6):e0128410.
20. World Health Organization. Antimicrobial resistance global report on surveillance 2014. Available at: http://www.google.com/url?sa=t&rct=j&q=&esrc=s&source=web&cd=2&ved=0CCoQFjABahUKEwjj3NCDvvfHAhXK04AKHecLAfQ&url=http%3A%2F%2Fwww.who.int%2Firis%2Fbitstream%2F10665%2F112642%2F1%2F9789241564748_eng.pdf&usg=AFQjCNEYHe6GdKBRHal2aksvCFRHTZsBig&sig2=4Cd65ehvmPmbrXO3IsDWzQ. Accessed September 14, 2015.
21. Park BJ, Wannemuehler KA, Marston BJ, et al. Estimation of the current global burden of cryptococcal meningitis among persons living with HIV/AIDS. AIDS 2009;23(4):525–30.
22. Mfinanga S, Chanda D, Kivuyo SL, et al. Cryptococcal meningitis screening and community-based early adherence support in people with advanced HIV infection starting antiretroviral therapy in Tanzania and Zambia: an open-label, randomised controlled trial. Lancet 2015;385(9983):2173–82.
23. Baddley JW, Perfect JR, Oster RA, et al. Pulmonary cryptococcosis in patients without HIV infection: factors associated with disseminated disease. Clin Microbiol Infect 2008;27(10):937–43.
24. Espinel-Ingroff A, Kidd SE. Current trends in the prevalence of *Cryptococcus gattii* in the United States and Canada. Infect Drug Resist 2015;8:89–97.
25. Morris A, Lundgren JD, Masur H, et al. Current epidemiology of *Pneumocystis pneumonia*. Emerg Infect Dis 2004;10(10):1713–20.
26. Roblot F, Le Moal G, Kauffmann-Lacroix C, et al. *Pneumocystis jirovecii* pneumonia in HIV-negative patients: a prospective study with focus on immunosuppressive drugs and markers of immune impairment. Scand J Infect Dis 2014;46(3):210–4.
27. Pappas PG, Alexander BD, Andes DR, et al. Invasive fungal infections among organ transplant recipients: results of the Transplant-Associated Infection Surveillance Network (TRANSNET). Clin Infect Dis 2010;50(8):1101–11.
28. Kontoyiannis DP, Marr KA, Park BJ, et al. Prospective surveillance for invasive fungal infections in hematopoietic stem cell transplant recipients, 2001-2006: overview of the Transplant-Associated Infection Surveillance Network (TRANSNET) Database. Clin Infect Dis 2010;50(8):1091–100.
29. Bitar D, Lortholary O, Le Strat Y, et al. Population-based analysis of invasive fungal infections, France, 2001-2010. Emerg Infect Dis 2014;20(7):1149–55.
30. Nucci M, Garnica M, Gloria AB, et al. Invasive fungal diseases in haematopoietic cell transplant recipients and in patients with acute myeloid leukaemia or myelodysplasia in Brazil. Clin Microbiol Infect 2013;19(8):745–51.
31. Warnock DW. Trends in the epidemiology of invasive fungal infections. Nihon Ishinkin Gakkai Zasshi 2007;48(1):1–12.
32. Cortez KJ, Roilides E, Quiroz-Telles F, et al. Infections caused by *Scedosporium* spp. Clin Microbiol Rev 2008;21(1):157–97.

33. Lamaris GA, Chamilos G, Lewis RE, et al. Scedosporium infection in a tertiary care cancer center: a review of 25 cases from 1989-2006. Clin Infect Dis 2006; 43(12):1580–4.
34. Dignani MC, Anaissie E. Human fusariosis. Clin Microbiol Rev 2004;10(Suppl 1): 67–75.
35. Myint T, Al-Hasan MN, Ribes JA, et al. Temporal trends, clinical characteristics, and outcomes of histoplasmosis in a tertiary care center in Kentucky, 2000 to 2009. J Int Assoc Provid AIDS Care 2014;13(2):100–5.
36. Kauffman CA, Freifeld AG, Andes DR, et al. Endemic fungal infections in solid organ and hematopoietic cell transplant recipients enrolled in the Transplant-Associated Infection Surveillance Network (TRANSNET). Transpl Infect Dis 2014;16(2):213–24.
37. Baddley JW, Winthrop KL, Patkar NM, et al. Geographic distribution of endemic fungal infections among older persons, United States. Emerg Infect Dis 2011; 17(9):1664–9.
38. Colombo AL, Tobon A, Restrepo A, et al. Epidemiology of endemic systemic fungal infections in Latin America. Med Mycol 2011;49(8):785–98.
39. Nacher M, Adenis A, Adriouch L, et al. What is AIDS in the Amazon and the Guianas? Establishing the burden of disseminated histoplasmosis. Am J Trop Med Hyg 2011;84(2):239–40.
40. Pan B, Chen M, Pan W, et al. Histoplasmosis: a new endemic fungal infection in China? Review and analysis of cases. Mycoses 2013;56(3):212–21.
41. Antinori S. *Histoplasma capsulatum*: more widespread than previously thought. Am J Trop Med Hyg 2014;90(6):982–3.
42. Gugnani HC, Muotoe-Okafor F. African histoplasmosis: a review. Rev Iberoam Micol 1997;14(4):155–9.
43. CDC. Increase in reported coccidioidomycosis—United States, 1998–2011. MMWR Morb Mortal Wkly Rep 2013;62(12):217–21.
44. Chang DC, Anderson S, Wannemuehler K, et al. Testing for coccidioidomycosis among patients with community-acquired pneumonia. Emerg Infect Dis 2008; 14(7):1053–9.
45. Padua y Gabriel A, Martinez-Ordaz VA, Velasco-Rodreguez VM, et al. Prevalence of skin reactivity to coccidioidin and associated risks factors in subjects living in a northern city of Mexico. Arch Med Res 1999;30(5):388–92.
46. Brown J, Benedict K, Park BJ, et al. Coccidioidomycosis: epidemiology. Clin Epidemiol 2013;5:185–97.
47. Queiroz-Telles F, Escuissato DL. Pulmonary paracoccidioidomycosis. Semin Respir Crit Care Med 2011;32(6):764–74.
48. Restrepo A, McEwen JG, Castañeda E. The habitat of *Paracoccidioides brasiliensis*: how far from solving the riddle? Med Mycol 2001;39(3):233–41.
49. Morris SK, Brophy J, Richardson SE, et al. Blastomycosis in Ontario, 1994-2003. Emerg Infect Dis 2006;12(2):274–9.
50. Benedict K, Roy M, Chiller T, et al. Epidemiologic and ecologic features of blastomycosis: a review. Curr Fungal Infect Rep 2012;6:327–35.
51. Reed KD, Meece JK, Archer JR, et al. Ecologic niche modeling of *Blastomyces dermatitidis* in Wisconsin. PLoS One 2008;3(4):e2034.
52. Supparatpinyo K, Khamwan C, Baosoung V, et al. Disseminated *Penicillium marneffei* infection in southeast Asia. Lancet 1994;344(8915):110–3.
53. Ranjana KH, Priyokumar K, Singh TJ, et al. Disseminated *Penicillium marneffei* infection among HIV-infected patients in Manipur state, India. J Infect 2002; 45(4):268–71.

54. Zheng J, Gui X, Cao Q, et al. A clinical study of acquired immunodeficiency syndrome associated *Penicillium marneffei* infection from a non-endemic area in China. PLoS One 2015;10(6):e0130376.
55. Wang YF, Xu HF, Han ZG, et al. Serological surveillance for *Penicillium marneffei* infection in HIV-infected patients during 2004-2011 in Guangzhou, China. Clin Microbiol Infect 2015;21(5):484–9.
56. Ahmed AOA, van Leeuwen W, Fahal A, et al. Mycetoma caused by *Madurella mycetomatis*: a neglected infectious burden. Lancet Infect Dis 2004;4(9):566–74.
57. Bonifaz A, Tirado-Sánchez A, Calderón L, et al. Mycetoma: experience of 482 cases in a single center in Mexico. PLoS Negl Trop Dis 2014;8(8):e3102.
58. van de Sande WW. Global burden of human mycetoma: a systematic review and meta-analysis. PLoS Negl Trop Dis 2013;7(11):e2550.
59. Kenyon C, Bonorchis K, Corcoran C, et al. A dimorphic fungus causing disseminated infection in South Africa. N Engl J Med 2013;369(15):1416–24.
60. Chowdhary A, Anil Kumar V, Sharma C, et al. Multidrug-resistant endemic clonal strain of *Candida auris* in India. Clin Microbiol Infect 2014;33(6):919–26.
61. Freitas DF, Valle AC, da Silva MB, et al. Sporotrichosis: an emerging neglected opportunistic infection in HIV-infected patients in Rio de Janeiro, Brazil. PLoS Negl Trop Dis 2014;8(8):e3110.
62. Vermeulen E, Lagrou K, Verweij PE. Azole resistance in *Aspergillus fumigatus*: a growing public health concern. Curr Opin Infect Dis 2013;26(6):493–500.

Update from the Laboratory

Clinical Identification and Susceptibility Testing of Fungi and Trends in Antifungal Resistance

Mohammad T. Albataineh, MD, PhD, Deanna A. Sutton, PhD,
Annette W. Fothergill, MA, MBA, MT, Nathan P. Wiederhold, PharmD*

KEYWORDS

- Fungal identification • Antifungal susceptibility testing • Antifungal resistance

KEY POINTS

- Proper identification of fungi to the species level requires more than morphologic/phenotypic assessment. Molecular and proteomic assays are now needed and are often used in combination with classic techniques.
- Antifungal susceptibility testing is a useful tool to provide information to clinicians to help guide therapy. Several commercially available assays, in addition to the Clinical and Laboratory Standards Institute (CLSI) and the European Union Committee on Antimicrobial Susceptibility Testing (EUCAST) broth microdilution methods, are available for testing against yeast. Clinical breakpoints have not been established, however, for each antifungal and each fungal species.
- Echinocandin resistance in *Candida glabrata* species is increasing at some US institutions. Many of these isolates may also be resistant to fluconazole. In addition, azole-resistant *Aspergillus fumigatus* is a growing concern worldwide. Treatment options against these resistant fungi are limited.

INTRODUCTION

Invasive fungal infections are associated with significant morbidity and mortality, because these infections are often difficult to diagnosis and treat. Fungi historically associated with invasive disease in humans include yeast within the genera *Candida*,

Disclosures: (N.P. Wiederhold) has received research support from Astellas, bioMérieux, Dow, F2G, Merck, Merz, Revolution Medicines, and Viamet and has served on advisory boards for Merck, Astellas, Toyama, and Viamet.
Fungus Testing Laboratory, Department of Pathology, University of Texas Health Science Center at San Antonio, 7703 Floyd Curl Drive, San Antonio, TX 78229, USA
* Corresponding author.
E-mail address: wiederholdn@uthscsa.edu

Infect Dis Clin N Am 30 (2016) 13–35
http://dx.doi.org/10.1016/j.idc.2015.10.014
0891-5520/16/$ – see front matter © 2016 Elsevier Inc. All rights reserved.
id.theclinics.com

Cryptococcus, and *Trichosporon;* the dimorphic fungi *Blastomyces dermatitidis, Coccidioides immitis/Coccidioides posadasii,* and *Histoplasma capsulatum;* molds, including limited species within the genera *Aspergillus, Fusarium,* and *Scedosporium;* and members of the order Mucorales. Over the past 2 decades there has been a significant increase in the number of fungal species associated with invasive disease in humans. Factors that have contributed to this increase include an increase in the number of immunocompromised patients at high risk for invasive fungal infections, such as HIV-AIDS patients, those receiving immunosuppressive chemotherapy for malignancies, and solid organ transplant recipients. Improvements in diagnostic assays and the clinical recognition of patients with risk factors for such infections, as well as improvements in the tools used to identify fungal species, have shortened the time to acquire a proper diagnosis. The treatment of invasive fungal infections can be challenging due to the limited number of clinically available drugs, in addition to drug interactions and toxicities associated with certain classes of antifungals that may limit their effectiveness. Although antifungal resistance has not reached the level of antibiotic resistance seen with some bacterial species, recent studies and publications indicate that this may be an emerging problem with some invasive fungal pathogens. The objectives of this article are to review the methods used for fungal identification in the clinical setting and to discuss methods for susceptibility testing and recent trends in antifungal resistance, including common pathogens that may develop multidrug resistance.

FUNGAL IDENTIFICATION IN THE CLINICAL SETTING
Identification by Morphologic/Phenotypic Characteristics and DNA Sequence Analysis

The identification of fungi in the clinical laboratory has historically relied on morphologic characteristics and physiologic traits. The description of the colony appearance and the microscopic features of the organism, including the reproductive structures, has been the hallmark for fungal identification for many years. Certain phenotypic/physiologic traits are also combined with the morphologic features to obtain the identities of fungal isolates. These include, but are not limited to, the ability of an organism to grow at certain temperatures, tolerance to cycloheximide and benomyl, nitrate assimilation, tolerance to different concentrations of sodium chloride, growth on trichophyton agar, and growth on urea agar.[1–4] Many of these phenotypic/physiologic assays are still used to identify an organism to the genus and possibly species level in clinical microbiology and reference mycology laboratories. Identification to the species level is clinically important because it provides clinicians with information that may be useful in the management of patients and guidance of antifungal therapy. Early identification and the initiation of appropriate therapy have been shown to influence patient outcomes whereas delaying appropriate therapy can be detrimental.[5–8] Identification to the species level is important in helping to guide appropriate therapy, because some fungi are intrinsically resistant to certain drugs. Furthermore, some species within the same species complex may have different antifungal susceptibility profiles and this can influence treatment.[9–11] Identification by morphologic/physiologic characteristics alone can be time consuming, and results may not be available in a timely fashion for clinical decisions. Morphologic identification can also be fraught with errors if done by those without proper training and experience. In addition, the morphologic features of fungi may be variable.[12,13] Different factors can affect these features, including the media used for subculture or exposure to external stressors, such as antifungal agents prior to recovery from clinical specimens that can often occur in patient groups at high risk for invasive fungal infections where empiric or preemptive antifungal therapy is often used.

The introduction of molecular tools, such as DNA sequence analysis, has dramatically changed how fungi are identified. These methods can both reduce the amount of time needed to determine the identity of an organism and reduce errors associated with morphologic variability. These methods, however, have their own limitations and do not eliminate the need for the morphologic evaluation of fungi in the clinical laboratory. For DNA sequence analysis, the results that are obtained must be compared with those deposited in databases from known organisms in order for an identity to be obtained. Publically available databases for DNA fungal sequence comparisons are available, including those at the National Center for Biotechnology Information (GenBank; www.ncbi.nlm.nih.gov/genbank/), the Centraalbureau voor Schimmelcultures Fungal Biodiversity Center in the Netherlands (CBS-KNAW; www.cbs.knaw.nl), the International Society of Human and Animal Mycology ITS Database (ISHAM; its.mycologylab.org), and the Fusarium-ID database (http://isolate.fusariumdb.org). Reference laboratories or clinical microbiology laboratories may also have their own databases. The use of sequence results can be extremely useful when compared with credible deposits. Not all fungal deposits within databases, however, have been confirmed to be from accurately identified organisms.[14-16] This can lead to erroneous results and the misidentification of the cultured specimen. In addition, the choice of the proper target sequence can be critical for the identification of fungi. Although the internal transcribed spacer (ITS) region has been put forth as a universal barcode for the identification of fungi,[17-19] this target cannot always be used alone to discriminate between closely related fungi. Several other DNA targets may be required to identify fungi in the clinical setting (**Table 1**), and the choice of targets depends on the suspected genus. Thus, an assessment of the morphology of the organism prior to sequence analysis can provide useful information as to which DNA targets to sequence for identification.

Matrix-Assisted Laser Desorption/Ionization Time-of-Flight Mass Spectrometry

Matrix-assisted laser desorption/ionization time-of-flight mass spectrometry (MALDI-TOF MS) offers a timely, accurate, and reproducible method that is increasingly used in place of conventional methods for identification of microbes to the species level.[20-23] In principle, the identification process relies on a comparison between the characteristic mass spectra of ribosomal proteins that are highly conserved among isolates of the same species but with interspecies variations. Samples for analysis are added to a metal slide and coated with an energy-absorbent compound termed the matrix (eg, α-cyano-4-hydroxycinnamic acid [CHCA]). Desorption and ionization by a laser beam

Table 1
DNA targets used for molecular sequence identification of fungi and examples of genera these targets may be used to identify

Targets	Genera
ITS	All genera
28S rDNA large subunit (D1/D2)	All genera
β-Tubulin	*Aspergillus*
Calmodulin	*Scedosporium*
Translation elongation factor	*Fusarium*
RNA polymerase	*Penicillium*
Glyceraldehyde-3-phosphate dehydrogenase	*Curvularia*

generates protonated ions that are accelerated and separated from each other based on their mass-to-charge ratio, which are detected by mass spectrometry.[24] The spectra that are obtained represent a unique fingerprint for each microorganism and are compared with a library of spectra of known species to make the identification.[25,26] Thus this technology is ideal for an accurate fungal identification at the species level, including differentiation of closely related species and subspecies. Mass spectrometry was first used in microbial testing in 1975, when bacteria with unique mass spectra signature were characterized for the first time.[27,28] The concept of laser desorption/ionization to analyze and characterize large-size proteins was established in the late 1980s.[29,30] Subsequently, many groups started analyzing protein profiles from intact bacterial and fungal cells as well as cell extracts using MALDI-TOF MS.[22,31–38] Currently, 2 systems, the Biotyper (Bruker, Billerica, Massachusetts, USA) and the Vitek MS (bioMérieux, Marcy-l'Etoile, France), have received approval from the US Food and Drug Administration (FDA) for use in bacterial and yeast identification.[39]

Several studies have evaluated the ability of MALDI-TOF MS for identification of yeast isolates, including but not limited to Candida, Cryptococcus, Saccharomyces, Pichia, Geotrichum, and Trichosporon species. In 1 large study, 1192 yeast isolates were tested using both the Biotyper and Vitek MS and compared with traditional phenotypic and biochemical techniques.[40] Overall, both systems performed similarly with 97.6% and 96.1% correct species identifications, respectively, by the Biotyper and Vitek MS, which were similar to conventional methods (96.9%). The MALDI-TOF MS systems, however, were able to discriminate between closely related species (eg, C orthopsilosis/C metapsilosis/C parapsilosis) whereas the traditional identification methods did not allow separation. The ability of MALDI-TOF MS to discriminate between closely related yeast species has also been reported.[41,42] Published studies have reported similar rates of correct species identification for yeast isolates (92%–99%) using this technology, with few isolates misidentified.[42–49] When no identification is made, this prompts the need of other means for species identification. MALDI-TOF MS has also been evaluated for the identification of mold isolates, with some studies reporting similar rates of correct species identification observed against yeasts, whereas others have reported lower rates.[34,50–55] Many of these studies, however, evaluated few mold species and relied on in-house supplementary databases that target only select pathogens commonly found in their patients. Due to the need of a standardized extraction protocols and comprehensive database to evaluate the ability of MALDI-TOF MS method to identify filamentous fungi, the National Institutes of Health mold database was created, which initially consisted of spectra from 249 reference isolates.[56] When evaluated against 421 clinical isolates, this database provided correct species identifications for 88.9% of the isolates tested with no misdentifications. This database also outperformed the one provided by the manufacturer, which correctly identified only 0.7% and 6.2% of the isolates to the species and genus levels, respectively.

IDENTIFICATION OF FUNGI WITH DIRECT SPECIMENS

One of the main limitations of assays used for the identification of fungi to the species level is the need for pure cultures. The culturing and growth of organisms for this purpose increases the turnaround time for results that may be useful to the clinicians in choosing or adjusting treatment. In addition, in many patients with invasive fungal infections, the infecting organism may never be recovered. Thus there is a need for assays that are able to detect and identify fungal organisms in direct patient specimens. These types of technologies have the ability to shorten the time for meaningful results to become available to clinicians. Two assays that have recently become available for clinical use on direct specimens include the T2 magnetic resonance (T2MR) test for *Candida* and a lateral flow assay for *Cryptococcus*.

T2 Magnetic Resonance Technology

Candida species are the fifth most common hospital-acquired pathogens and rank fourth among nosocomial bloodstream infections.[57–59] Bloodstream infections caused by *Candida* species are associated with significant morbidity, with rates approaching 40%.[57,60] Delaying the initiation of antifungal therapy in patients with invasive candidiasis has been shown to result in higher mortality rates.[5,7] The use of systemic antifungals, however, is not without risk due to drug interactions and adverse effects/toxicities that may be associated with different agents and the requirement of blood cultures for the diagnosis of invasive candidiasis that are limited by suboptimal sensitivity. A new technology for the diagnosis of invasive candidiasis is T2MR measurement. This technology can be used for the detection of a variety of biological targets, such as drugs, enzymes, proteins, and tumor cells.[61,62] For the detection of *Candida* species in whole blood, the T2Candida assay (T2Biosystems, Lexington, MA, USA) combines nuclear magnetic resonance spectroscopy with polymerase chain reaction. In this automated assay, red blood cells are first lysed allowing the pathogen cells and debris to be concentrated.[63,64] The *Candida* cells are then lysed via mechanical means, and the DNA is amplified using pan-*Candida* primers directed at the ITS2 region. The amplified product is then hybridized to supramagnetic nanoparticles that agglomerate, disrupting the microscopic magnetic fields experienced by the surrounding water molecules, which in turn alters the magnetic resonance signal that can be measured.[65] This system has received FDA market authorization in the United States and has the ability to detect 5 common *Candida* species, including *C albicans*, *C glabrata*, *C krusei*, *C parapsilosis*, and *C tropicalis*. In this assay, the detection of *C albicans* is grouped with *C tropicalis*, and *C glabrata* with *C krusei*, based on typical antifungal susceptibilities patterns of each species.[66] Some centers still use fluconazole for the treatment of *C glabrata* infections in relatively stable, nonimmunosuppressed hosts. Thus, the coupling of *C glabrata* and *C krusei*, a species that is intrinsically resistant to fluconazole, may be problematic for antifungal stewardship in blood culture–negative patients where the T2Candida assay is positive for this pair.

Studies have demonstrated excellent analytical sensitivity for the T2Candida assay, with ranges between 1 colony-forming unit (CFU)/mL and 3 CFUs/mL for the common species that this assay detects.[63,64,66] Excellent clinical specificity has also been reported in 1 study.[64] In this study, blood was collected from 1801 patients with a vast majority not having invasive candidiasis. The overall clinical specificity was 99.4% and was 98.9% for *C albicans*/*C tropicalis*, 99.3% for *C parapsilosis*, and 99.9% for *C krusei*/*C glabrata*. The mean time to negativity for the T2Candida assay was 4.2 hours compared with greater than or equal to 120 hours for blood cultures. The sensitivity in blood samples spike with known amounts of *Candida* cells ranged from 88.1% to 94.2%. Thus, the T2Candida assay may be able to rapidly and accurately exclude the possibility of candidemia and thus limit inappropriate use of antifungal agents in the absence of this disease. In this study, however, only 6 prospectively collected samples were positive for *Candida* species. Thus, the clinical sensitivity of this assay remains unknown.

Cryptococcal Antigen Lateral Flow Assay

The detection of cryptococcal antigen (CRAG) in cerebral spinal fluid (CSF) or serum is useful for the detection of cryptococcosis. Several assays are available for this purpose, and these detect the glucuronoxylomannan component of the *Cryptococcus* capsule. These include latex agglutination (LA) assays, enzyme immunoassays (EIAs), and lateral flow immunoassays (LFAs). In addition to diagnosis, these assays can be used to monitor patients with cryptococcosis. Studies have demonstrated that high serum and CSF CRAG titers are correlated with mycological failure and the risk of death,[67–70] whereas higher CSF titers may predict relapse during therapy in HIV positive patients.[71] Higher serum titers may also be used to help predict HIV positive individuals at risk of developing cryptococcal meningitis immune reconstitution inflammatory syndrome after starting antiretroviral therapy.[72]

The LA and EIA CRAG assays have been available for clinical use the longest. Overall, the sensitivity and specificity of both the LA and EIA tests range between 93% and 100%.[73–75] False-negative and false-positive results, however, have been reported with both systems, and titer determinations should not be used interchangeably between these assays or between different LA kits. In addition, cross-reactivity with *Trichosporon* species may occur with the EIA,[76] and interpretation of LA assay results may be subjective with variability between operators.[77] Other disadvantages of these assays include the need for refrigeration of reagents, the processing of samples using either enzymes or heat, and the need for experienced laboratory personnel.[77,78]

The IMMY CrAg LFA (Immuno-Mycologics, Norman, OK, USA) is now available and approved for the detection of CRAG in serum and CSF samples. Studies have reported that this assay is also suitable for use on plasma and urine.[77–80] This is a rapid point-of-care dipstick test in which gold-conjugated monoclonal antibodies against CRAG are impregnated on an immunochromatographic strip. The gold-conjugated–monoclonal antibody–CRAG complex then migrates along the dipstick via capillary action and interacts with immobilized monoclonal antibodies to CRAG to form a red line.[78] This assay is capable of detecting *Cryptococcal* serotypes A, B, C, and D, and 1 study has reported the successful detection of CRAG with the LFA in *Cryptococcus gattii*–infected patients.[77] The LFA assay is easy to perform, does not require refrigeration, cold-chain shipping, or laboratory equipment, and results are available within 10 to 20 minutes.[77,78] Because of these characteristics, the World Health Organization recommends that the LFA be used to screen HIV-positive individuals for cryptococcosis. In addition, this assay largely meets the Affordable, Sensitive, Specific, User-friendly, Rapid and robust, Equipment-free, and Deliverable to end users (ASSURED) criteria for point-of-care testing.[77,81] The sensitivity and specificity of the LFA in both serum and CSF have ranged between 98% to 100% and 92% and 100%, respectively.[77–80,82–84] Studies that have compared the performance of the cryptococcal LFA to that of the LA and EIA assays have reported excellent concordance between the assays.[77,78,80,82–84] The titers that are obtained by the LFA, however, may be higher than those observed by LA assays or EIAs. Although it has been suggested that the ratio of CRAG titers measured by LA compared with LFA is consistently 1:5,[85] other investigators have found more variable results, suggesting that titers obtained by the LFA assay should not be directly translated into equivalent results obtained by LA assays or EIAs.[77]

ANTIFUNGAL SUSCEPTIBILITY TESTING
Clinical and Laboratory Standards Institute and European Union Committee on Antimicrobial Susceptibility Testing Reference Standards

When a fungal pathogen is isolated from a patient with a fungal infection, antifungal susceptibility testing may be performed to help determine the potential suitability of antifungal agents for treatment. Antifungal susceptibility testing is a means to provide an estimate of the in vitro potency of an agent against a pathogen of interest, and the results may then be correlated with in vivo activity observed in clinical studies or animal models of infection to predict the likely outcome of therapy.[86–88] Susceptibility testing may be of value because elevated antifungal minimum inhibitory concentration (MIC) values, representing decreased vitro activity, are associated with poor outcomes and breakthrough infections,[89] whereas reductions in overall treatment costs due to de-escalation in therapy from an echinocandin to fluconazole in patients with infections due to susceptible *Candida* species have also been reported.[90] Antifungal susceptibility testing is also used as a means to survey the development of resistance and to predict the therapeutic potential and spectrum of activity of investigational agents.[86–88] For antifungal susceptibility testing to be clinically useful, however, it must reliably predict the likelihood of clinical success. There are several factors that also influence outcomes in patients with fungal infections other than antifungal susceptibility. These include (1) the host's immune response, (2) the severity of the underlying disease and other comorbidities, (3) drug interactions, and (4) the pharmacokinetics of the agents and concentrations achieved at the site of infection.[86,87,91]

Two organizations that establish methods for antifungal susceptibility testing and antifungal clinical breakpoints are the CLSI in the United States and the EUCAST. The broth microdilution methods set by these organizations serve as the gold standards for susceptibility testing and use 96-well cell culture trays to allow multiple tests to be performed simultaneously for both yeast and molds. This is more convenient and efficient than macrobroth susceptibility testing, although this method should still be used for certain species (eg, *Coccidioides* spp, *Blastomyces dermatitidis*, and *H capsulatum*) by reference laboratories.[92] Over the past several years, there have been efforts to harmonize the methods and clinical breakpoints for antifungal susceptibility testing between these 2 groups. Some differences do exist, including the starting inoculum density (0.5–2.5×10^3 cells/mL [CLSI] vs 0.5 to 2.5×10^5 cells/mL [EUCAST]), glucose content (0.2% [CLSI] vs 2% [EUCAST]), microtiter well types (round-bottom [CLSI] vs flat-bottom [EUCAST]), and endpoint determinations (visual [CLSI] vs spectrophotometric [EUCAST]).[93,94] Despite the method differences, the results are comparable.[95–97] One issue with both the CLSI and EUCAST broth microdilution susceptibility testing that has been identified is the problem of interlaboratory variability for caspofungin MICs, with some laboratories reporting low values whereas others report high values for this echinocandin.[98] This variability seems to be greatest for *C glabrata* and *C krusei* and may lead to falsely classifying susceptible isolates as resistant to the echinocandins. Because of this, EUCAST does not recommend susceptibility testing with caspofungin but instead recommends the use of micafungin or anidulafungin MICs as surrogate markers for caspofungin susceptibilty or resistance.[94] Studies have clearly demonstrated high concordance rates for anidulafungin and micafungin MICs in detecting mutations within the *FKS* gene that confer echinocandin resistance in multiple *Candida* species.[99,100]

There are also differences in the clinical breakpoints that define resistance as set by CLSI and EUCAST (**Tables 2** and **3**). Despite the differences in methods, the categorical agreement that is obtained is comparable,[95–97,101] although some differences have been reported.[95] Clinical breakpoints have not been set for each antifungal agent against each type of fungus. The CLSI has only established breakpoints for fluconazole, voriconazole, and the echinocandins against certain *Candida* species, and no breakpoints have been set against molds or endemic fungi. In contrast, EUCAST has established breakpoints for certain antifungals against yeast and some molds, including *Aspergillus* species. The decision by the CLSI Subcommittee on Antifungal

Table 2
Clinical and Laboratory Standards Institute clinical breakpoints against Candida spp

Azoles	Candida albicans			Candida glabrata			Candida krusei			Candida parapsilosis			Candida tropicalis			Candida guilliermondii		
Species	S (≤)	SDD	R (≥)	S (≤)	SDD	R (≥)	S (≤)	SDD	R (≥)	S (≤)	SDD	R (≥)	S (≤)	SDD	R (≥)	S (≤)	SDD	R (≥)
FLU	2	4	8	—	≤32	64	—[a]	—	—	2	4	8	2	4	8	—	—	—
VOR	0.12	0.25–0.5	1	—	—	—	0.5	1	2	0.12	0.25–0.5	1	0.12	0.25–0.5	1	—	—	—

Echinocandins	Candida albicans			Candida glabrata			Candida krusei			Candida parapsilosis			Candida tropicalis			Candida guilliermondii		
Species	S (≤)	I	R (≥)	S (≤)	I	R (≥)	S (≤)	I	R (≥)	S (≤)	I	R (≥)	S (≤)	I	R (≥)	S (≤)	I	R (≥)
AFG	0.25	0.5	1	0.12	0.25	0.5	0.25	0.5	1	2	4	8	0.25	0.5	1	2	4	8
CAS	0.25	0.5	1	0.12	0.25	0.5	0.25	0.5	1	2	4	8	0.25	0.5	1	2	4	8
MFG	0.25	0.5	1	0.06	0.12	0.25	0.25	0.5	1	2	4	8	0.25	0.5	1	2	4	8

Abbreviations: AFG, anidulafungin; CAS, caspofungin; FLU, fluconazole; I, intermediate; MFG, micafungin; R, resistant; S, susceptible; SDD, susceptible dose-dependent; VOR, voriconazole.

[a] C krusei considered resistant to fluconazole despite MIC values. No CLSI clinical breakpoints set for fluconazole against C guilliermondii or for voriconazole against C glabrata or C guilliermondii. CLSI has not set breakpoints for amphotericin B, itraconazole, or posaconazole in the M27-S4 supplement.

Table 3
European Union Committee on Antimicrobial Susceptibility Testing clinical breakpoints against Candida spp

Species	Candida albicans		Candida glabrata		Candida krusei		Candida parapsilosis		Candida tropicalis		Candida guilliermondii	
	S (≤)	R (>)	S (≤)	R (>)	S (≤)	R (>)	S (≤)	R (>)	S (≤)	R (>)	S (≤)	R (>)
AMB	1	1	1	1	1	1	1	1	1	1	—	—
FLU	2	4	0.002	32	—	—	2	4	2	4	—	—
ITR	0.06	0.06	—	—	—	—	0.12	0.12	0.12	0.12	—	—
POS	0.06	0.06	—	—	—	—	0.06	0.06	0.06	0.06	—	—
VOR	0.12	0.12	—	—	—	—	0.12	0.12	0.12	0.12	—	—
AFG	0.03	0.03	0.06	0.06	0.06	0.06	0.002	4	0.06	0.06	—	—
MFG	0.016	0.016	0.03	0.03	—	—	0.002	2	—	—	—	—

EUCAST has not set clinical breakpoints for caspofungin against *Candida* spp.
Abbreviations: AFG, anidulafungin; AMB, amphotericin B; FLU, fluconazole; ITR, itraconazole; MFG, micafungin; POS, posaconazole; R, resistant; S, susceptible; VOR, voriconazole.

Susceptibility Testing to not set breakpoints for certain drugs and against certain fungi is primarily based on the lack of clinical evidence demonstrating outcomes associated with the results of in vitro susceptibility testing.

In the absence of clinical breakpoints, guidance may be provided by epidemiologic cutoff values (ECVs or ECOFFs). ECVs are statistically derived MIC thresholds that allow for the discrimination between wild-type strains and non–wild-type strains (ie, isolates with acquired resistance mechanisms).[88,102] There are various means to determine the ECV, but in general the ECV encompasses approximately 95% to 99% of the isolates within the wild-type MIC distribution. ECVs should be both drug specific and species specific and can be used as a means to identify isolates less likely to respond to therapy due to acquired resistance mechanisms when clinical breakpoints are unavailable.[88,102] ECVs are also an effective means of tracking the emergence of resistance and serve as an important component in establishing species-specific clinical breakpoints. ECVs were a major component of evidence used to revise the CLSI antifungal clinical breakpoints and establish drug-specific and species-specific breakpoints.[103] ECVs do not predict or correlate with clinical outcome. Instead, they can be used to alert clinicians that mechanisms of drug resistance are present in a given isolate.

Commercially Available Antifungal Susceptibility Assays

In addition to the methods set by CLSI and EUCAST, commercially available tests are available for antifungal susceptibility testing. These include colorimetric and gradient diffusions assays as well as automated tests. The YeastOne Sensititre test (Thermo Scientific, Waltham, MA, USA formerly TREK Diagnostic Systems) is a broth microdilution assay format that uses the blue colorimetric dye resazurin (alamarBlue) that is converted to by metabolically active cells to resorufin. Several studies of the YeastOne assay, including multicenter evaluations, have demonstrated excellent reproducibility and very good agreement with the broth microdilution reference methods.[104–111] When previously published results were reanalyzed using the new CLSI echinocandin clinical breakpoints (revised in 2012), excellent essential agreement (100% within 2 dilutions) was observed against *Candida* species.[108] Overall categorical agreement, however, was somewhat lower for caspofungin than micafungin (93.6% vs 99.6%) between the YeastOne assay and the CLSI broth microdilution method, and this was driven by the low categorical agreement for caspofungin against *C glabrata* (89.7%) and *C krusei* (69.1%) between the 2 methods. A multilaboratory study also reported a high percentage of *C glabrata* and *C krusei* isolates that were classified as intermediate to caspofungin when MICs were measured using this assay.[112] The clinical relevance of this finding is unknown, because some investigators have suggested that infections caused by isolates that are intermediate to caspofungin respond favorably to treatment with this agent.[113]

The antifungal MIC agar-based assay Etest (bioMérieux) uses a plastic strip that contains a concentration gradient of a particular antifungal agent. The strip is placed onto the surface of an agar plate that has been inoculated with a fungal isolate, and antifungal agent then diffuses into the agar. The MIC is read after a period of incubation at the concentration where the elliptical zone of inhibition intersects the strip. This method is commonly used for susceptibility testing against various *Candida* species and is also considered a sensitive and reliable method for detecting decreased susceptibility to amphotericin B among *Candida* isolates and *Cryptococcus neoformans*.[114–116] Several studies have reported very good essential agreement (>90%) between the Etest assay and the CLSI and EUCAST broth microdilution reference methods.[104,105] Others have reported less than optimal categorical agreement between the Etest assay and the CLSI broth microdilution method for caspofungin against *C glabrata* and *C krusei* based on the revised CLSI echinocandin clinical breakpoints.[117,118] In addition, a recent study reported poor overall agreement between Etest and EUCAST MICs for amphotericin B and posaconazole (75.1%) when used to measure activity against members of the order Mucorales, the causative agents of mucormycosis, and recommended that the Etest assay not be used against these fungi.[119] The quality and reliability of Etest MIC results may also be influenced by operator technique in applying the strips as well as the trailing affect that may be observed with the azoles against some yeast species. Similar to what has been observed with the YeastOne colorimetric assay, 1 study has also reported a high incidence of *C glabrata* and *C krusei* isolates with intermediate caspofungin MICs with this assay.[117]

The yeast susceptibility test, Vitek 2 (bioMérieux), is a fully automated assay for performing antifungal susceptibility testing. Several studies have reported reproducible and accurate results compared with the CLSI broth micordilution method.[105,120–125] Recent studies have also demonstrated that this assay was comparable to the CLSI broth microdilution assay for fluconazole susceptibility testing with good categorical agreement using the revised and lower CLSI clinical breakpoints.[124,126] In the United States, only fluconazole, voriconazole, and caspofungin are approved by the FDA for antifungal susceptibility testing by Vitek 2, although additional agents are available for testing in other countries.[122,123,127,128] One of the limitations of this system for caspofungin is that the lower end of the concentration range is 0.25 μg/mL, making correct discrimination between susceptible and intermediate categories for *C glabrata* isolates impossible. In addition, 1 study reported that 19.4% of caspofungin-resistant *Candida* isolates with known mechanisms of resistance (mutations in *FKS* hotspot regions) were misclassified as susceptible to caspofungin.[129]

TRENDS IN ANTIFUNGAL RESISTANCE
Echinocandin Resistance in Candida glabrata

The detection of resistance may be the most important function of antifungal susceptibility testing, because the use of drugs to which the infecting organism is resistant is more likely to result in clinical failure.[88] Overall, the rates of antifungal resistance are low compared with what is observed with antibiotic resistance. There are some interesting trends, however, in the area of antifungal resistance. Recent studies from institutions in the United States have focused on the development of echinocandin resistance in *Candida* species, in particular *C glabrata*. Breakthrough *Candida* infections in immunocompromised individuals (bone marrow transplant and solid organ transplant recipients) who received micafungin prophylaxis were reported at 1 institution where the rate of echinocandin-resistant *C glabrata* increased from 4.9% to 12.3% over a 10-year period.[130,131] High rates of echinocandin resistance in this species have also been reported at other medical centers, although regional differences may be present.[132,133] There is also evidence that many echinocandin-resistant *C glabrata* isolates are also resistant to fluconazole.[133,134] Because treatment options are limited in the setting of resistance to multiple antifungal classes, this development is concerning.

Because of the variability that can occur with broth microdilution susceptibility testing, it has been suggested that hotspot regions with in the *FKS* genes be sequenced to identify resistant isolates. Some studies have shown that the presence of an *FKS* mutation is an independent risk factor for therapeutic failure in patients with invasive candidiasis caused by *C glabrata* and that echinocandin MICs were not independently associated with poor outcomes.[113,135] *FKS* mutations, however, have not been independent risk factors for clinical failure in all studies.[132] Instead, a consistent factor associated with therapeutic failure and/or the development of *FKS* mutations various studies has been prior echinocandin exposure.[113,131,132,135] In addition, not all *FKS* mutations are created equal. Two studies have reported higher echinocandin MICs and persistent or breakthrough infections in patients with infections caused by *C glabrata* isolates harboring the S663F or S663P amino acid substitutions due to mutations within *FKS* hotspots as opposed to other mutations in these regions.[104,132] These observations are consistent with in vitro results that have demonstrated differences in echinocandin potency in inhibiting the $(1,3)$-β-D-glucan synthase enzyme and changes in in vivo efficacy with echinocandin therapy in experimental models between isolates harboring different mutations.[136,137]

Azole Resistance in Aspergillus fumigatus

Azole resistance in *A fumigatus* has also recently gained increased attention. It has been known that in patients with chronic exposure to azoles, such as those with chronic pulmonary aspergillosis, resistance to this class of agents can develop in *A fumigatus*. The first reports came from isolates collected from patients in the United States and Sweden in the 1990s who had been treated with itraconazole.[138,139] As with *Candida* species, resistance in *Aspergillus* can occur due to point mutations in the *CYP51A* gene, which encodes the enzyme responsible for the demethylation of lanosterol in the final step in ergosterol biosynthesis. The location of the point mutation with in the *CYP51A* gene and the corresponding amino acid change may lead to different resistance patterns. This is consistent with the predicted structural properties of the Cyp51 enzyme and its interactions with the different structures found within this class.[140] Some point mutations may specifically affect certain members of this class, whereas others result in pan-azole resistance.

Globally, the rates of azole resistance in *A fumigatus* have been reported to be between 4% and 5%.[141–144] Recently, increases in the incidence of azole resistance in *A fumigatus* have been noted the United Kingdom and the Netherlands. In the United Kingdom, an increase in the rates of azole resistance from 5% to 7% to up to 20% was reported between 2004 and 2009, with these isolates primarily coming from patients with chronic pulmonary aspergillosis combined with long-term azole exposure.[140,145] In the Netherlands, similar rates of resistance have been reported.[146] Documented invasive aspergillosis, however, due to azole-resistant *A fumigatus* isolates has also been reported in patients without previous azole exposure. In these individuals, the isolates also contain tandem repeats in the promoter region of *CYP51A* in addition to point mutations within this gene. These include the TR_{34}/L98H and the TR_{46}/Y121F/T289A mutations, and isolates with these changes have also been recovered from the environment, including the indoor environment of hospitals and areas in direct proximity to the medical centers (eg, flower beds), as well as in areas where azole fungicides are used in agriculture.[147–149] Isolates with these mutations have now been reported in different countries in Europe, China, Asia, Africa, and Australia.[141,150–153] A recent study has also reported the discovery of these mutations in isolates collected from patients in the United States with invasive aspergillosis.[154] The rise in azole resistance rates in *A fumigatus* isolates in some countries and the discovery of mechanisms of resistance associated with environmental exposure are concerning, because treatment options may be limited, and infections due to resistant isolates may be associated with a higher probability of treatment failure.[149,155,156] For both treatment and epidemiologic purposes, it is important that correct species identification is made. Although usually distinguishable from other *Aspergillus* species, such as *A terreus*, *A niger,* and *A flavus*, based on morphologic and phenotypic characteristics, *A fumigatus* is a member of the section *Fumigati,* which consists of at least 51 phylogentically distinct species.[157] Discrimination between members of this section is difficult due to the morphologic instability but important because several species within this section are refractory to antifungal therapy.[158–160] Species identification cannot always be made, however, because isolates are not always recovered from patients with invasive disease. Although assays have been developed to detect azole resistance in direct specimens, the true clinical utility of these diagnostic tools is unknown.[140,161]

SUMMARY

The introduction of new assays for the identification of fungi, including molecular and proteomic tools and technologies for the detection of fungi in direct specimens, is improving the information that is provided to clinicians by clinical microbiology laboratories. The correct identification of the species that is causing infection is important and can help guide therapy and ensure the use of appropriate antifungal agents. The availability of approved assays for the detection and identification of fungi on direct specimens may also improve treatment in patients with invasive fungal infections, because they can make results available to clinicians more rapidly. Antifungal susceptibility testing also provides valuable information to clinicians when isolates are available for testing. These results can assist in guiding therapy and in surveillance studies can help to identify changes in resistance patterns. Such observations have recently been made for echinocandin resistance in *C glabrata* and azole resistance in *A fumigatus*.

REFERENCES

1. Nelson PD, Toussoun TA, Marasas WFO. Growing fusarium species for identification. In: Nelson PD, Toussoun TA, Marassas WFO, editors. Fusarium species: an illustrated manual for identification. University Park (PA): Pennsylvania State University Press; 1983. p. 13–4.
2. Pincus DH, Salkin IF, Hurd NJ, et al. Modification of potassium nitrate assimilation test for identification of clinically important yeasts. J Clin Microbiol 1988;26: 366–8.
3. Kane J, Summerbell R, Sigler L, et al. Physiological and other special tests for identifying dermatophyes. In: Kane J, editor. Laboratory handbook of dermatophytes. Belmont (CA): Star Publishing Co; 1997. p. 45–79.
4. Summerbell RC. The benomyl test as a fundamental diagnostic method for medical mycology. J Clin Microbiol 1993;31:572–7.
5. Morrell M, Fraser VJ, Kollef MH. Delaying the empiric treatment of *Candida* bloodstream infection until positive blood culture results are obtained: a potential risk factor for hospital mortality. Antimicrob Agents Chemother 2005;49: 3640–5.
6. Greene RE, Schlamm HT, Oestmann JW, et al. Imaging findings in acute invasive pulmonary aspergillosis: clinical significance of the halo sign. Clin Infect Dis 2007;44:373–9.
7. Garey KW, Rege M, Pai MP, et al. Time to initiation of fluconazole therapy impacts mortality in patients with candidemia: a multi-institutional study. Clin Infect Dis 2006;43:25–31.
8. Chamilos G, Lewis RE, Kontoyiannis DP. Delaying amphotericin B-based frontline therapy significantly increases mortality among patients with hematologic malignancy who have zygomycosis. Clin Infect Dis 2008;47:503–9.

9. Balajee SA, Gribskov JL, Hanley E, et al. *Aspergillus lentulus* sp. nov., a new sibling species of *A. fumigatus*. Eukary Cell 2005;4:625–32.
10. Gilgado F, Serena C, Cano J, et al. Antifungal susceptibilities of the species of the *Pseudallescheria boydii* complex. Antimicrob Agents Chemother 2006;50: 4211–3.
11. Lackner M, de Hoog GS, Verweij PE, et al. Species-specific antifungal susceptibility patterns of *Scedosporium* and *Pseudallescheria* species. Antimicrob Agents Chemother 2012;56:2635–42.
12. Balajee SA, Houbraken J, Verweij PE, et al. *Aspergillus* species identification in the clinical setting. Stud Mycol 2007;59:39–46.
13. Balajee SA, Nickle D, Varga J, et al. Molecular studies reveal frequent misidentification of *Aspergillus fumigatus* by morphotyping. Eukary Cell 2006;5: 1705–12.
14. Bridge PD, Roberts PJ, Spooner BM, et al. On the unreliability of published DNA sequences. New Phytol 2003;160:43–8.
15. Deckert RJ, Hsiang T, Peterson RL. Genetic relationships of endophytic *Lophodermium nitens* isolates from needles of *Pinus strobus*. Mycol Res 2002;106: 305–13.
16. Crous PW. Adhering to good cultural practice (GCP). Mycol Res 2002;106: 1378–9.
17. Schoch CL, Seifert KA, Huhndorf S, et al, Fungal Barcoding Consortium, Fungal Barcoding Consortium Author List. Nuclear ribosomal internal transcribed spacer (ITS) region as a universal DNA barcode marker for Fungi. Proc Natl Acad Sci U S A 2012;109:6241–6.
18. Seifert KA. Progress towards DNA barcoding of fungi. Mol Ecol Resour 2009; 9(Suppl 1):83–9.
19. Petti CA. Detection and identification of microorganisms by gene amplification and sequencing. Clin Infect Dis 2007;44:1108–14.
20. Saenz AJ, Petersen CE, Valentine NB, et al. Reproducibility of matrix-assisted laser desorption/ionization time-of-flight mass spectrometry for replicate bacterial culture analysis. Rapid Commun Mass Spectrom 1999;13:1580–5.
21. Walker J, Fox AJ, Edwards-Jones V, et al. Intact cell mass spectrometry (ICMS) used to type methicillin-resistant *Staphylococcus aureus*: media effects and inter-laboratory reproducibility. J Microbiol Methods 2002;48:117–26.
22. Bernardo K, Pakulat N, Macht M, et al. Identification and discrimination of Staphylococcus aureus strains using matrix-assisted laser desorption/ionization-time of flight mass spectrometry. Proteomics 2002;2:747–53.
23. Seng P, Drancourt M, Gouriet F, et al. Ongoing revolution in bacteriology: routine identification of bacteria by matrix-assisted laser desorption ionization time-of-flight mass spectrometry. Clin Infect Dis 2009;49:543–51.
24. Singhal N, Kumar M, Kanaujia PK, et al. MALDI-TOF mass spectrometry: an emerging technology for microbial identification and diagnosis. Front Microbiol 2015;6:791.
25. Nomura F. Proteome-based bacterial identification using matrix-assisted laser desorption ionization-time of flight mass spectrometry (MALDI-TOF MS): A revolutionary shift in clinical diagnostic microbiology. Biochim Biophys Acta 2015; 1854:528–37.
26. Croxatto A, Prod'hom G, Greub G. Applications of MALDI-TOF mass spectrometry in clinical diagnostic microbiology. FEMS Microbiol Rev 2012;36:380–407.
27. Anhalt JP, Fenselau C. Identification of bacteria using mass-spectrometry. Anal Chem 1975;47:219–25.

28. Risby TH, Yergey AL. Identification of bacteria using linear programmed thermal-degradation mass-spectrometry - preliminary investigation. J Phys Chem 1976;80(26):2839–45.

29. Karas M, Hillenkamp F. Laser desorption ionization of proteins with molecular masses exceeding 10,000 daltons. Anal Chem 1988;60:2299–301.

30. Sauer S. Typing of single nucleotide polymorphisms by MALDI mass spectrometry: principles and diagnostic applications. Clin Chim Acta 2006;363:95–105.

31. Claydon MA, Davey SN, EdwardsJones V, et al. The rapid identification of intact microorganisms using mass spectrometry. Nat Biotechnol 1996;14:1584–6.

32. Girault S, Chassaing G, Blais JC, et al. Coupling of MALDI-TOF mass analysis to the separation of biotinylated peptides by magnetic streptavidin beads. Anal Chem 1996;68:2122–6.

33. Liang XL, Zheng KF, Qian MG, et al. Determination of bacterial protein profiles by matrix-assisted laser desorption/ionization mass spectrometry with high-performance liquid chromatography. Rapid Commun Mass Spectrom 1996; 10:1219–26.

34. Li TY, Liu BH, Chen YC. Characterization of *Aspergillus* spores by matrix-assisted laser desorption/ionization time-of-flight mass spectrometry. Rapid Commun Mass Spectrom 2000;14:2393–400.

35. Holland RD, Wilkes JG, Rafii F, et al. Rapid identification of intact whole bacteria based on spectral patterns using matrix-assisted laser desorption/ionization with time-of-flight mass spectrometry. Rapid Commun Mass Spectrom 1996; 10:1227–32.

36. Krishnamurthy T, Ross PL, Rajamani U. Detection of pathogenic and non-pathogenic bacteria by matrix-assisted laser desorption/ionization time-of-flight mass spectrometry. Rapid Commun Mass Spectrom 1996;10:883–8.

37. Cain TC, Lubman DM, Weber WJ. Differentiation of bacteria using protein profiles from matrix-assisted laser-desorption ionization time-of-flight mass-spectrometry. Rapid Commun Mass Spectrom 1994;8:1026–30.

38. Amiri-Eliasi BJ, Fenselau C. Characterization of protein biomarkers desorbed by MALDI from whole fungal cells. Anal Chem 2001;73:5228–31.

39. Yvonne Shea MS. Successful validation and clearance of MALDI-ToF MS for microorganism identification. FDA; 2014. Available at: http://www.fda.gov/downloads/MedicalDevices/NewsEvents/WorkshopsConferences/UCM401483.pdf. Accessed November 11, 2015..

40. Bader O, Weig M, Taverne-Ghadwal L, et al. Improved clinical laboratory identification of human pathogenic yeasts by matrix-assisted laser desorption ionization time-of-flight mass spectrometry. Clin Microbiol Infect 2011;17:1359–65.

41. Pinto A, Halliday C, Zahra M, et al. Matrix-assisted laser desorption ionization-time of flight mass spectrometry identification of yeasts is contingent on robust reference spectra. PLoS One 2011;6:e25712.

42. Posteraro B, Vella A, Cogliati M, et al. Matrix-assisted laser desorption ionization-time of flight mass spectrometry-based method for discrimination between molecular types of *Cryptococcus neoformans* and *Cryptococcus gattii*. J Clin Microbiol 2012;50:2472–6.

43. Marklein G, Josten M, Klanke U, et al. Matrix-assisted laser desorption ionization-time of flight mass spectrometry for fast and reliable identification of clinical yeast isolates. J Clin Microbiol 2009;47:2912–7.

44. Bizzini A, Greub G. Matrix-assisted laser desorption ionization time-of-flight mass spectrometry, a revolution in clinical microbial identification. Clin Microbiol Infect 2010;16:1614–9.

45. van Veen SQ, Claas ECJ, Kuijper EJ. High-throughput identification of bacteria and yeast by matrix-assisted laser desorption ionization-time of flight mass spectrometry in conventional medical microbiology laboratories. J Clin Microbiol 2010;48:900–7.

46. Westblade LF, Jennemann R, Branda JA, et al. Multicenter study evaluating the Vitek MS system for identification of medically important yeasts. J Clin Microbiol 2013;51:2267–72.

47. Pence MA, McElvania TeKippe E, Wallace MA, et al. Comparison and optimization of two MALDI-TOF MS platforms for the identification of medically relevant yeast species. Eur J Clin Microbiol Infect Dis 2014; 33:1703–12.

48. Mancini N, De Carolis E, Infurnari L, et al. Comparative evaluation of the Bruker Biotyper and Vitek MS matrix-assisted laser desorption ionization-time of flight (MALDI-TOF) mass spectrometry systems for identification of yeasts of medical importance. J Clin Microbiol 2013;51:2453–7.

49. Stevenson LG, Drake SK, Shea YR, et al. Evaluation of matrix-assisted laser desorption ionization-time of flight mass spectrometry for identification of clinically important yeast species. J Clin Microbiol 2010;48:3482–6.

50. Santos C, Paterson RRM, Venancio A, et al. Filamentous fungal characterizations by matrix-assisted laser desorption/ionization time-of-flight mass spectrometry. J Appl Microbiol 2010;108:375–85.

51. Hettick JM, Green BJ, Buskirk AD, et al. Discrimination of Penicillium isolates by matrix-assisted laser desorption/ionization time-of-flight mass spectrometry fingerprinting. Rapid Commun Mass Spectrom 2008;22:2555–60.

52. Chen HY, Chen YC. Characterization of intact *Penicillium* spores by matrix-assisted laser desorption/ionization mass spectrometry. Rapid Commun Mass Spectrom 2005;19:3564–8.

53. Marinach-Patrice C, Lethuillier A, Marly A, et al. Use of mass spectrometry to identify clinical *Fusarium* isolates. Clin Microbiol Infect 2009;15:634–42.

54. De Carolis E, Posteraro B, Lass-Florl C, et al. Species identification of *Aspergillus, Fusarium* and *Mucorales* with direct surface analysis by matrix-assisted laser desorption ionization time-of-flight mass spectrometry. Clin Microbiol Infect 2012;18:475–84.

55. Becker PT, de Bel A, Martiny D, et al. Identification of filamentous fungi isolates by MALDI-TOF mass spectrometry: clinical evaluation of an extended reference spectra library. Med Mycol 2014;52:826–34.

56. Lau AF, Drake SK, Calhoun LB, et al. Development of a clinically comprehensive database and a simple procedure for identification of molds from solid media by matrix-assisted laser desorption ionization-time of flight mass spectrometry. J Clin Microbiol 2013;51:828–34.

57. Wisplinghoff H, Bischoff T, Tallent SM, et al. Nosocomial bloodstream infections in US hospitals: analysis of 24,179 cases from a prospective nationwide surveillance study. Clin Infect Dis 2004;39:309–17.

58. Sievert DM, Ricks P, Edwards JR, et al, National Healthcare Safety Network(NHSN) Team and Participating NHSN Facilities. Antimicrobial-resistant pathogens associated with healthcare-associated infections: summary of data reported to the National Healthcare Safety Network at the Centers for Disease Control and Prevention, 2009-2010. Infect Control Hosp Epidemiol 2013;34: 1–14.

59. Yapar N. Epidemiology and risk factors for invasive candidiasis. Ther Clin Risk Manag 2014;10:95–105.

60. Pappas PG, Rex JH, Lee J, et al. A prospective observational study of candidemia: epidemiology, therapy, and influences on mortality in hospitalized adult and pediatric patients. Clin Infect Dis 2003;37:634–43.

61. Lee H, Sun E, Ham D, et al. Chip-NMR biosensor for detection and molecular analysis of cells. Nat Med 2008;14:869–74.

62. Haun JB, Castro CM, Wang R, et al. Micro-NMR for rapid molecular analysis of human tumor samples. Sci Transl Med 2011;3:71ra16.

63. Neely LA, Audeh M, Phung NA, et al. T2 magnetic resonance enables nanoparticle-mediated rapid detection of candidemia in whole blood. Sci Transl Med 2013;5:182ra154.

64. Mylonakis E, Clancy CJ, Ostrosky-Zeichner L, et al. T2 magnetic resonance assay for the rapid diagnosis of candidemia in whole blood: a clinical trial. Clin Infect Dis 2015;60:892–9.

65. Technology Behind-T2candida. 2015. Available at: http://www.t2biosystems.com/t2candida/technology-behind-t2candida/. Accessed October 16, 2015.

66. Beyda ND, Alam MJ, Garey KW. Comparison of the T2Dx instrument with T2Candida assay and automated blood culture in the detection of Candida species using seeded blood samples. Diagn Microbiol Infect Dis 2013;77:324–6.

67. Dromer F, Mathoulin-Pelissier S, Launay O, et al, French Cryptococcosis Study Group. Determinants of disease presentation and outcome during cryptococcosis: the CryptoA/D study. PLoS Med 2007;4:e21.

68. Brouwer AE, Teparrukkul P, Pinpraphaporn S, et al. Baseline correlation and comparative kinetics of cerebrospinal fluid colony-forming unit counts and antigen titers in cryptococcal meningitis. J Infect Dis 2005;192:681–4.

69. Diamond RD, Bennett JE. Prognostic factors in cryptococcal meningitis. A study in 111 cases. Ann Intern Med 1974;80:176–81.

70. Kabanda T, Siedner MJ, Klausner JD, et al. Point-of-care diagnosis and prognostication of cryptococcal meningitis with the cryptococcal antigen lateral flow assay on cerebrospinal fluid. Clin Infect Dis 2014;58:113–6.

71. Lortholary O, Poizat G, Zeller V, et al. Long-term outcome of AIDS-associated cryptococcosis in the era of combination antiretroviral therapy. AIDS 2006;20:2183–91.

72. Boulware DR, Meya DB, Bergemann TL, et al. Clinical features and serum biomarkers in HIV immune reconstitution inflammatory syndrome after cryptococcal meningitis: a prospective cohort study. PLoS Med 2010;7:e1000384.

73. Jaye DL, Waites KB, Parker B, et al. Comparison of two rapid latex agglutination tests for detection of cryptococcal capsular polysaccharide. Am J Clin Pathol 1998;109:634–41.

74. Kiska DL, Orkiszewski DR, Howell D, et al. Evaluation of new monoclonal antibody-based latex agglutination test for detection of cryptococcal polysaccharide antigen in serum and cerebrospinal fluid. J Clin Microbiol 1994;32:2309–11.

75. Tanner DC, Weinstein MP, Fedorciw B, et al. Comparison of commercial kits for detection of cryptococcal antigen. J Clin Microbiol 1994;32:1680–4.

76. Gade W, Hinnefeld SW, Babcock LS, et al. Comparison of the PREMIER cryptococcal antigen enzyme immunoassay and the latex agglutination assay for detection of cryptococcal antigens. J Clin Microbiol 1991;29:1616–9.

77. McMullan BJ, Halliday C, Sorrell TC, et al. Clinical utility of the cryptococcal antigen lateral flow assay in a diagnostic mycology laboratory. PLoS One 2012;7:e49541.

78. Boulware DR, Rolfes MA, Rajasingham R, et al. Multisite validation of crypto-coccal antigen lateral flow assay and quantification by laser thermal contrast. Emerg Infect Dis 2014;20:45–53.

79. Lindsley MD, Mekha N, Baggett HC, et al. Evaluation of a newly developed lateral flow immunoassay for the diagnosis of cryptococcosis. Clin Infect Dis 2011;53:321–5.

80. Jarvis JN, Percival A, Bauman S, et al. Evaluation of a novel point-of-care cryp-tococcal antigen test on serum, plasma, and urine from patients with HIV-associated cryptococcal meningitis. Clin Infect Dis 2011;53:1019–23.

81. WHO. Rapid advice: diagnosis, prevention and management of cryptococcal disease in HIV-infected adults, adolescents and children. Geneva (Switzerland): WHO press; 2011.

82. Binnicker MJ, Jespersen DJ, Bestrom JE, et al. Comparison of four assays for the detection of cryptococcal antigen. Clin Vaccine Immunol 2012;19: 1988–90.

83. Suwantarat N, Dalton JB, Lee R, et al. Large-scale clinical validation of a lateral flow immunoassay for detection of cryptococcal antigen in serum and cerebro-spinal fluid specimens. Diagn Microbiol Infect Dis 2015;82:54–6.

84. Hansen J, Slechta ES, Gates-Hollingsworth MA, et al. Large-scale evaluation of the immuno-mycologics lateral flow and enzyme-linked immunoassays for detection of cryptococcal antigen in serum and cerebrospinal fluid. Clin Vaccine Immunol 2013;20:52–5.

85. Rajasingham R, Meya DB, Boulware DR. Integrating cryptococcal antigen screening and pre-emptive treatment into routine HIV care. J Acquir Immune Defic Syndr 2012;59:e85–91.

86. Pfaller MA, Rex JH, Rinaldi MG. Antifungal susceptibility testing: technical ad-vances and potential clinical applications. Clin Infect Dis 1997;24:776–84.

87. Rex JH, Pfaller MA. Has antifungal susceptibility testing come of age? Clin Infect Dis 2002;35:982–9.

88. Pfaller MA, Diekema DJ. Progress in antifungal susceptibility testing of Candida spp. by use of Clinical and Laboratory Standards Institute broth microdilution methods, 2010 to 2012. J Clin Microbiol 2012;50:2846–56.

89. Baddley JW, Patel M, Bhavnani SM, et al. Association of fluconazole pharmaco-dynamics with mortality in patients with candidemia. Antimicrob Agents Chemo-ther 2008;52:3022–8.

90. Collins CD, Eschenauer GA, Salo SL, et al. To test or not to test: a cost minimi-zation analysis of susceptibility testing for patients with documented Candida glabrata fungemias. J Clin Microbiol 2007;45:1884–8.

91. Pappas PG, Rex JH, Sobel JD, et al, French Cryptococcosis Study Group. Guidelines for treatment of candidiasis. Clin Infect Dis 2004;38:161–89.

92. Chryssanthou E, Gronfors C, Khanna N. Comparison of broth macrodilution, broth microdilution and E-test susceptibility tests of Cryptococcus neoformans for fluconazole. Mycoses 1997;40:423–7.

93. CLSI. Reference method for broth dilution antifungal susceptibility testing of yeasts; approved standard - third edition. CLSI Document M27-A3. Wayne (PA): Clinical and Laboratory Standards Institute; 2008.

94. Arendrup MC, Cuenca-Estrella M, Lass-Florl C, et al. EUCAST technical note on the EUCAST definitive document EDef 7.2: method for the determi-nation of broth dilution minimum inhibitory concentrations of antifungal agents for yeasts EDef 7.2 (EUCAST-AFST). Clin Microbiol Infect 2012;18: E246–7.

95. Pfaller MA, Castanheira M, Diekema DJ, et al. Comparison of European Committee on Antimicrobial Susceptibility Testing (EUCAST) and Etest methods with the CLSI broth microdilution method for echinocandin susceptibility testing of Candida species. J Clin Microbiol 2010;48:1592–9.
96. Pfaller MA, Andes D, Diekema DJ, et al, CLSI Subcommittee for Antifungal Susceptibility Testing. Wild-type MIC distributions, epidemiological cutoff values and species-specific clinical breakpoints for fluconazole and Candida: time for harmonization of CLSI and EUCAST broth microdilution methods. Drug Resist Updat 2010;13:180–95.
97. Arendrup MC, Garcia-Effron G, Lass-Florl C, et al. Echinocandin susceptibility testing of Candida species: comparison of EUCAST EDef 7.1, CLSI M27-A3, Etest, disk diffusion, and agar dilution methods with RPMI and isosensitest media. Antimicrob Agents Chemother 2010;54:426–39.
98. Espinel-Ingroff A, Arendrup MC, Pfaller MA, et al. Interlaboratory variability of Caspofungin MICs for Candida spp. Using CLSI and EUCAST methods: should the clinical laboratory be testing this agent? Antimicrob Agents Chemother 2013;57:5836–42.
99. Pfaller MA, Diekema DJ, Jones RN, et al. Use of anidulafungin as a surrogate marker to predict susceptibility and resistance to caspofungin among 4,290 clinical isolates of Candida by using CLSI methods and interpretive criteria. J Clin Microbiol 2014;52:3223–9.
100. Pfaller MA, Messer SA, Diekema DJ, et al. Use of micafungin as a surrogate marker to predict susceptibility and resistance to caspofungin among 3,764 clinical isolates of Candida by use of CLSI methods and interpretive criteria. J Clin Microbiol 2014;52:108–14.
101. Pfaller MA, Castanheira M, Messer SA, et al. Comparison of EUCAST and CLSI broth microdilution methods for the susceptibility testing of 10 Systemically active antifungal agents when tested against Candida spp. Diagn Microbiol Infect Dis 2014;79:198–204.
102. Turnidge J, Paterson DL. Setting and revising antibacterial susceptibility breakpoints. Clin Microbiol Rev 2007;20:391–408.
103. CLSI. Reference method for broth dilution antifungal susceptibility testing of yeasts; fourth informational supplement. CLSI document M27-S4. Wayne (PA): Clinical and Laboratory Standards Institute; 2012.
104. Alexander BD, Byrne TC, Smith KL, et al. Comparative evaluation of etest and sensititre YeastOne panels against the clinical and laboratory standards institute M27-A2 reference broth microdilution method for testing Candida susceptibility to seven antifungal agents. J Clin Microbiol 2007;45:698–706.
105. Cuenca-Estrella M, Gomez-Lopez A, Alastruey-Izquierdo A, et al. Comparison of the Vitek 2 antifungal susceptibility system with the clinical and laboratory standards institute (CLSI) and European Committee on Antimicrobial Susceptibility Testing (EUCAST) Broth Microdilution Reference Methods and with the Sensititre YeastOne and Etest techniques for in vitro detection of antifungal resistance in yeast isolates. J Clin Microbiol 2010;48:1782–6.
106. Espinel-Ingroff A, Pfaller M, Messer SA, et al. Multicenter comparison of the Sensititre YeastOne colorimetric antifungal panel with the NCCLS M27-A2 reference method for testing new antifungal agents against clinical isolates of Candida spp. J Clin Microbiol 2004;42:718–21.
107. Espinel-Ingroff A, Pfaller M, Messer SA, et al. Multicenter comparison of the sensititre YeastOne Colorimetric Antifungal Panel with the National Committee for Clinical Laboratory standards M27-A reference method for testing clinical

isolates of common and emerging *Candida* spp., *Cryptococcus* spp., and other yeasts and yeast-like organisms. J Clin Microbiol 1999;37:591–5.

108. Pfaller MA, Chaturvedi V, Diekema DJ, et al. Comparison of the Sensititre YeastOne colorimetric antifungal panel with CLSI microdilution for antifungal susceptibility testing of the echinocandins against *Candida* spp., using new clinical breakpoints and epidemiological cutoff values. Diagn Microbiol Infect Dis 2012;73:365–8.

109. Pfaller MA, Chaturvedi V, Diekema DJ, et al. Clinical evaluation of the Sensititre YeastOne colorimetric antifungal panel for antifungal susceptibility testing of the echinocandins anidulafungin, caspofungin, and micafungin. J Clin Microbiol 2008;46:2155–9.

110. Pfaller MA, Espinel-Ingroff A, Jones RN. Clinical evaluation of the sensititre YeastOne colorimetric antifungal plate for antifungal susceptibility testing of the new triazoles voriconazole, posaconazole, and ravuconazole. J Clin Microbiol 2004; 42:4577–80.

111. Pfaller MA, Jones RN, Microbiology Resource Committee, College of American Pathologists. Performance accuracy of antibacterial and antifungal susceptibility test methods: report from the College of American Pathologists Microbiology Surveys Program (2001-2003). Arch Pathol Lab Med 2006;130:767–78.

112. Eschenauer GA, Nguyen MH, Shoham S, et al. Real-world experience with echinocandin MICs against *Candida* species in a multicenter study of hospitals that routinely perform susceptibility testing of bloodstream isolates. Antimicrob Agents Chemother 2014;58:1897–906.

113. Shields RK, Nguyen MH, Press EG, et al. The presence of an FKS mutation rather than MIC is an independent risk factor for failure of echinocandin therapy among patients with invasive candidiasis due to *Candida glabrata*. Antimicrob Agents Chemother 2012;56:4862–9.

114. Wanger A, Mills K, Nelson PW, et al. Comparison of etest and national-committee-for-clinical-laboratory-standards broth macrodilution method for antifungal susceptibility testing - enhanced ability to detect amphotericin B-resistant *Candida* isolates. Antimicrob Agents Chemother 1995;39:2520–2.

115. Baker CN, Stocker SA, Culver DH, et al. Comparison of the E-test to agar dilution, broth microdilution, and agar diffusion susceptibility testing techniques by using a special challenge set of bacteria. J Clin Microbiol 1991; 29:533–8.

116. Lozano-Chiu M, Paetznick VL, Ghannoum MA, et al. Detection of resistance to amphotericin B among *Cryptococcus neoformans* clinical isolates: performances of three different media assessed by using E-test and National Committee for Clinical Laboratory Standards M27-A methodologies. J Clin Microbiol 1998;36:2817–22.

117. Arendrup MC, Pfaller MA, Danish Fungaemia Study Group. Caspofungin Etest susceptibility testing of Candida species: risk of misclassification of susceptible isolates of *C. glabrata* and *C. krusei* when adopting the revised CLSI caspofungin breakpoints. Antimicrob Agents Chemother 2012;56:3965–8.

118. Bourgeois N, Laurens C, Bertout S, et al. Assessment of caspofungin susceptibility of *Candida glabrata* by the Etest(R), CLSI, and EUCAST methods, and detection of FKS1 and FKS2 mutations. Eur J Clin Microbiol Infect Dis 2014; 33:1247–52.

119. Caramalho R, Maurer E, Binder U, et al. Etest cannot be recommended for in vitro susceptibility testing of mucorales. Antimicrob Agents Chemother 2015;59:3663–5.

120. Borghi E, Iatta R, Sciota R, et al. Comparative evaluation of the Vitek 2 yeast susceptibility test and CLSI broth microdilution reference method for testing antifungal susceptibility of invasive fungal isolates in Italy: the GISIA3 study. J Clin Microbiol 2010;48:3153–7.
121. Bourgeois N, Dehandschoewercker L, Bertout S, et al. Antifungal susceptibility of 205 *Candida* spp. isolated primarily during invasive Candidiasis and comparison of the Vitek 2 system with the CLSI broth microdilution and Etest methods. J Clin Microbiol 2010;48:154–61.
122. Pfaller MA, Diekema DJ, Procop GW, et al. Multicenter comparison of the VITEK 2 antifungal susceptibility test with the CLSI broth microdilution reference method for testing amphotericin B, flucytosine, and voriconazole against *Candida* spp. J Clin Microbiol 2007;45:3522–8.
123. Pfaller MA, Diekema DJ, Procop GW, et al. Multicenter comparison of the VITEK 2 yeast susceptibility test with the CLSI broth microdilution reference method for testing fluconazole against *Candida* spp. J Clin Microbiol 2007; 45:796–802.
124. Pfaller MA, Diekema DJ, Procop GW, et al. Comparison of the Vitek 2 yeast susceptibility system with CLSI microdilution for antifungal susceptibility testing of fluconazole and voriconazole against *Candida* spp., using new clinical breakpoints and epidemiological cutoff values. Diagn Microbiol Infect Dis 2013;77: 37–40.
125. Posteraro B, Martucci R, La Sorda M, et al. Reliability of the Vitek 2 yeast susceptibility test for detection of in vitro resistance to fluconazole and voriconazole in clinical isolates of *Candida albicans* and *Candida glabrata*. J Clin Microbiol 2009;47:1927–30.
126. Pfaller MA, Diekema DJ, Procop GW, et al. Multicenter evaluation of the new Vitek 2 yeast susceptibility test using new CLSI clinical breakpoints for fluconazole. J Clin Microbiol 2014;52:2126–30.
127. Aubertine CL, Rivera M, Rohan SM, et al. Comparative study of the new colorimetric VITEK 2 yeast identification card versus the older fluorometric card and of CHROMagar *Candida* as a source medium with the new card. J Clin Microbiol 2006;44:227–8.
128. Peterson JF, Pfaller MA, Diekema DJ, et al. Multicenter Comparison of the vitek 2 antifungal susceptibility test with the CLSI broth microdilution reference method for testing caspofungin, micafungin, and posaconazole against *Candida* spp. J Clin Microbiol 2011;49:1765–71.
129. Astvad KM, Perlin DS, Johansen HK, et al. Evaluation of caspofungin susceptibility testing by the new vitek 2 AST-YS06 yeast card using a unique collection of FKS wild-type and hot spot mutant isolates, including the five most common *Candida* Species. Antimicrob Agents Chemother 2013;57:177–82.
130. Pfeiffer CD, Garcia-Effron G, Zaas AK, et al. Breakthrough invasive candidiasis in patients on micafungin. J Clin Microbiol 2010;48:2373–80.
131. Alexander BD, Johnson MD, Pfeiffer CD, et al. Increasing echinocandin resistance in *Candida glabrata*: clinical failure correlates with presence of FKS mutations and elevated minimum inhibitory concentrations. Clin Infect Dis 2013; 56:1724–32.
132. Beyda ND, John J, Kilic A, et al. FKS mutant Candida glabrata: risk factors and outcomes in patients with candidemia. Clin Infect Dis 2014;59:819–25.
133. Pham CD, Bolden CB, Kuykendall RJ, et al. Development of a Luminex-based multiplex assay for detection of mutations conferring resistance to Echinocandins in *Candida glabrata*. J Clin Microbiol 2014;52:790–5.

134. Pfaller MA, Castanheira M, Lockhart SR, et al. Frequency of decreased susceptibility and resistance to echinocandins among fluconazole-resistant bloodstream isolates of *Candida glabrata*. J Clin Microbiol 2012;50: 1199–203.

135. Shields RK, Nguyen MH, Press EG, et al. Anidulafungin and micafungin MIC breakpoints are superior to that of caspofungin for identifying FKS mutant *Candida glabrata* strains and Echinocandin resistance. Antimicrob Agents Chemother 2013;57:6361–5.

136. Garcia-Effron G, Lee S, Park S, et al. Effect of *Candida glabrata* FKS1 and FKS2 mutations on echinocandin sensitivity and kinetics of 1,3-beta-D-glucan synthase: implication for the existing susceptibility breakpoint. Antimicrob Agents Chemother 2009;53:3690–9.

137. Arendrup MC, Perlin DS, Jensen RH, et al. Differential in vivo activities of anidulafungin, caspofungin, and micafungin against *Candida glabrata* isolates with and without FKS resistance mutations. Antimicrob Agents Chemother 2012;56: 2435–42.

138. Chryssanthou E. In vitro susceptibility of respiratory isolates of *Aspergillus* species to itraconazole and amphotericin B. acquired resistance to itraconazole. Scand J Infect Dis 1997;29:509–12.

139. Denning DW, Venkateswarlu K, Oakley KL, et al. Itraconazole resistance in *Aspergillus fumigatus*. Antimicrob Agents Chemother 1997;41:1364–8.

140. Howard SJ, Cerar D, Anderson MJ, et al. Frequency and evolution of Azole resistance in *Aspergillus fumigatus* associated with treatment failure. Emerg Infect Dis 2009;15:1068–76.

141. Lockhart SR, Frade JP, Etienne KA, et al. Azole resistance in *Aspergillus fumigatus* isolates from the ARTEMIS global surveillance study is primarily due to the TR/L98H mutation in the cyp51A gene. Antimicrob Agents Chemother 2011; 55:4465–8.

142. Baddley JW, Marr KA, Andes DR, et al. Patterns of susceptibility of *Aspergillus* isolates recovered from patients enrolled in the Transplant-Associated Infection Surveillance Network. J Clin Microbiol 2009;47:3271–5.

143. Pfaller M, Boyken L, Hollis R, et al. Use of epidemiological cutoff values to examine 9-year trends in susceptibility of *Aspergillus* species to the triazoles. J Clin Microbiol 2011;49:586–90.

144. Pfaller MA, Diekema DJ, Ghannoum MA, et al, Clinical and Laboratory Standards Institute Antifungal Testing Subcommittee. Wild-type MIC distribution and epidemiological cutoff values for *Aspergillus fumigatus* and three triazoles as determined by the Clinical and Laboratory Standards Institute broth microdilution methods. J Clin Microbiol 2009;47:3142–6.

145. Bueid A, Howard SJ, Moore CB, et al. Azole antifungal resistance in *Aspergillus fumigatus*: 2008 and 2009. J Antimicrob Chemother 2010;65: 2116–8.

146. Snelders E, van der Lee HA, Kuijpers J, et al. Emergence of azole resistance in *Aspergillus fumigatus* and spread of a single resistance mechanism. PLoS Med 2008;5:e219.

147. Snelders E, Huis In 't Veld RA, Rijs AJ, et al. Possible environmental origin of resistance of *Aspergillus fumigatus* to medical triazoles. Appl Environ Microbiol 2009;75:4053–7.

148. Chowdhary A, Sharma C, Kathuria S, et al. Azole-resistant *Aspergillus fumigatus* with the environmental TR46/Y121F/T289A mutation in India. J Antimicrob Chemother 2014;69:555–7.

149. van der Linden JW, Camps SM, Kampinga GA, et al. Aspergillosis due to vori-conazole highly resistant *Aspergillus fumigatus* and recovery of genetically related resistant isolates from domiciles. Clin Infect Dis 2013;57:513–20.
150. Chowdhary A, Kathuria S, Xu J, et al. Clonal expansion and emergence of environmental multiple-triazole-resistant *Aspergillus fumigatus* strains car-rying the TR(3)(4)/L98H mutations in the cyp51A gene in India. PLoS One 2012;7:e52871.
151. Seyedmousavi S, Hashemi SJ, Zibafar E, et al. Azole-resistant *Aspergillus fumi-gatus*, Iran. Emerg Infect Dis 2013;19:832–4.
152. Badali H, Vaezi A, Haghani I, et al. Environmental study of azole-resistant *Asper-gillus fumigatus* with TR34/L98H mutations in the cyp51A gene in Iran. Mycoses 2013;56:659–63.
153. Chowdhary A, Sharma C, van den Boom M, et al. Multi-azole-resistant *Asper-gillus fumigatus* in the environment in Tanzania. J Antimicrob Chemother 2014;69:2979–83.
154. Wiederhold NP, Garcia Gil V, Gutierrez F, et al. First detection of TR34/L98H and TR46/Y121F/T289A Cyp51 mutations in *Aspergillus fumigatus* isolates in the United States. J Clin Microbiol 2015. [Epub ahead of print].
155. Seyedmousavi S, Mouton JW, Melchers WJ, et al. The role of azoles in the man-agement of azole-resistant aspergillosis: from the bench to the bedside. Drug Resist Updat 2014;17:37–50.
156. van der Linden JW, Snelders E, Kampinga GA, et al. Clinical implications of azole resistance in *Aspergillus fumigatus*, The Netherlands, 2007-2009. Emerg Infect Dis 2011;17:1846–54.
157. Sugui JA, Peterson SW, Figat A, et al. Genetic relatedness versus biological compatibility between *Aspergillus fumigatu*s and related species. J Clin Micro-biol 2014;52:3707–21.
158. Barrs VR, van Doorn TM, Houbraken J, et al. Aspergillus felis sp. nov., an emerging agent of invasive aspergillosis in humans, cats, and dogs. PLoS One 2013;8:e64871.
159. Zbinden A, Imhof A, Wilhelm MJ, et al. Fatal outcome after heart transplantation caused by *Aspergillus lentulus*. Transpl Infect Dis 2012;14:E60–3.
160. Vinh DC, Shea YR, Jones PA, et al. Chronic invasive aspergillosis caused by *Aspergillus viridinutans*. Emerg Infect Dis 2009;15:1292–4.
161. Vermeulen E, Lagrou K, Verweij PE. Azole resistance in *Aspergillus fumigatus*: a growing public health concern. Curr Opin Infect Dis 2013;26:493–500.

Nonculture Diagnostics in Fungal Disease

Margaret V. Powers-Fletcher, PhD[a], Kimberly E. Hanson, MD, MHS[b,c],*

KEYWORDS

- Laboratory diagnosis of invasive fungal infection • Fungal antigen detection
- Fungal serology • Molecular detection of fungi • Clinical mycology

KEY POINTS

- The direct detection of fungal components in clinical specimens can expedite the diagnosis of an invasive infection. Molecular diagnostics in particular have the potential for high sensitivity and specificity with a rapid turnaround time.
- Serial surveillance with fungal cell wall biomarkers and/or polymerase chain reaction is useful to guide preemptive and targeted therapy in at-risk stem cell transplant and hematologic malignancy patients.
- Because of the ubiquitous nature of fungi in the environment, false-positive test results are possible and results should be interpreted in the context of the patients and the clinical setting.

INTRODUCTION

Isolation of fungi in culture is a critical component of the diagnostic process and is required for phenotypic susceptibility testing. However, laboratory techniques that do not require growing the organism in culture (eg, fungal antibody, antigen, nucleic acid, and/or histology-based detection) also play an important role in the diagnosis of invasive fungal infection (IFI) and have potential advantages that supplement traditional culture-based methods. The purpose of this review is to discuss the test characteristics of nonculture diagnostics, to summarize their associated advantages and disadvantages (**Box 1**), and highlight the ways in which these nonculture assays have been integrated into clinical algorithms for the diagnosis and management of IFI (**Fig. 1**).

Disclosure statement: The authors have nothing to disclose.
[a] ARUP Laboratories, 500 Chipeta Way, Salt Lake City, UT 84108, USA; [b] Department of Medicine, Division of Infectious Diseases, University of Utah School of Medicine, 30 N 1900E, Room 4B319, Salt Lake City, UT 84132, USA; [c] Department of Pathology, University of Utah School of Medicine, 15 N Medical Drive East, Suite 1100, Salt Lake City, UT 84122, USA
* Corresponding author. University of Utah School of Medicine, 30 North 1900 East, Room 4B319, Salt Lake City, UT 84132.
E-mail address: kim.hanson@hsc.utah.edu

Infect Dis Clin N Am 30 (2016) 37–49
http://dx.doi.org/10.1016/j.idc.2015.10.005
0891-5520/16/$ – see front matter © 2016 Elsevier Inc. All rights reserved.

id.theclinics.com

Box 1
Advantages and limitations of nonculture diagnostic techniques for fungi

Antibody detection

+ It provides evidence of previous exposure and identifies at-risk patient populations.

+ It supports the diagnosis of certain infections (ie, histoplasmosis, coccidioidomycosis, or chronic and allergic aspergillosis) and is useful for following the response to therapy.

− It does not consistently differentiate between previous exposure and active disease.

Antigen detection[a]

+ Serial surveillance of at-risk patients may identify fungal infections sooner than traditional methods and has utility for preemptive therapeutic strategies.

+ It may be useful as a prognostic indicator and for following the response to therapy.

− Utility of a single test result for diagnosis is limited, and repeated positives are required to define a positive result.

− Cross reactivity between related organisms limits specificity, and false-positive tests are common.

Histology and special stains

+ It is the gold standard for diagnosis of IFI.

+ It allows differentiation of organisms into broad categories of potential pathogens.

− There is limited specificity for genus- and species-level identification.

− Sensitivity depends on the adequacy of sample collection.

− It requires invasive procedures to obtain a specimen.

Nucleic acid detection

+ There is potential for high sensitivity and specificity using a variety of specimen types.

+ It produces more rapid results than traditional methods.

− There is a lack of standardization between laboratory-developed assays.

− It does not differentiate invasive infection from colonization or contamination.

− Most assays require specialized equipment and expertise.

− Sequencing based–tests can be expensive.

+, Advantages; −, limitations.
[a] Comments are focused on the *Aspergillus* galactomannan and (1, 3)-β-D-glucan assays.

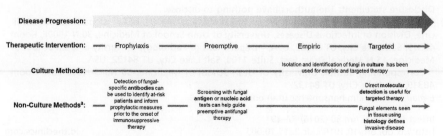

Fig. 1. The diagnostic and therapeutic continuum of IFI.[1]

ANTIBODY DETECTION

Fungi are ubiquitous in the environment, and human exposure to potential pathogens is unavoidable. Previously exposed individuals may have detectable serum antibodies directed to fungal antigens, which does not necessarily indicate an active or recent infection. Serologic testing is not recommended for the diagnosis of IFIs other than histoplasmosis, blastomycosis, coccidioidomycosis, and the chronic or allergic forms of aspergillosis. For example, an increase in total serum immunoglobulin E (IgE) or *Aspergillus*-specific IgE can contribute to a diagnosis of allergic bronchopulmonary aspergillosis.[2] Detection of fungal-specific antibodies can also provide evidence of previous exposure to endemic fungi, which can help identify the etiologic agent of an ongoing disease or identify a patient that is at risk for developing fulminant disease in the future, as is the case for patients undergoing immunosuppressive therapy. Details outlining the test characteristics of commonly used antibody assays for histoplasmosis, blastomycosis, and coccidioidomycosis are described in **Box 2**.

ANTIGEN DETECTION

The ability to detect fungal antigens in patient samples has substantially augmented the approach to IFI diagnosis. These biomarkers, which largely include components of the fungal cell wall, are shed during fungal growth. Their detection can suggest invasive infection in the appropriate patient population, often before other clinical signs or symptoms of disease are present. The cell wall biomarkers should be used in conjunction with other laboratory and clinical findings. The characteristics of different antigen detection assays are described in the text below, with details on assay performance summarized in **Box 3**.

(1, 3)-β-D-Glucan

The cell wall component (1, 3)-β-D-glucan (BDG) is found in many organisms, including *Candida* species, *Pneumocystis jiroveci*, and multiple filamentous fungi, such as *Aspergillus* spp, *Fusarium* spp, and *Acremonium* spp; notable exceptions are *Cryptococcus* spp, the *Mucorales*, and the yeast phase of *Blastomyces dermatitidis*.[7] There is currently one Food and Drug Administration (FDA)–approved assay for the detection of BDG in clinical samples (Fungitell Assay, Associates of Cape Code Inc; Falmouth, MA). This assay is only approved for use with serum specimens, but other specimen types have been used and potentially validated for off-label use by individual laboratories. BDG has been used both for serial surveillance in at-risk patients[8] and as an adjunct to the diagnosis of established IFI.[9] When used for serial screening, sampling rates of 2 to 3 times a week is recommended.[7] The assay has also been used to diagnose infections caused by dimorphic fungi[6,10,11] and on cerebrospinal fluid (CSF) specimens for the diagnosis of fungal meningitis due to *Exserohilum rostratum*.[12]

Aspergillus Galactomannan

Another cell wall biomarker for IFI is galactomannan (GM). GM is produced by a variety of fungi, including *Aspergillus* spp, *Penicillium* spp, *Paecilomyces spp/Purpureocillium licacinum*, and *Histoplasma* spp. There is currently one FDA-approved assay for the detection of *Aspergillus* GM (Platelia Aspergillus EIA, Bio-Rad; Marnes-la-Coquette, France) using both serum and bronchoalveolar lavage (BAL) specimens; additional specimen types, such as CSF, have also been used in clinical practice.[13]

Sequential GM testing has been used to guide preemptive antifungal therapy during the neutropenic period following hematopoietic stem cell transplantation or cytotoxic chemotherapy for hematologic malignancy. A range of testing frequencies has been

Box 2
Characteristics of antibody detection assays for the dimorphic fungi

Complement Fixation

General Information
- CF is predicated on the ability of free complement to lyse sensitized RBCs
  - Positive result
    - Ab present in the patient sample interacts with fungal Ag in the reaction well.
    - The Ab-Ag complex binds free complement.
    - No RBC lysis occurs, and the cells settle to the bottom of the well.
  - Negative result
    - Lack of Ab-Ag complexes results in remaining free complement.
    - RBCs are lysed, producing a red pigment throughout the well.
- Titrations of the patient sample are performed to determine antibody titer.

Histoplasma[3,4]
- Two separate Ags are used (yeast and mycelial).
- Diagnosis is based on fourfold increase in Ab titer.
  - A single titer of 1:32 or greater is suggestive of active infection but not diagnostic.
- Antibodies persist for years after infection.
- It is cross reactive with related fungi and other granulomatous processes.

Blastomyces[4]
- It is frequently cross reactive with *Histoplasma* and *Coccidioides*.
- CF results are positive in approximately 16% to 25% of cases of pulmonary blastomycosis.

Coccidioides[5,6]
- Detectable Abs usually develop within 4 to 6 weeks after exposure and reach a maximum response within 2 to 3 months.
- Any titer suggests past or current infection.
  - A titer of 1:32 or greater may indicate disseminated disease, whereas less than 1:32 suggests past infection or self-limited disease.
  - Positive results should be further defined using immunodiffusion
- Titers are used to follow therapy.

Immunodiffusion

General Information
- Based on the bandlike precipitate that forms when patient Abs and test Ags are combined:
  - Abs (control and patient sample) and soluble fungal Ags are placed in separate wells and allowed to diffuse outward into the test medium.
  - Visible line formation (precipitate) correlating with the positive control suggests target Abs are present.

Histoplasma[3]
- It detects Abs to M and H glycoprotein.
  - The M band is found in both acute and chronic cases and can persist for months to years after infection.
  - The H band is less common and rarely observed without the M band.
- It is more specific but less sensitive than CF.

Blastomyces[4]
- It uses partially purified A antigen of *B dermatitidis*.
- Results of ID are positive in approximately 28% to 40% of cases of pulmonary blastomycosis.

Coccidioides[5,6]
- It can detect Abs that correlate with CF (using an ID-CF antigen) or a tube precipitin (using an ID-TP antigen).
  - ID-TP detects IgM Abs, whereas ID-CF detects IgG antibodies.
- Serum precipitins can be detected within 1 to 3 weeks after the onset of primary infection but are rarely detected 6 months after infection.
  - Precipitins may reappear with relapse or persist in disseminated disease.

Abbreviations: Abs, antibodies; Ag, antigen; RBC, red blood cell; TP, tube precipitin.

Box 3
Characteristics of antigen detection assays

(1, 3)-β-D-glucan

- There is limited specificity for individual fungal pathogens.

- Performance varies based on the organism.
  - Greatest sensitivity (96%) and specificity (84%) for *Pneumocystis* pneumonia[31]
  - Similar sensitivity compared with serum galactomannan for *Aspergillus* spp[32]
  - Increased sensitivity compared with blood culture for invasive candidiasis, with adequate specificity (63%–73%)[33]

- False positives have been associated with the following:
  - Certain hemodialysis dialysis membranes[8]
  - Intravenous immunoglobulin[34]
  - Surgical sponges and gauze products[35]
  - Lung transplantation, possibly as a result of underlying airway colonization[36]
  - Beta-lactam antibiotics may be less problematic than previously thought.[37]

- The optimal cutoff to define a positive test has not been defined for pediatric patients.[38]

Aspergillus galactomannan

- Performance varies by patient population and disease prevalence.[39]
  - The best sensitivity (70%–89%) and specificity (85%–92%) was observed in the HM/HSCT setting.[39]

- Sensitivity increased in BAL relative to serum for pulmonary IA after HM/HSCT and SOT.[40]

- False positives have been associated with the following:
  - Other filamentous fungi
  - Coadministration of certain antibiotics (but piperacillin/tazobactam may no longer be a concern)[41]
  - Certain food stuffs (eg, milk formulas or popsicles)[42]
  - Translocation of *Bifidobacterium* from the guts of neonates[43]

- Detection of GM in BAL does not differentiate colonization from invasive disease.

Histoplasma Antigen

- There is high clinical specificity for an endemic mycosis.
  - Cross reactivity among the dimorphic fungi is possible.[44,45]

- For disseminated disease, antigenuria is the most sensitive.[26]
  - Urine antigen sensitivity: nonimmunosuppressed (80%), immunosuppressed (82%), and patients with AIDS (95%)
  - Serum antigen sensitivity: nonimmunosuppressed (67%), immunosuppressed (60%), and patients with AIDS (86%)
  - Combined urine/serum sensitivity: nonimmunosuppressed (82%), immunosuppressed (82%), and patients with AIDS (95%)

Cryptococcal antigen

- It is highly sensitive and specific, especially for meningoencephalitis and disseminated disease.
  - The following is found in patients with documented or suspected cryptococcal meningitis[28]:

    - Pooled sensitivity and specificity using serum are 97.6% and 98.1%, respectively.

    - Pooled sensitivity and specificity using CSF are 98.9% and 98.9%, respectively.

    - Lower pooled sensitivity for urine specimens is 85.0% (specificity not calculated).

- Available assays vary in their ability to detect serotype C (ie, *Cryptococcus gattii*).[46]

- Titers obtained by different laboratories or methods may not necessarily be comparable.[47]

Abbreviations: BAL, bronchoalveolar lavage; GM, galactomannan; HM, hematologic malignancy; HSCT, hematopoietic stem cell transplantation; IA, invasive aspergillosis; SOT, solid organ transplantation.

studied,[14,15] but most experts agree that testing twice weekly is appropriate to balance the need for both rapid detection of invasive aspergillosis (IA) and cost containment.[16] Twice-weekly testing for patients at risk for IA is also recommended by the manufacturers.[17]

Serial surveillance using GM detection can reduce antifungal use in at-risk patients without affecting overall mortality, thereby decreasing antifungal drug toxicity and cost. In a study evaluating sequential serum GM testing combined with protocol-driven computed tomography scans, Maertens and colleagues[14] demonstrated a 78% reduction (from 35% to 8%) in the use of antifungals among 41 neutropenic patients who would otherwise have qualified for empirical antifungal treatment based on persistent or recurrent fever, without compromising outcomes. Similar results were observed in a randomized controlled trial that evaluated the use of GM serial surveillance along with other clinical and laboratory findings to guide preemptive antifungal treatment in febrile neutropenic patients. Although the preemptive approach resulted in an increased incidence of IFI (mostly due to Candida spp in patients not receiving fluconazole prophylaxis), the overall survival between groups was equivalent. Furthermore, antifungal use was significantly lower in the preemptive arm.[18]

In addition to its application in serial surveillance, GM detection can also be used for monitoring treatment response and as a predictor of outcomes in cases of IA. In a multi-center analysis of patients with IA, Chai and colleagues[19] found that GM measurements within the first 2 weeks of antifungal therapy could be used to predict clinical outcomes; a reduction of greater than 35% between baseline and week one predicted a satisfactory clinical response, whereas increasing GM levels indicated a poor clinical outcome.

Antigen Detection for Dimorphic Fungi

Detection of circulating Histoplasma, Blastomyces, and Coccidioides antigens also has established clinical utility. Although specific assays for the detection of individual dimorphic organisms have been developed,[20,21] the most widely used and well studied of these detect Histoplasma. A single test has been approved by the FDA for in vitro diagnostic use (Alpha Histoplasma Antigen enzyme immunoassay [EIA]; IMMY, Norman, OK) using urine specimens[22]; but studies have also shown that Histoplasma antigen can be reliably detected in serum, CSF, and BAL fluid as well.[23-25] Antigen detection is useful for the diagnosis of both acute pulmonary and disseminated histoplasmosis, especially in immunosuppressed patients.[26] The assay can also be used to monitor patient response to antifungal therapy, as antigen levels in urine generally decline following treatment. The rate of this reduction varies depending on the assay.[27]

Cryptococcal Antigen

Both Cryptococcus neoformans and Cryptococcus gattii shed a polysaccharide capsular antigen that can be detected in infected patients. There are multiple commercially available, FDA-approved assays for the detection of this cryptococcal antigen (CrAg), which use latex agglutination, EIA, or lateral flow assay methodologies. These tests are FDA approved for use on CSF and/or serum specimens, and studies have shown that CrAg can also be detected in urine.[28]

Detection of CrAg can be used to facilitate the diagnosis of invasive cryptococcosis in symptomatic patients or for screening of asymptomatic patients with AIDS (CD4 <100 cells/mm^3) to guide preemptive antifungal therapy before the initiation of antiretroviral therapy.[29] Screening has primarily been used in the high prevalence areas of sub-Saharan Africa.[30] Of note, antigen detection may persist beyond clinical resolution, and monitoring titers to determine treatment efficacy or relapse during the maintenance phase of treatment is not recommended.[29]

Histology and Special Stains

The diagnostic gold standard for IFI is demonstration of fungal elements in tissue or normally sterile body fluid using a variety of histopathology stains. The utility of histopathology or cytology to identify the infecting fungus beyond generalized terms, however, varies based on the organism.[48] Additional limitations include the requirement for an invasive procedure to obtain the specimen as well as the potential for sampling bias. An excellent overview of the morphologic features of fungi in tissue was recently published[48] and is beyond the scope of this review. However, a brief description of the common histopathology stains and general identifying characteristics of fungi is provided in **Box 4**.

NUCLEIC ACID DETECTION TECHNIQUES

The direct detection of fungal nucleic acid in patient specimens is a potentially rapid and accurate way to identify invasive fungal pathogens. A variety of molecular techniques have been adapted for fungal diagnostics, with assays designed to detect either a broad range of organisms or specific pathogens within a genera or species. Important molecular diagnostic considerations are highlighted in **Box 5**.

Box 4
Direct staining of fungi in tissue and body fluid

Nonspecific stains

- *Calcofluor white* is a fluorochrome that binds β-glucans and chitin within the fungal cell wall. Fluorescence increases the sensitivity of staining, but there is limited specificity because of cross reactivity with other chitin- and cellulose-containing structures.

- *Periodic acid-Schiff* stains the polysaccharide component of fungal cell walls magenta, thus allowing better distinction of fungal elements from surrounding tissue.

- *Grocott methenamine silver* stains fungal cell walls black. A light green counterstain produces contrast between fungi and surrounding tissue.

Targeted stains

- *India ink* is a negative staining technique whereby the stain particles are excluded from the thick polysaccharide capsule of *Cryptococcus* in CSF.

- *Mucicarmine* (mucin stain) stains acidic mucins pink. It can be used to stain the capsule of *Cryptococcus* in tissue.

- *Fontana-Masson* silver stain is used to detect the melanin pigment in *Cryptococcus* as well as in dematiaceous fungi.

- *Fluorescence in situ hybridization* techniques use fluorescently labeled, fungal-targeted oligonucleotides to detect and identify specific fungi in clinical specimens.

General identification characteristics

- *Dimorphic fungi* have characteristic features in vivo, such as the intracellular yeast forms of histoplasmosis and spherules in coccidioidomycosis.

- *Dematiaceous fungi* have melanin pigment in their cell wall.

- *Mucorales* appear as broad, ribbonlike hyphae that are pauci-septate.

- *Hyaline Hyphomycetes* are difficult to distinguish from one another in clinical specimens. Describing all septate hyphae with dichotomous branching as being consistent with *Aspergillus* can be misleading to the clinician and results in misidentification 20% of the time.[49]

Box 5
Molecular detection techniques for IFIs

Pan-fungal approaches

- Use of multi-copy gene targets, with both conserved and variable regions, facilitates detection and identification.

- Sequence databases lack well-curated fungal references, and a thorough adjudication of references is required for accurate identification.

- Contamination of specimens, collection devices, and reagents is a significant concern.

Genus/species-specific approaches

- Gene target selection influences assay sensitivity and specificity.

- The nucleic acid extraction method also has a significant impact on test performance.

- PCR is the most common method in clinical practice.

  Candida

  - The FDA-approved T2Candida assay has a sensitivity that approximates blood culture.

  - Performance of direct-detection techniques in patients with invasive candidiasis but who have negative blood culture is poorly defined.

  Aspergillus

  - There are no FDA-approved assays.

  - Current tests are laboratory developed.

  - PCR is useful to guide preemptive and targeted therapy.

Abbreviation: PCR, polymerase chain reaction.

Pan-Fungal Approaches

A variety of methods, including DNA sequencing, microarrays, and polymerase chain reaction (PCR)–electrospray ionization mass spectrometry, have been used to develop broad-range molecular detection assays. The most common approach for pan-fungal detection is PCR followed by Sanger sequencing. Typically, the ribosomal RNA gene cluster, with both highly conserved (18S and 28S) and variable (Internal Transcribed Spacer [ITS] and D1/D2) regions, is used as the fungal target; sequence analysis of the amplicon is used to determine organism identification. Pan-fungal PCR with amplicon sequencing may be particularly useful when fungal culture was either negative or not requested at the time tissue biopsy was performed. The diagnostic sensitivity of this approach applied to formalin-fixed, paraffin-embedded tissue ranges from 86% to 94% in culture-proven cases and 64% to 89% in histopathology-confirmed cases.[50–53] Importantly, contamination of specimens, collection devices,[54] and reagents[55] with fungal nucleic acid is a significant concern that should be monitored by the laboratory as well as considered by the clinician.

Genus/Species-Specific Approaches

Although laboratory-developed tests (LDTs) specifically targeting the endemic mycoses[56] and *Mucorales*[57] exist, organism-specific nucleic acid amplification tests have been most well studied for *Candida* and *Aspergillus*. Similar to pan-fungal approaches, these assays often use PCR technology; but the gene target is either genus or species specific.

For *Candida*, direct detection assays have been applied for diagnosis of both superficial infections[58] and invasive candidiasis (IC).[59] Recently, the FDA approved the first direct detection *Candida* nucleic acid test (T2Candida T2 Biosystems, Inc; Lexington, MA). This assay combines targeted PCR with T2 magnetic resonance to allow for the detection of the 5 most common *Candida* species directly from blood specimens with an overall specificity of 99.4% (95% confidence interval [CI], 99.1%–99.6%) and overall sensitivity of 91.1% (95% CI, 86.9%–94.2%) compared with blood culture.[60] Although this assay has the potential to significantly improve the diagnosis and management of suspected IC, further evaluation is required to determine how it can be most cost-effectively implemented.

Molecular diagnostic tests for the detection of *Aspergillus* spp are also becoming more widely used, especially in Europe.[16] LDTs have been applied to multiple specimen types (eg, BAL, tissue, and the various fractions of blood) and in many different testing algorithms. For example, the results of a comprehensive meta-analysis demonstrated that a single *Aspergillus* PCR performed using whole blood, plasma, or serum had a sensitivity of 88% and specificity of 75% for proven/probable IA and that specificity was increased to 87% when 2 consecutive PCR tests were required to define a positive test result.[61] In addition, a meta-analysis of 15 different studies using BAL specimens demonstrated a pooled sensitivity and specificity of 79% and 94%, respectively, for proven/probable IA.[62] The ability to differentiate airway colonization from invasive disease using direct nucleic acid detection from BAL specimens, is limited,[63] but high fungal burdens determined by quantitative PCR seem to be more suggestive of invasion.[64]

Both meta-analyses highlighted the significant heterogeneity that exists among current LDTs. To help address the issue of standardization, the European *Aspergillus* PCR Initiative completed a multicenter comparison of existing *Aspergillus* PCR protocols using whole blood; the findings of this study are highlighted in **Box 6**.

Detection of Molecular Markers of Resistance

As the molecular basis for antifungal drug resistance is becoming better understood, genotypic testing may also provide more rapid susceptibility information compared with traditional phenotypic methods. Azole resistance in *Aspergillus* spp is often caused by mutations in *Cyp51a*, which lead to a mutated enzyme involved in ergosterol

---

Box 6
EAPCRI evaluation of PCR protocols for *Aspergillus* nucleic acid detection in whole blood

Factors associated with optimal assay sensitivity

- Specimen volume ($\geq$3 mL)
- Method of mechanical disruption of fungal cell walls (bead beating)
- Use of a white cell lysis buffer
- Inclusion of an internal control
- Elution volumes (<100 µL)

Based on these results, the EAPCRI proposed a standardized whole-blood fungal DNA extraction protocol[65] for direct detection of *Aspergillus*.

Abbreviation: EAPCRI, European *Aspergillus* PCR Initiative.
  Data from White PL, Bretagne S, Klingspor L, et al. Aspergillus PCR: one step closer to standardization. J Clin Microbiol 2010;48(4):1231–40.

synthesis.[66] Mutations in the FKS gene of *Candida* are responsible for resistance to echinocandin drugs.[67] LDTs designed to detect these mutations have been developed but to date have primarily been applied to cultured isolates as a part of epidemiologic drug resistance surveillance studies.[68]

SUMMARY

Nonculture diagnostic techniques have become an essential component of the evaluation for suspected IFI. As a group, these assays can help to identify patients with IFIs earlier than is possible with culture, are often more sensitive than traditional laboratory methods, and can be used as a guide for targeted therapeutic interventions as well as additional diagnostic studies. There are challenges associated with these methods, however, including the risk of false-positive results due to contamination or cross reactivity as well as false negatives owing to imperfect assay sensitivity. As a general rule, no laboratory diagnostic test should be used as a stand-alone test for the diagnosis of IFI. Current fungal diagnostic tests should be used in combination with assessments of the host and radiographic features to optimally manage at-risk patients.

REFERENCES

1. Miller R, Assi M. Endemic fungal infections in solid organ transplantation. Am J Transplantant 2013;13(Suppl 4):250–61.
2. Knutsen AP, Bush RK, Demain JG, et al. Fungi and allergic lower respiratory tract diseases. J Allergy Clin Immunol 2012;129(2):280–91 [quiz: 292–83].
3. Kauffman CA. Histoplasmosis: a clinical and laboratory update. Clin Microbiol Rev 2007;20(1):115–32.
4. Wheat LJ. Approach to the diagnosis of the endemic mycoses. Clin Chest Med 2009;30(2):379–89, viii.
5. Pappagianis D, Zimmer BL. Serology of coccidioidomycosis. Clin Microbiol Rev 1990;3(3):247–68.
6. Saubolle MA, McKellar PP, Sussland D. Epidemiologic, clinical, and diagnostic aspects of coccidioidomycosis. J Clin Microbiol 2007;45(1):26–30.
7. Associates of Cape Cod Inc. Assay for (1, 3)-beta-D-Glucan in serum: fungitell instructions for use. In: Associates of Cape Cod I, editor. Falmouth (MA): 2011.
8. Hanson KE, Pfeiffer CD, Lease ED, et al. beta-D-glucan surveillance with preemptive anidulafungin for invasive candidiasis in intensive care unit patients: a randomized pilot study. PLoS One 2012;7(8):e42282.
9. He S, Hang JP, Zhang L, et al. A systematic review and meta-analysis of diagnostic accuracy of serum 1,3-beta-d-glucan for invasive fungal infection: focus on cutoff levels. J Microbiol Immunol Infect 2015;48(4):351–61.
10. Egan L, Connolly P, Wheat LJ, et al. Histoplasmosis as a cause for a positive Fungitell (1–> 3)-beta-D-glucan test. Med Mycol 2008;46(1):93–5.
11. Thompson GR 3rd, Bays DJ, Johnson SM, et al. Serum (1->3)-beta-D-glucan measurement in coccidioidomycosis. J Clin Microbiol 2012;50(9):3060–2.
12. Litvintseva AP, Lindsley MD, Gade L, et al. Utility of (1–3)-beta-D-glucan testing for diagnostics and monitoring response to treatment during the multistate outbreak of fungal meningitis and other infections. Clin Infect Dis 2014;58(5):622–30.
13. Machetti M, Zotti M, Veroni L, et al. Antigen detection in the diagnosis and management of a patient with probable cerebral aspergillosis treated with voriconazole. Transpl Infect Dis 2000;2(3):140–4.
14. Maertens J, Theunissen K, Verhoef G, et al. Galactomannan and computed tomography-based preemptive antifungal therapy in neutropenic patients at

high risk for invasive fungal infection: a prospective feasibility study. Clin Infect Dis 2005;41(9):1242–50.

15. Husain S, Kwak EJ, Obman A, et al. Prospective assessment of Platelia Aspergillus galactomannan antigen for the diagnosis of invasive aspergillosis in lung transplant recipients. Am J Transplant 2004;4(5):796–802.

16. Schelenz S, Barnes RA, Barton RC, et al. British Society for Medical Mycology best practice recommendations for the diagnosis of serious fungal diseases. Lancet Infect Dis 2015;15(4):461–74.

17. Bio-Rad. PlateliaTM Aspergillus EIA [package insert]. In: Bio-Rad, editor. Marnes La Coquette (France): 2009.

18. Cordonnier C, Pautas C, Maury S, et al. Empirical versus preemptive antifungal therapy for high-risk, febrile, neutropenic patients: a randomized, controlled trial. Clin Infect Dis 2009;48(8):1042–51.

19. Chai LY, Kullberg BJ, Johnson EM, et al. Early serum galactomannan trend as a predictor of outcome of invasive aspergillosis. J Clin Microbiol 2012;50(7):2330–6.

20. Connolly P, Hage CA, Bariola JR, et al. Blastomyces dermatitidis antigen detection by quantitative enzyme immunoassay. Clin Vaccine Immunol 2012;19(1):53–6.

21. Durkin M, Connolly P, Kuberski T, et al. Diagnosis of coccidioidomycosis with use of the Coccidioides antigen enzyme immunoassay. Clin Infect Dis 2008;47(8): e69–73.

22. IMMY. ALPHA histoplasma EIA test kit: for the detection of histoplasma antigen. In: IMMY, editor. Norman (OK): 2011.

23. Wheat LJ, Kohler RB, Tewari RP, et al. Significance of Histoplasma antigen in the cerebrospinal fluid of patients with meningitis. Arch Intern Med 1989;149(2): 302–4.

24. Hage CA, Davis TE, Fuller D, et al. Diagnosis of histoplasmosis by antigen detection in BAL fluid. Chest 2010;137(3):623–8.

25. Riddell JT, Kauffman CA, Smith JA, et al. Histoplasma capsulatum endocarditis: multicenter case series with review of current diagnostic techniques and treatment. Medicine (Baltimore) 2014;93(5):186–93.

26. Wheat JL. Current diagnosis of histoplasmosis. Trends Microbiol 2003;11(10): 488–94.

27. Zhang X, Gibson B Jr, Daly TM. Evaluation of commercially available reagents for diagnosis of histoplasmosis infection in immunocompromised patients. J Clin Microbiol 2013;51(12):4095–101.

28. Huang HR, Fan LC, Rajbanshi B, et al. Evaluation of a new cryptococcal antigen lateral flow immunoassay in serum, cerebrospinal fluid and urine for the diagnosis of cryptococcosis: a meta-analysis and systematic review. PLoS One 2015;10(5): e0127117.

29. Perfect JR, Dismukes WE, Dromer F, et al. Clinical practice guidelines for the management of cryptococcal disease: 2010 update by the Infectious Diseases Society of America. Clin Infect Dis 2010;50(3):291–322.

30. WHO Guidelines Approved by the Guidelines Review Committee. Rapid advice: diagnosis, prevention and management of cryptococcal disease in HIV-infected adults, adolescents and children. Geneva (Switzerland): World Health Organization; 2011.

31. Onishi A, Sugiyama D, Kogata Y, et al. Diagnostic accuracy of serum 1,3-beta-D-glucan for pneumocystis jiroveci pneumonia, invasive candidiasis, and invasive aspergillosis: systematic review and meta-analysis. J Clin Microbiol 2012;50(1):7–15.

32. Marty FM, Koo S. Role of (1->3)-beta-D-glucan in the diagnosis of invasive aspergillosis. Med Mycol 2009;47(Suppl 1):S233–40.

33. Nguyen MH, Wissel MC, Shields RK, et al. Performance of Candida real-time polymerase chain reaction, beta-D-glucan assay, and blood cultures in the diagnosis of invasive candidiasis. Clin Infect Dis 2012;54(9):1240–8.

34. Ikemura K, Ikegami K, Shimazu T, et al. False-positive result in limulus test caused by Limulus amebocyte lysate-reactive material in immunoglobulin products. J Clin Microbiol 1989;27(9):1965–8.

35. Kanamori H, Kanemitsu K, Miyasaka T, et al. Measurement of (1-3)-beta-D-glucan derived from different gauze types. Tohoku J Exp Med 2009;217(2):117–21.

36. Alexander BD, Smith PB, Davis RD, et al. The (1,3){beta}-D-glucan test as an aid to early diagnosis of invasive fungal infections following lung transplantation. J Clin Microbiol 2010;48(11):4083–8.

37. Penack O, Schwartz S, Thiel E, et al. Lack of evidence that false-positive Aspergillus galactomannan antigen test results are due to treatment with piperacillin-tazobactam. Clin Infect Dis 2004;39(9):1401–2 [author reply: 1402–3].

38. Smith PB, Benjamin DK Jr, Alexander BD, et al. Quantification of 1,3-beta-D-glucan levels in children: preliminary data for diagnostic use of the beta-glucan assay in a pediatric setting. Clin Vaccine Immunol 2007;14(7):924–5.

39. Pfeiffer CD, Fine JP, Safdar N. Diagnosis of invasive aspergillosis using a galactomannan assay: a meta-analysis. Clin Infect Dis 2006;42(10):1417–27.

40. Fisher CE, Stevens AM, Leisenring W, et al. Independent contribution of bronchoalveolar lavage and serum galactomannan in the diagnosis of invasive pulmonary aspergillosis. Transpl Infect Dis 2014;16(3):505–10.

41. Mikulska M, Furfaro E, Del Bono V, et al. Piperacillin/tazobactam (Tazocin) seems to be no longer responsible for false-positive results of the galactomannan assay. J Antimicrob Chemother 2012;67(7):1746–8.

42. Guigue N, Menotti J, Ribaud P. False positive galactomannan test after ice-pop ingestion. N Engl J Med 2013;369(1):97–8.

43. Mennink-Kersten MA, Donnelly JP, Verweij PE. Detection of circulating galactomannan for the diagnosis and management of invasive aspergillosis. Lancet Infect Dis 2004;4(6):349–57.

44. Kuberski T, Myers R, Wheat LJ, et al. Diagnosis of coccidioidomycosis by antigen detection using cross-reaction with a Histoplasma antigen. Clin Infect Dis 2007; 44(5):e50–54.

45. Wheat J, Wheat H, Connolly P, et al. Cross-reactivity in Histoplasma capsulatum variety capsulatum antigen assays of urine samples from patients with endemic mycoses. Clin Infect Dis 1997;24(6):1169–71.

46. Percival A, Thorkildson P, Kozel TR. Monoclonal antibodies specific for immunorecessive epitopes of glucuronoxylomannan, the major capsular polysaccharide of Cryptococcus neoformans, reduce serotype bias in an immunoassay for cryptococcal antigen. Clin Vaccine Immunol 2011;18(8):1292–6.

47. McMullan BJ, Halliday C, Sorrell TC, et al. Clinical utility of the cryptococcal antigen lateral flow assay in a diagnostic mycology laboratory. PLoS One 2012; 7(11):e49541.

48. Guarner J, Brandt ME. Histopathologic diagnosis of fungal infections in the 21st century. Clin Microbiol Rev 2011;24(2):247–80.

49. Sangoi AR, Rogers WM, Longacre TA, et al. Challenges and pitfalls of morphologic identification of fungal infections in histologic and cytologic specimens: a ten-year retrospective review at a single institution. Am J Clin Pathol 2009;131(3):364–75.

50. Munoz-Cadavid C, Rudd S, Zaki SR, et al. Improving molecular detection of fungal DNA in formalin-fixed paraffin-embedded tissues: comparison of five tissue DNA extraction methods using panfungal PCR. J Clin Microbiol 2010;48(6):2147–53.

51. Lau A, Chen S, Sorrell T, et al. Development and clinical application of a panfungal PCR assay to detect and identify fungal DNA in tissue specimens. J Clin Microbiol 2007;45(2):380–5.
52. Buitrago MJ, Aguado JM, Ballen A, et al. Efficacy of DNA amplification in tissue biopsy samples to improve the detection of invasive fungal disease. Clin Microbiol Infect 2013;19(6):E271–7.
53. Rickerts V, Khot PD, Myerson D, et al. Comparison of quantitative real time PCR with sequencing and ribosomal RNA-FISH for the identification of fungi in formalin fixed, paraffin-embedded tissue specimens. BMC Infect Dis 2011;11:202.
54. Harrison E, Stalhberger T, Whelan R, et al. Aspergillus DNA contamination in blood collection tubes. Diagn Microbiol Infect Dis 2010;67(4):392–4.
55. Loeffler J, Hebart H, Bialek R, et al. Contaminations occurring in fungal PCR assays. J Clin Microbiol 1999;37(4):1200–2.
56. Babady NE, Buckwalter SP, Hall L, et al. Detection of Blastomyces dermatitidis and Histoplasma capsulatum from culture isolates and clinical specimens by use of real-time PCR. J Clin Microbiol 2011;49(9):3204–8.
57. Simner PJ, Uhl JR, Hall L, et al. Broad-range direct detection and identification of fungi by use of the PLEX-ID PCR-Electrospray Ionization Mass Spectrometry (ESI-MS) System. J Clin Microbiol 2013;51(6):1699–706.
58. Han HW, Hsu MM, Choi JS, et al. Rapid detection of dermatophytes and Candida albicans in onychomycosis specimens by an oligonucleotide array. BMC Infect Dis 2014;14:581.
59. Avni T, Leibovici L, Paul M. PCR diagnosis of invasive candidiasis: systematic review and meta-analysis. J Clin Microbiol 2011;49(2):665–70.
60. Mylonakis E, Clancy CJ, Ostrosky-Zeichner L, et al. T2 magnetic resonance assay for the rapid diagnosis of candidemia in whole blood: a clinical trial. Clin Infect Dis 2015;60(6):892–9.
61. Mengoli C, Cruciani M, Barnes RA, et al. Use of PCR for diagnosis of invasive aspergillosis: systematic review and meta-analysis. Lancet Infect Dis 2009;9(2):89–96.
62. Tuon FF. A systematic literature review on the diagnosis of invasive aspergillosis using polymerase chain reaction (PCR) from bronchoalveolar lavage clinical samples. Rev Iberoam Micol 2007;24(2):89–94.
63. Hayette MP, Vaira D, Susin F, et al. Detection of Aspergillus species DNA by PCR in bronchoalveolar lavage fluid. J Clin Microbiol 2001;39(6):2338–40.
64. Luong ML, Clancy CJ, Vadnerkar A, et al. Comparison of an Aspergillus real-time polymerase chain reaction assay with galactomannan testing of bronchoalveolar lavage fluid for the diagnosis of invasive pulmonary aspergillosis in lung transplant recipients. Clin Infect Dis 2011;52(10):1218–26.
65. White PL, Perry MD, Loeffler J, et al. Critical stages of extracting DNA from Aspergillus fumigatus in whole-blood specimens. J Clin Microbiol 2010;48(10):3753–5.
66. Bader O, Weig M, Reichard U, et al. cyp51A-Based mechanisms of Aspergillus fumigatus azole drug resistance present in clinical samples from Germany. Antimicrobial Agents Chemother 2013;57(8):3513–7.
67. Dudiuk C, Gamarra S, Jimenez-Ortigosa C, et al. Quick detection of FKS1 mutations responsible for clinical echinocandin resistance in Candida albicans. J Clin Microbiol 2015;53(7):2037–41.
68. van der Linden JW, Arendrup MC, Warris A, et al. Prospective multicenter international surveillance of azole resistance in Aspergillus fumigatus. Emerg Infect Dis 2015;21(6):1041–4.

Antifungal Agents

Spectrum of Activity, Pharmacology, and Clinical Indications

Jeniel E. Nett, MD, PhD[a,b], David R. Andes, MD[a,b],*

KEYWORDS

- Antifungal • Spectrum of activity • Azole • Echinocandins • Amphotericin B
- Pharmacokinetics • Indications • Toxicity

KEY POINTS

- The currently available antifungal agents vary significantly in terms of spectrum of activity. The echinocandins exhibit potent activity against *Candida*, whereas the newer triazoles offer an extended spectrum of activity that includes *Aspergillus* and emerging filamentous pathogens.
- The pharmacokinetic properties differ among the antifungal drugs. Important considerations include absorption, tissue site penetration, impact of organ dysfunction on dosing, routes of metabolism, and the need for therapeutic drug monitoring.
- Many triazoles are metabolized via hepatic CYP450 enzymes. Drug–drug interactions are frequent and common enzyme polymorphisms may lead to unpredictable drug levels.
- Drug dosing and Food and Drug Administration–approved clinical indications for individual antifungal drugs are reviewed.

INTRODUCTION: THE EVOLUTION OF ANTIFUNGAL DRUG THERAPY

Continued advancement of medical science offers life-saving treatment options for a variety of hematologic, oncologic, and rheumatologic conditions. Immunosuppression, a common therapeutic side-effect, predisposes patients to invasive fungal infections, which are escalating in prevalence.[1,2] The development of effective, well-tolerated antifungals has lagged behind the advances of antibacterial therapy. Amphotericin B deoxycholate, an antifungal developed in the 1950s, marked a major therapeutic advance (**Box 1**). Although very effective for the treatment of numerous

Disclosure Statement: The authors have nothing to disclose.
[a] Department of Medicine, University of Wisconsin, Madison, WI 53705, USA; [b] Department of Medical Microbiology & Immunology, University of Wisconsin, Madison, WI 53705, USA
* Corresponding author. 5211 UW Medical Foundation Centennial Building, 1685 Highland Avenue, Madison, WI 53705.
E-mail address: dra@medicine.wisc.edu

> **Box 1**
> **History of antifungal therapy**
>
> - The first antifungal, amphotericin B deoxycholate, was introduced in 1958. It offers potent, broad-spectrum antifungal activity but is associated with significant renal toxicity and infusion reactions.
> - Flucytosine, a pyrimidine analogue introduced in 1973, is active against *Candida* and *Cryptococcus*. Its use is limited by emergence of drug resistance and toxicity.
> - The first-generation azole drugs, including fluconazole and itraconazole, became available in the 1990s. These agents offer the advantage of oral administration and have good activity against yeast pathogens. Due to CYP450 interactions, there are many drug–drug interactions.
> - Lipid-based amphotericin B formulations were introduced in the 1990s and maintain the potent, broad-spectrum activity of the deoxycholate formulation with less toxicity.
> - The echinocandin drugs became available in the 2000s and offer excellent activity against *Candida* with few drug–drug interactions; however, they are available in parenteral form only.
> - The second-generation of azole drugs, including voriconazole, posaconazole, and isavuconazole, were brought to market beginning in the 2000s. The major advantage of these agents is the extended spectrum of activity against filamentous fungi.

invasive fungal infections, it is not without cost. Side-effects, including renal failure, electrolyte abnormalities, and infusion reactions, often limit its use.[3] However, for many years, amphotericin B remained the sole option for the treatment of invasive mycosis. In the 1970s, flucytosine, a pyrimidine analogue, was introduced. Its use has been limited by rapid emergence of resistance when used alone, as well as associated toxicities, including bone marrow suppression. In the mid-1990s, new lipid-based amphotericin B formulations were brought to market. Compared with the initial deoxycholate formulation, these have improved side-effect profiles with reduced nephrotoxicity and remain the mainstay for treatment of many life-threatening fungal infections.

In addition to the advent of the lipid-based amphotericin B formulations, another major advance of the 1990s was the addition of the triazole drug class (see **Box 1**). Compared with the amphotericin B formulations, the azole drugs are significantly better tolerated. The first-generation azole drugs (fluconazole-1990, itraconazole-1992) demonstrate excellent activity against *Candida* spp. The spectrum of itraconazole activity also includes endemic fungi, such as histoplasmosis. However, the original triazoles agents are inferior to amphotericin B for treatment of invasive filamentous fungal infections, such as aspergillosis and mucormycosis. The second-generation azole drugs (voriconazole-2002, posaconazole-2006) are broad-spectrum agents, with additional activity against filamentous fungi while retaining anti-*Candida* activity.[4,5] The newest azole released in 2015 (isavuconazole) has similarly broad activity with more favorable pharmacologic properties, allowing for improved bioavailability, more predictable drug levels, and fewer drug interactions.

The newest antifungal class, the echinocandins, was introduced in 2001 with caspofungin. Micafungin and anidulafungin were soon to follow. These agents exhibit potent activity against *Candida* spp, including many azole-resistant organisms and *C glabrata*. In addition, they demonstrate modest activity against *Aspergillus* spp. Favorable attributes of the echinocandin drugs include their excellent side-effect profiles and few drug–drug interactions. However, only parental formulations are available for this drug class.

PHARMACOLOGIC CONSIDERATIONS

Numerous obstacles are encountered on delivery of an antimicrobial compound to the site of fungal infection. Important pharmacokinetic factors include absorption in the gastrointestinal tract (for oral formulations), anatomic distribution, metabolism, and elimination. For example, amphotericin B and the echinocandin drugs have minimal gastrointestinal absorption and are solely available as parenteral formulations. Conversely, the azole drugs are able to be absorbed through the gastrointestinal mucosa, although the extent varies by individual antifungal. For example, fluconazole and isavuconazole are readily absorbed with high bioavailability, whereas absorption of posaconazole is limited and saturable.[6,7] The newer posaconazole capsule formulation circumvents this limitation by delayed release of the compound, resulting in higher bioavailability with more predictable drug levels.[8] Another important variable to consider is drug metabolism. For example, polymorphisms are common in the CYP2C19 enzyme that metabolizes voriconazole. Variable metabolism leads to unpredictable drug levels, which may place patients at risk for toxicity or therapeutic failure.[9] The anatomic distribution also varies among the antifungals. An example of an important clinical consideration is the limited penetration of the echinocandins into the cerebrospinal fluid, eye, and urine.[10,11]

POLYENES

Polyenes are natural products of *Streptomyces nodosus*, a soil actinomycete (**Fig. 1**).[12] A single agent, amphotericin B, is available for treatment of systemic fungal infections; however, there are multiple formulations. The deoxycholate formulation was initially developed and 3 lipid-based formulations have been designed and developed to limit toxicity and improve tolerability. Amphotericin B exerts its activity through hydrophobic interactions with cell membrane ergosterol, subsequently disrupting membrane function. Pores formation allows the efflux of potassium, leading to cell death.[13]

Spectrum of Activity and Resistance

Amphotericin B is one of the most potent antifungals, demonstrating activity against an array of yeast and filamentous fungal pathogens (**Table 1**).

Amphotericin B exhibits activity against *Cryptococcus* spp and most *Candida* spp, with the exception of *Candida lusitaniae*, which routinely is found to have higher minimal inhibitory concentrations (MICs).[14–16] It also demonstrates activity against *Aspergillus* spp, with the major exception of *Aspergillus terreus*, which is often resistant.[17] In addition, the amphotericin B formulations are active against the dimorphic fungi, including *Histoplasma capsulatum*, *Blastomyces dermatitidis*, *Coccidioides immitis* and *posadasii*, and *Paracoccidioides* spp.[17–19] Amphotericin B is active against many pathogenic organisms of the Mucorales group. However, *Scedosporium* spp and *Fusarium* spp, often have higher MICs.[15,17,20,21] In general, acquired resistance to amphotericin B is exceedingly uncommon despite its multiple decades of clinical use.

Pharmacology

Amphotericin B is available as the original deoxycholate formulation and as 2 lipid-based formulations: liposomal amphotericin B (L-AmB) and amphotericin B lipid complex (ABLC). A fourth formulation, amphotericin B colloidal dispersion (ABCD), is not currently being manufactured. Given the limited solubility of amphotericin B and its poor oral bioavailability, all formulations are parenteral. The drug can be dosed daily

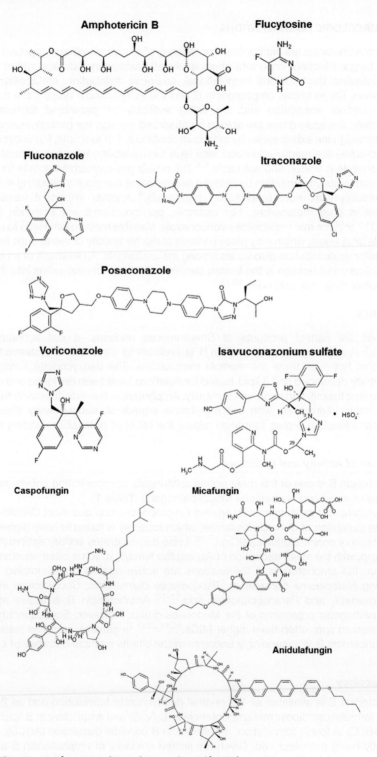

Fig. 1. Structures of commonly used systemic antifungal agents.

Table 1
Spectrum of activity for systemic antifungal agents

	AMB	5FC	FLU	ITR	VOR	POS	ISA	CAS	MICA	ANI
Candida albicans	++	++	++	++	++	++	++	++	++	++
Candida glabrata	++	++	+	+	++	++	++	+	+	+
Candida parapsilosis	++	++	++	++	++	++	++	++	++	++
Candida tropicalis	++	++	++	++	++	++	++	++	++	++
Candida krusei	++	+	–	+	++	++	++	++	++	++
Candida lusitaniae	–	++	++	++	++	++	++	++	++	++
Aspergillus fumigatus	++	–	–	+	++	++	++	+	+	+
Cryptococcus neoformans	++	++	++	++	++	++	++	–	–	–
Mucorales	++	–	–	–	–	++	++	–	–	–
Fusarium spp	+	–	–	+	++	++	++	–	–	–
Scedosporium spp	+	–	–	+	+	+	+	–	–	–
Blastomyces dermatitidis	++	–	+	++	++	++	++	–	–	–
Coccidioides immitis	++	–	++	++	++	++	++	–	–	–
Histoplasma capsulatum	++	–	+	++	++	++	++	–	–	–

Abbreviations: 5FC, flucytosine; AMB, amphotericin B; ANI, anidulafungin; CAS, caspofungin; FLU, fluconazole; ISA, isavuconazole; ITR, itraconazole; MICA, micafungin; POS, posaconazole; VOR, voriconazole.

given its long half-life.[22,23] Animal studies have shown the lipid formulations of amphotericin B to be less potent than amphotericin B deoxycholate on a weight (mg/kg) basis.[24] Approximately 4-fold to 5-fold higher concentrations of the lipid-based formulations are required to achieve efficacy similar to the deoxycholate formulation. This is consistent with the higher clinical dosing of these formulations (L-AmB 3–6 mg/kg/d, ABLC 3–6 mg/kg/d, and ABCD 3–4 mg/kg/d) compared with the conventional deoxycholate formulation (0.7–1 mg/kg/d) (**Table 2**).

Amphotericin B is widely distributed throughout the host. Although drug levels in the cerebrospinal fluid are nearly undetectable, it remains the drug of choice for the treatment of cryptococcal meningitis.[25,26] Given the high protein binding of amphotericin B, it is assumed that the drug accumulates in the brain parenchyma, with the relatively low cerebral spinal fluid levels not predicting the drug's activity at this site. The pharmacokinetic properties vary among the individual amphotericin B formulations. For example, L-AmB demonstrates enhanced central nervous system penetration, achieving 4-fold to 7-fold higher brain parenchyma concentrations compared with the other formulations. In an animal model of meningitis, this characteristic was found to correlate with greater efficacy.[13,27] One similarity among the lipid-based amphotericin B formulations is the ability of the carrier molecules to decrease renal tubular cell binding, significantly reducing (10-fold–20-fold) the propensity for renal toxicity.

Amphotericin B exhibits a long elimination half-life (>15 days). The drug accumulates most highly in the liver and spleen and to a lesser extent in the kidney, lung, myocardium, and brain. In addition, it has not been shown to be metabolized.[28,29] Amphotericin B deoxycholate is excreted as unchanged drug into the feces (43%) and urine (21%).[29] The liposomal formulation is also excreted as unchanged drug. However, only 10% of the L-AmB formulation was found to be excreted in the urine or feces. It is suspected that the liposome carrier enhances tissue sequestration, decreasing the rate of elimination.

Table 2
Dosing regimens and clinical indications for frequently used systemic antifungal agents

	Clinical Indications	Dosing: Adult			Dosing: Pediatric
		IV	Oral	Notes	
Amphotericin B	Aspergillosis Candidiasis, invasive Candidiasis, mucosal Cryptococcosis Coccidioidomycosis Blastomycosis Histoplasmosis Mucormycosis Penicilliosis Phaeohyphomycosis Sporotrichosis	0.7–1 mg/kg/d[a]	NA	—	0.7–1 mg/kg/d[a]
Flucytosine	Cryptococcosis (in combination therapy) Second-line: Candidiasis	NA	25 mg/kg 4×/d	GFR <50: Decrease dosing interval to q 12–48 h	25 mg/kg 4×/d
Fluconazole	Candidiasis, invasive Candidiasis, mucosal[c] Cryptococcosis Prophylaxis, candidiasis	400–800 mg/d 100–200 mg/d[c]	400–800 mg/d 100–200 mg/d[c]	CrCl <50:Decrease dose by 50%	3–12 mg/kg/d
Itraconazole	Blastomycosis Candidiasis, mucosal Coccidioidomycosis Histoplasmosis Onychomycosis Paracoccidioidomycosis Sporotrichosis Second-line: Aspergillosis	NA	200 mg 1–3×/d	NA	2.5–5 mg/kg 2–3×/d

Drug	Indication				
Voriconazole	Aspergillosis Candidiasis, invasive Candidiasis, mucosal Fusariosis Scedosporiosis	6 mg/kg for 2 doses, then 4 mg/kg q 12 h	400 mg bid for 2 doses, then 200 mg q 12 h	CrCl <50: Avoid IV formulation Hepatic impairment: Consider 50% reduction	4–7 mg/kg q 12 h
Posaconazole	Candidiasis, mucosal Prophylaxis, invasive fungal infection	300 mg/d	Suspension: 800 mg/d divided Tablet: 300 mg bid for 2 doses, then 300 mg/d	GFR <50: Avoid IV formulation	Age ≥13: Suspension: 200 mg tid Tablet: 300 mg bid for 2 doses, then 300 mg/d
Isavuconazole	Aspergillosis Mucormycosis	372 mg q 8 h for 6 doses, then 372 mg/d	372 mg IV q 8 h for 6 doses, then 372 mg/d	Severe hepatic impairment: caution	NA
Caspofungin	Candidiasis, invasive Candidiasis, mucosal Empiric therapy[b] Second-line: Aspergillosis	70 mg for 1 dose, then 50 mg/d	NA	Moderate hepatic impairment: 35 mg/d	50 mg/m²/d
Micafungin	Candidiasis, invasive Candidiasis, mucosal Prophylaxis, invasive[c] fungal infection	100–150 mg/d 50 mg/d[c]	NA	NA	1–3 mg/kg/d
Anidulafungin	Candidiasis, invasive Candidiasis, mucosal	100–200 mg for 1 dose, then 50–200 mg/d	NA	NA	Age >16: 100–200 mg for 1 dose, then 50–100 mg/d

Abbreviations: CrCl, creatinine clearance; GFR, glomerular filtration rate; IV, intravenous.

[a] Dosing is listed for the amphotericin B deoxycholate formulation. Dosages for the lipid formulations are higher, L-AmB 3 to 6 mg/kg/d, ABLC 3 to 6 mg/kg/d, and ABCD 3 to 4 mg/kg/d.

[b] For patients with febrile neutropenia.

[c] Lower doses can be administered for the specified indication.

Clinical Indications

Amphotericin B was the first antifungal drug developed and is approved for the treatment of many invasive fungal infections including candidiasis, aspergillosis, cryptococcosis, blastomycosis, histoplasmosis, mucormycosis, and sporotrichosis (see **Table 2**). It is associated with significant renal toxicity, particularly the deoxycholate formulation, which may its limit use or result in dose reduction, ultimately leading to treatment failure.[30] The lipid-based preparations of amphotericin B have an improved toxicity profile and are commonly used as first-line agents for many of the approved indications.[30,31]

Amphotericin B is approved for the treatment of candidemia and invasive candidiasis based on multiple trials demonstrating effectiveness.[12,32–34] The current Infectious Diseases Society of America (IDSA) guidelines list the lipid-based amphotericin B formulations as second-line therapies with the deoxycholate formulation as a third-line alternative in resource limited areas.[2] However, given the efficacy and safety of alternative agents, such as the echinocandins, amphotericin B is not commonly used for this indication. Of note, the deoxycholate formulation is well-tolerated in neonates and remains first-line for the treatment of disseminated candidiasis in this patient population.[2,35] Given its enhanced ability to penetrate the central nervous system, L-AmB is the preferred formulation for the treatment of *Candida* meningitis or endophthalmitis.[2,36]

The amphotericin B formulations are recommended for initial treatment of many endemic fungal infections, particularly for patients with severe, life-threatening infections.[25,37–39] Amphotericin B is first-line therapy for the treatment of cryptococcal meningitis and is administered in combination with flucytosine during the induction period.[39–41] The lipid-based formulations are preferred for organ transplant recipients. Amphotericin B is approved for the treatment of coccidioidomycosis, histoplasmosis, and blastomycosis. It is recommended as initial therapy for the treatment of severe infections.[25,37,38] The liposomal formulation of amphotericin B is recommended as first-line for the treatment of mucormycosis.[42] L-AmB is also an option for treatment of sporotrichosis, particularly patients with disseminated or severe disease.[43] Amphotericin B has an indication for the treatment of aspergillosis. However, voriconazole is the preferred therapy for aspergillosis based on efficacy in a multicenter trial.[44,45] An important role for amphotericin B is the treatment of mycoses in pregnant patients because the triazole class is contraindicated due to established teratogenicity.[46]

Toxicities

Although amphotericin B demonstrates potent antifungal activity, its use is often limited by significant toxicities. Common adverse effects include renal toxicity, infusion reactions, electrolyte abnormalities, and hepatotoxicity.[3,47] Renal toxicity is mediated by both direct tubular damage and rapid vasoconstriction via tubuloglomerular feedback from osmotic changes.[48] Intravenous fluid is commonly administered to help reduce renal damage. The risk of renal toxicity is dose-dependent, increasing with the total cumulative dose. Acute renal failure occurs in approximately 30% of patients and is associated with a mortality rate of more than 50% in this setting.[3] Surprisingly, the rate of nephrotoxicity is significantly lower in children and neonates.[2,35] The deoxycholate formulation of amphotericin B is commonly used in these patient populations with minimal toxicity. The lipid-based formulations are associated with significantly less nephrotoxicity.[13,49] However, infusion-related reactions often occur. These reactions seem to be induced by toll-like receptor (TLR)-2 activation, resulting in a proinflammatory cytokine response.[31] Pretreatment with nonsteroidal anti-inflammatory agents, antihistamines, and corticosteroids may be helpful. The hepatotoxicity associated with amphotericin B is uncommon and generally mild.[50]

Drug–Drug Interactions

Amphotericin B is not metabolized by hepatic CYP450 enzymes and has very few drug–drug interactions (**Box 2**). The pertinent drug–drug interactions for amphotericin B are related to the nephrotoxicity and electrolyte disturbance that may be augmented by other drugs with similar renal side effects. One common example is the coadministration of amphotericin B with immunosuppressants, such as tacrolimus or cyclosporine, in transplant recipients. This combination is associated with increased risk of kidney injury and electrolyte disturbances.[51]

FLUCYTOSINE

Flucytosine is a fluorinated pyrimidine (5-fluorocytosine) (see **Fig. 1**). As a pyrimidine analogue, it is imported by fungal cytosine permease and converted to fluorouracil by cytosine deaminase. Fluorouracil impairs nucleic acid synthesis, ultimately interfering with protein synthesis as well.[52]

Spectrum of Activity and Resistance

The activity of flucytosine is limited to the common pathogenic yeasts (see **Table 1**). Its spectrum includes many *Candida* spp, including *C albicans*, *C glabrata*, *C parapsilosis*, and *C tropicalis*. *C krusei* and *C lusitaniae* are also included in the spectrum but MICs are higher. Despite this activity, flucytosine is rarely used for the treatment of candidiasis alone because resistance rapidly develops with monotherapy.[2,53] Flucytosine demonstrates activity against *Cryptococcus* spp and is commonly administered in conjunction with amphotericin B.[16] It is not active against the dimorphic fungi or filamentous fungal pathogens.[21,54] Resistance to *Candida albicans* is reported to be near 10%, often related to decreased drug

---

Box 2
Summary of drug–drug interactions for systemic antifungal agents

- Amphotericin B has few significant drug–drug interactions. The main concerns arise from drugs with the potential for additive nephrotoxicity.

- Absorption of 2 triazole formulations—the itraconazole oral capsules and the posaconazole oral solution—is affected by gastric acidity. Medications that alter gastric pH, such as proton pump inhibitors and histamine-2 blockers, should be avoided.

- The azole drugs act as substrates and inhibitors of the CYP450 enzymes (CYP3A4, CYP2C19, CYP 2C9) and the affinities for each enzyme vary significantly by individual drug.

- Given the hundreds of potential drug–drug interactions for azoles, a patient's medication list should be carefully examined with initiation and discontinuation of azoles.

- Some of the common drug–drug interactions for azoles include antiarrhythmics, antipsychotics, immunosuppressants, migraine medications, antibiotics, anticoagulants, antidepressants, antiepileptics, antiretrovirals, chemotherapeutics, antihypertensives, lipid-lowering agents, narcotics, sedatives, hormonal therapies, and medications for diabetes.

- The echinocandin drugs have relatively few drug–drug interactions. A unique aspect for caspofungin is that it uses the OATP-1B1 transporter and may interact with immunosuppressants, antiepileptics, antiretrovirals, and rifampin.

uptake by the cytosine permease.[55,56] During therapy, mutations in enzymes converting flucytosine to the toxic metabolites 5-fluorouracil and 5-fluorouridine monophosphate may also lead to resistance.

Pharmacology

Flucytosine is highly bioavailable (80%–90%) and the only formulation available in the United States is an oral capsule.[57] It is dosed frequently, 4 times daily, due to its short half-life and pharmacodynamic characteristics.[58,59]

Flucytosine accumulates ubiquitously throughout host compartments. Specifically, high cerebrospinal fluid and vitreal fluid levels are achievable.[58,59] The drug is not significantly metabolized. The drug is primarily excreted renally and the unchanged drug exhibits excellent antifungal activity in the urine.[10,57] Patients with renal insufficiency have impaired drug clearance. Therefore, a 2-fold to 4-fold longer dosing interval is recommended for patients with a glomerular filtration rate (GFR) less than 50 (see **Table 2**). These dosing changes are guided by therapeutic drug monitoring with peak concentration targets ranging from 30 to 100 mg/L.

Clinical Indications

Flucytosine is a first-line therapy for the treatment of cryptococcal meningitis. It is administered with amphotericin B during the induction period.[39–41] Although flucytosine exhibits activity against most Candida spp, resistance develops quickly during use, limiting its treatment potential as a single agent.[2,53] To prevent emergence of resistance, flucytosine can be coadministered with an additional antifungal drug, such as amphotericin B, in select situations. Of note, flucytosine monotherapy may be an option for treatment of Candida cystitis given the high urinary concentrations of flucytosine and the relatively short course of therapy.[17,49,58]

Toxicities

Flucytosine is associated with 2 main toxicities: bone marrow suppression and liver toxicity. Bone marrow toxicity, in particular, can be limiting, leading to the lowering of the drug dose or drug discontinuation.[58] Cytopenias, including anemia, leukopenia, and thrombocytopenia, are dose-dependent, occurring more frequently with serum flucytosine concentrations of 125 μg/mL or greater.[60] Considering the renal clearance of flucytosine, patients with renal insufficiency are at high risk for toxicity. Both peak drug levels and cell counts should be monitored during therapy. Dose reductions are often needed. Flucytosine administration can also be associated with gastrointestinal upset and rash. Animal studies demonstrate teratogenic effects and flucytosine is contraindicated in pregnancy.[61]

Drug–Drug Interactions

Flucytosine is not a substrate or inhibitor of the CYP450 enzymes (see **Box 2**). There are very few drug–drug interactions. Because flucytosine is renally cleared, medications altering renal function may affect drug levels and the risk of toxicity.

AZOLES

The antifungal azole drug class is composed of imidazoles (clotrimazole, ketoconazole, miconazole) and triazoles (fluconazole, itraconazole, voriconazole, posaconazole, isavuconazole) that are named according to the number of nitrogen atoms in the azole ring.[62] These agents impair ergosterol synthesis by inhibiting C14-α sterol demethylase. Cell membrane integrity is disrupted by the accumulation of sterol precursors and the reduction of ergosterol.[63–68] The original azole drugs (ketoconazole, miconazole) exhibit significant toxicity during systemic administration. However, the newer triazoles (fluconazole, itraconazole, posaconazole, voriconazole, isavuconazole) have an improved safety panel (see **Fig. 1**).[63] Many azole drugs (ketoconazole, miconazole, clotrimazole, butoconazole, tioconazole, terconazole) are also available as topical preparations for the treatment of vaginal candidiasis or cutaneous fungal infection.[2]

Spectrum of Activity and Resistance

Fluconazole
Fluconazole is active against many medically important *Candida* spp, including *C albicans*, *C parapsilosis*, *C tropicalis*, *C lusitaniae*, and *C dubliniensis* (see **Table 1**).[69] MICs are higher for *Candida* spp, including *C glabrata*, *C guilliermondii*, and *C rugosa*.[14] Of note, fluconazole is not active against *Candida krusei*. Fluconazole displays excellent activity against *Cryptococcus neoformans*.[16,70] Although the spectrum of activity includes dimorphic pathogens *B dermatitidis*, *Coccidioides immitis*, and *H capsulatum*, MICs are significantly higher for fluconazole compared with other available azoles (itraconazole, posaconazole, voriconazole, isavuconazole) and fluconazole is less commonly used for the treatment of these infections, with the exception of coccidioidomycosis.[71] Fluconazole is not active against *Aspergillus* spp, *Fusarium* spp, *Scedosporium* spp, or the Mucorales.[17,21,71–74]

Itraconazole
Like fluconazole, itraconazole demonstrates activity against most *Candida* spp, with higher MICs for *C glabrata* and *C krusei* (see **Table 1**).[70,75,76] The spectrum of activity also includes the dimorphic fungal pathogens *B dermatitidis*, *H capsulatum*, *Coccidioides* spp, *Paracoccidioides* spp, and *Sporothrix schenckii* (see **Table 1**).[18,19,71,77] Itraconazole is also active against many *Aspergillus* spp, including *A fumigatus*, *A flavus*, *A nidulans*, and *A terreus*.[15] Itraconazole exhibits minimal activity against *Fusarium* spp and the Mucorales.

Voriconazole
Voriconazole offers anti-*Candida* activity in many ways similar to fluconazole and itraconazole (see **Table 1**).[76,78] In addition, voriconazole displays activity against a subset of fluconazole-resistant *C glabrata* strains.[79,80] Voriconazole is also active *Cryptococcus* spp and the dimorphic fungal pathogens *B dermatitidis*, *Coccidioides immitis*, and *H capsulatum* (see **Table 1**).[4,16,18,69] It exhibits potent activity against most *Aspergillus* spp, including amphotericin B–resistant *A terreus*.[15,71] The spectrum of activity of voriconazole also includes *Fusarium* spp *and Scedosporium* spp; however, activity against the Mucorales is minimal.[15,20,71,81]

Posaconazole
Posaconazole is active against most *Candida* spp, including *C albicans*, *C parapsilosis*, *C tropicalis*, and *C lusitaniae*, with higher MICs for *C krusei*, *C glabrata*, and *C guilliermondii* (see **Table 1**).[17,70,82] Like voriconazole, posaconazole also displays activity against a subset of fluconazole-resistant isolates but higher MICs are observed for these organisms.[14] The spectrum of activity of posaconazole includes *Cryptococcus* spp, *Coccidioides immitis*, *B dermatitidis*, and *H capsulatum*[70,71,83] (see **Table 1**). Posaconazole demonstrates potent activity against *Aspergillus* spp, including *A fumigatus*, *A flavus*, *A niger*, and *A terreus*.[15,17] Posaconazole also exhibits activity against several of the Mucorales.[15,81]

Isavuconazole

The spectrum of activity of isavuconazole includes most *Candida* spp, including *C glabrata* and *C krusei* (see **Table 1**).[84,85] Isavuconazole is active against most common *Aspergillus* spp, including *A fumigatus*, *A flavus*, and *A terreus*. MICs are similar to those observed for voriconazole and are higher than those observed for posaconazole.[86,87] Isavuconazole exhibits potent activity against *Cryptococcus* spp, as well as the dimorphic fungal pathogens *B dermatitidis*, *Coccidioides immitis*, and *H capsulatum*.[85,88,89] Isavuconazole further demonstrates activity against a subset of *Scedosporium* spp and organisms in the Mucorales group.[89,90]

Resistance

The term resistance includes both intrinsic resistance, as discussed in the spectrum of activity, and extrinsic resistance, which is acquired. The rate of extrinsic triazole resistance has been increasing, particularly for *C glabrata*. During the past decade, the frequency of fluconazole-resistant *C glabrata* has increased from 9% to 14%.[91,92] Azole cross-resistance is common, with most fluconazole-resistant isolates exhibiting resistance to voriconazole as well. In recent years, the rate of azole-resistant *A fumigatus* has also been rising significantly, particularly in Europe, where rates are reported as high as 20%, although they vary by geographic region.[93,94] The higher resistance rates in certain areas have been linked to antifungal use in agriculture. Azole-resistant invasive aspergillosis has a very poor prognosis, with mortality rates above 80%.[94] The main mechanism of azole resistance for *Aspergillus*, *Candida*, and *Cryptococcus* spp involves the mutation of the azole drug target, lanosterol 14α-demethylase.[93] For *Aspergillus* spp, this commonly leads to resistance to all azole drugs. However, for *Candida* spp, the modification of this drug target may lead to resistance to fluconazole alone, azole pan-resistance, or resistance to a subset of azoles. A second mechanism of resistance, the upregulation of efflux pumps, has also been shown to promote drug resistance via a decrease in intracellular drug levels.

Pharmacology

Fluconazole

The pharmacokinetic characteristics of the individual azole drugs are distinct due to their variation in molecular weight, solubility, and protein binding. Fluconazole is unique due to its low molecular weight and high aqueous solubility. It demonstrates high bioavailability, approximately 90%, and its absorption is not affected by gastric acidity or food.[6,95,96] Currently, there are 2 oral formulations, a tablet and a powder for suspension, and an intravenous solution. The recommended dosages are not affected by the route of administration (see **Table 2**). Due to its relatively long half-life and pharmacodynamic pattern of activity, fluconazole is dosed daily.

Fluconazole effectively penetrates most host body tissues, including the central nervous system. Therapeutic concentrations can be achieved in the cerebrospinal fluid and ocular compartments.[97] Fluconazole achieves high urinary concentrations because it is primarily renally cleared with approximately 66% to 76% of unchanged fluconazole secreted into the urine.[98,99] Dose reductions are thus recommended for patients with advanced renal insufficiency.[100] Fluconazole is removed by hemodialysis and should be administered following hemodialysis.[101,102] Unlike other triazole drugs, fluconazole is not extensively metabolized in the liver. Dose adjustments are not necessary for patients with hepatic impairment.

Itraconazole

Itraconazole is currently available in 2 oral preparations: a capsule and an oral solution complexed with hydroxypropyl-β-cyclodextrin. It has also been formulated with cyclodextrin for intravenous use but this preparation is not currently available. The absorption and bioavailability of the 2 itraconazole oral formulations vary. Absorption of the capsule formulation is approximately 55% but it is improved with gastric acidity and food intake.[6,103,104] Therefore, it is recommended to be administered with an acidic beverage and food. Medications that reduce gastric acidity, such as proton pump inhibitors and histamine-2 blockers, should be avoided. The oral solution exhibits superior bioavailability, near 80%, and the absorption of itraconazole is not affected by gastric acidity or food intake.[105] Interpatient variability is less with this formulation and serum concentrations are typically 30% higher than for the tablet formulation.

Several clinical studies have examined the relationship between itraconazole serum levels and therapeutic response for a variety of fungal infections.[106–109] Itraconazole levels can be measured by either high-performance liquid chromatography (HPLC) or bioassay. The former measures the concentrations of 2 active compounds, the parent drug and the active hydroxyitraconazole metabolite.[110] Based on available data, an itraconazole level greater than 0.5 µg/mL is suggested for treatment of oral candidiasis or prophylaxis for fungal infections.[111] However, for treatment of invasive fungal infection, an itraconazole concentration of 1 to 2 µg/ml has been linked to treatment success.[108]

Itraconazole is highly protein bound (99%).[112] Unlike fluconazole and voriconazole, only low levels of the drug are found in the cerebrospinal fluid and fluid compartments of the eye.[112,113] Thus, the use of itraconazole for the treatment of infections involving the central nervous system or the eye is not commonly recommended. A unique pharmacokinetic observation is the accumulation of itraconazole in the skin and nail tissues. With levels reaching nearly 20-fold higher concentrations than those measured in the plasma, it is an ideal agent for the treatment of cutaneous and nail mycoses.[114–116] Itraconazole is metabolized, primarily by the CYP450 isoenzyme 3A4, to the active metabolite hydroxyitraconazole and several inactive metabolites.[114] Although metabolites can be found in both the urine and feces, the urinary metabolites are inactive and itraconazole is not useful for the treatment of infections involving the lower urinary tract.[114,117] Dose reductions are not required for renal failure or dialysis.[118,119] However, itraconazole is hepatically metabolized and dose reduction is recommended for patients with hepatic impairment (see **Table 2**).[114,120]

Voriconazole

Voriconazole is formulated as an oral tablet, an oral suspension, and an intravenous solution (complexed with sulfobutylether β-cyclodextrin). The bioavailability for both oral formulations is quite high, greater than 90%.[10,121] Absorption is not affected by gastric acidity and is optimal in the fasted state. Loading doses for the first 24 hours are recommended to more rapidly achieve therapeutic levels (see **Table 2**).[4,63] Given its shorter half-life (6 hours), voriconazole is dosed twice daily.

Serum levels of voriconazole may vary widely among patients, primarily due to differences in metabolism. Voriconazole is extensively metabolized by the CYP450 enzymes and polymorphisms are common in the primary enzyme CYP2C19.[122,123] Patients can possess polymorphisms that lead to either slow or rapid metabolism, placing them at risk for toxicity or therapeutic failure, respectively.[124–127] Clinical studies show therapeutic success is associated with voriconazole serum trough concentrations ranging from 1 to 2 µg/mL.[128,129] However, higher voriconazole concentrations, those exceeding 6 µg/mL, have been linked to adverse drug events, including hepatitis and delirium. Given the variability in metabolism of voriconazole among patients, therapeutic drug monitoring is recommended during treatment of invasive fungal infections.[9]

Voriconazole is 58% protein bound.[4] Similar to fluconazole, levels in the cerebrospinal fluid and ocular compartments reach greater than 50% of serum concentrations, allowing for the treatment of infections of the central nervous system and eye.[130–132] Voriconazole is metabolized via the hepatic CYP450 isoenzymes CYP2C9, CYP2C19, and CYP3A4; dose reduction is recommend for patients with impaired liver function.[133] Because minimal active drug is secreted into the urine, voriconazole is not useful for the treatment of fungal urinary tract infections.[122,133] Although voriconazole is not significantly renally cleared, the cyclodextrin component of the intravenous formulation may accumulate in patients with renal insufficiency. Although studies have not identified cyclodextrin toxicity, the intravenous formulation is not commonly recommended for patients with a GFR less than 50 if other treatment options are available.[134]

Posaconazole

Posaconazole is currently available as an oral suspension, a delayed release tablet, and an intravenous solution that is complexed with sulfobutylether β-cyclodextrin (see **Table 2**). Absorption and bioavailability differ between the 2 oral formulations. For the oral solution, absorption highly depends on food intake with high-fat meals best promoting absorption.[135] Like itraconazole, the absorption depends on gastric acidity and is reduced by proton pump inhibitors and histamine-2 blockers.[136–138] Posaconazole exhibits saturable absorption, requiring the oral suspension to be dosed multiple times daily, despite its relative long half-life (>24 hours).[10,139] The newer tablet formulation incorporates a pH-dependent polymer matrix that allows for delayed drug release. This circumvents the saturable absorption limitation of the oral solution and allows for once-daily dosing. Absorption of the tablet formulation is not significantly influenced by food intake or gastric acidity, allowing for improved bioavailability (54%) and more reliable serum concentrations.[82]

Similar to studies with itraconazole and voriconazole, clinical studies suggest therapeutic drug monitoring is of benefit for posaconazole, particularly for the oral suspension formulation.[140–144] For patients receiving posaconazole for treatment of refractory aspergillosis, the greatest efficacy was observed in those with steady state concentrations greater than 1.25 μg/mL, whereas those with levels less than 0.5 μg/mL had the lowest success rate. In studies examining the efficacy for prophylaxis, posaconazole concentrations greater than 0.5 μg/mL or greater than 0.7 μg/mL were associated with fewer breakthrough fungal infections.

Posaconazole is highly protein bound (98%). Available data from clinical investigations and animal studies show poor penetration of posaconazole into the cerebrospinal fluid and ocular compartments; posaconazole is not recommended for treatment of endophthalmitis or infections of the central nervous system.[10,83,145–147] Posaconazole undergoes metabolism by uridine diphosphate (UDP)-glucuronidation and is excreted via the bile and feces.[148] Dose adjustments are not necessary for patients with renal insufficiency. However, similar to voriconazole, the intravenous formulation is complexed with a cyclodextrin that may accumulate with renal impairment.[149] Therefore, the intravenous formulation is not recommended for patients with a GFR less than 50.

Isavuconazole

Isavuconazonium, the water-soluble prodrug of isavuconazole, is available as an oral capsule and an intravenous solution. In contrast to the intravenous formulations for voriconazole and posaconazole, the isavuconazonium intravenous formulation does not contain the sulfobutylether β-cyclodextrin vehicle that may accumulate with renal insufficiency. Isavuconazole exhibits a prolonged half-life (>75 hours) and is dosed daily following a 2-day loading period (see **Table 2**).[150] The oral formulation is highly bioavailable and the absorption is not significantly affected by food intake or gastric acidity.[85,150] Preliminary patient pharmacokinetic data have thus far not demonstrated utility for therapeutic drug monitoring for isavuconazole. Given the high bioavailability and relatively consistent metabolism, the interpatient variability in drug levels is expected to be lower than that observed for posaconazole, itraconazole, and voriconazole.

Isavuconazole is highly protein bound (>99%). The distribution of isavuconazole has not been extensively studied but drug levels in the cerebral spinal fluid and eye compartments are predicted to be low.[85] However, brain parenchymal concentrations in animal studies are higher than those observed in serum. Isavuconazole is metabolized by hepatic CYP450 enzymes and metabolites are excreted in the feces.[150] Because minimal active drug is excreted in the urine, treatment of fungal urinary tract infections is not recommended. Because hepatic metabolism and drug clearance have shown to be slowed in patients with liver impairment, a 50% dose reduction is recommended.[151] Dose reductions are not required for patients with renal insufficiency or dialysis.

Clinical Indications

Fluconazole
Fluconazole has indications for the treatment of both mucosal and systemic candidiasis, the treatment of cryptococcosis, and prophylaxis for candidiasis (see **Table 2**). Clinical trials have shown fluconazole to be effective for the treatment of invasive candidiasis in non-neutropenic patients.[152–155] However, recent meta-analysis suggests the triazoles are inferior to echinocandins as initial therapy for invasive disease.[156] The current IDSA guidelines recommend fluconazole as a first-line therapy for treatment of mucosal candidiasis and as a first-line option for step-down therapy for invasive candidiasis due to susceptible *Candida* isolates.[2] Multiple trials have confirmed the efficacy and tolerability of fluconazole for the treatment of oropharyngeal and esophageal candidiasis.[157–165] Fluconazole remains a first-line therapy for the treatment of patients with mucosal candidiasis, including those with human immunodeficiency virus (HIV). Fluconazole is also indicated for the treatment of vulvovaginal candidiasis in nonpregnant women.[2] Clinical trials have found a single dose of oral fluconazole to be as effective as topical therapy for uncomplicated vaginal candidiasis treatment.[166–168] In addition, weekly therapy has proven useful for disease prevention in patients with recurrent vulvovaginal candidiasis.[169]

Fluconazole is approved for the treatment of cryptococcosis.[41,170,171] Currently, it is recommended for initial treatment of mild-to-moderate pulmonary disease.[39] It is also first-line for consolidation therapy in patients with severe cryptococcosis or cryptococcal meningitis following successful induction therapy with an amphotericin B–containing regimen. At a lower dose, fluconazole is used for maintenance or suppressive therapy to prevent relapse. Fluconazole is approved for prophylaxis against fungal infections in neutropenic patients.[2,172,173] Compared with the azoles with activity against mold pathogens and amphotericin B, fluconazole is solely effective at preventing candidiasis.[144,174,175] When compared with posaconazole, clinical trials found fluconazole to be less effective for prevention of invasive aspergillosis.[144,175]

Itraconazole
Itraconazole is approved for the treatment of numerous mycoses, including blastomycosis, mucosal candidiasis, coccidioidomycosis, cryptococcosis, histoplasmosis,

onychomycosis, and sporotrichosis (see **Table 2**). It is also approved for empiric treatment of fungal infection in neutropenic patients and as second-line treatment of aspergillosis. For treatment of endemic fungal pathogens, it is primarily used as initial therapy for mild-to-moderate disease. For severe blastomycosis, histoplasmosis, coccidioidomycosis, paracoccidioidomycosis, and sporotrichosis, amphotericin B is recommended for initial therapy. Itraconazole can be administered for step-down therapy but it is not ideal for the treatment of mycoses involving the central nervous system due to its poor central nervous system penetration.[25,37,38,176–179] Although it has an indication for the treatment of cryptococcosis, it is not a preferred agent for consolidation or maintenance therapy given its poor cerebrospinal fluid penetration and higher reported failure rate.[39]

Itraconazole has been shown to be effective for the treatment of oropharyngeal, esophageal, and vaginal candidiasis but it is not currently recommended as first-line therapy for these infections.[2,180] It does not offer clear benefit compared with fluconazole treatment of mucosal candidiasis and is associated with more side-effects, variable gastric absorption, and less predictable drug levels.[157–159,181] Itraconazole does remain a treatment option for patients with these infections who are not responding to fluconazole. It is not approved for treatment of candidemia or invasive candidiasis.

Itraconazole effectively prevents invasive fungal infection in patients with hematologic malignancy or autologous bone marrow transplantation.[182–184] However, it is not as well tolerated as fluconazole, often leading to discontinuation due to gastrointestinal side effects, and it is not commonly used for this indication.[174] Although it likely offers protection against filamentous fungal infections, the activity spectrum for itraconazole does not include the Mucorales organisms.[21] Itraconazole is also approved as salvage therapy for the treatment of invasive aspergillosis. However, it has not been compared with voriconazole or amphotericin B. It is only recommended for patients who are unable to tolerate these preferred agents.[45,185] Conversely, itraconazole is commonly used for chronic pulmonary aspergillosis and allergic bronchopulmonary aspergillosis treatment.[186,187]

Voriconazole

Voriconazole is approved for the treatment of invasive aspergillosis, esophageal candidiasis, invasive candidiasis, scedosporiosis, and fusariosis (see **Table 2**). In a large randomized trial, voriconazole was found to be superior to amphotericin B for the treatment of invasive pulmonary aspergillosis and is currently recommended as first-line therapy.[44,45] It is also the drug of choice for most invasive forms of aspergillosis, including sinusitis, brain abscess, endocarditis, osteomyelitis, and septic arthritis. Additionally, it is also recommended for the treatment of fungal infections caused by *Scedosporium* spp or *Fusarium* spp based on salvage therapy trials and retrospective analysis.[4,188,189]

Voriconazole is approved for the treatment of both mucosal and invasive candidiasis. It was found to be as effective as a regimen of amphotericin B followed by fluconazole for treatment of candidemia in a randomized clinical trial.[154] However, voriconazole is not recommended as first-line therapy for the treatment of invasive candidiasis for most patient groups because there is little advantage when compared with fluconazole. The circumstances in which voriconazole should be considered in place of fluconazole include infection with *Candida krusei*, infection with fluconazole-resistant *Candida glabrata* (susceptible to fluconazole), intolerance to fluconazole, or if antifungal coverage for mold infection is warranted.[2] Likewise, voriconazole is approved for the treatment of esophageal candidiasis but is not commonly used for this indication with the exception of candidiasis due to fluconazole-resistant organisms.[160]

Posaconazole

Posaconazole is approved for the treatment of oropharyngeal candidiasis and prophylaxis for invasive fungal infection (see **Table 2**). Clinical trials have shown posaconazole to be as effective or more effective for prevention of invasive fungal infection, when compared with fluconazole or itraconazole.[144,175] Studies have included stem cell transplant recipients with graft-versus-host disease and neutropenic patients. Given its extended spectrum of activity, posaconazole protects against many filamentous fungal pathogens in addition to invasive candidiasis. Posaconazole is also approved for treatment of oropharyngeal candidiasis based on noninferiority to fluconazole and effectiveness for azole-refractory cases.[164,190,191] It is not recommended as first-line therapy but may be an alternative for patients intolerant of other medications or with infection caused by resistant organisms. A randomized trial examining the utility of posaconazole for treatment of invasive aspergillosis is ongoing.

Isavuconazole

Isavuconazole is approved for the treatment of invasive aspergillosis and invasive mucormycosis (see **Table 2**). The indication for treatment of aspergillosis is based on results of a large randomized, controlled trial comparing isavuconazole and voriconazole for treatment of invasive aspergillosis and other mold infections (www.fda.gov). For all subjects and the subset with aspergillosis, both all-cause mortality and treatment success were similar and isavuconazole met noninferiority criteria. Isavuconazole is also approved for treatment of mucormycosis based on an open-label noncomparative trial which included subjects with refractory mucormycosis and subjects who had not received prior therapy (www.fda.gov). When examining overall response and all-cause mortality, results for isavuconazole-treated subjects (31% and 38%, respectively) were similar to those reported in prior investigations for amphotericin B and posaconazole.

Toxicities

In general, the triazole drugs are fairly well-tolerated. As a drug class, the most common side-effects include rash, headache, or gastrointestinal upset.[172,192,193] Hepatotoxicity, marked by elevation of liver chemistry tests and, less commonly, liver failure, is the most common and serious class effect. Voriconazole poses the highest risk (31%), whereas itraconazole, posaconazole, and isavuconazole present lower risks (10%–20%). Monitoring of liver chemistry tests during azole use is recommended but infrequently results in drug discontinuation.[50] Voriconazole has several unique side-effects, including a photosensitive skin rash, reversible visual changes (photopsia), and fluoride-associated bone toxicity.[44] The former has also been linked to skin malignancy in the setting of prolonged use. With the exception of isavuconazole, the azole drugs cause QT prolongation, presenting a risk for arrhythmia, especially in the setting of drug–drug interactions.[51] In contrast, isavuconazole is associated with QT shortening and is contraindicated for patients with familial short QT syndrome.[85] The azole drugs are contraindicated in pregnancy due to an established link to birth defects.[46,61]

Drug–drug interactions

Of the antifungal drug classes, the triazole drugs have the highest potential for serious drug–drug reactions. They are substrates and inhibitors of various hepatic CYP450 metabolic enzymes and have the potential for hundreds of drug–drug interactions.

The possible drug–drug interactions vary by individual drug because each has a variable affinity for the isoenzymes (CYP2C19, CYP3A4, CYP2C9).[194] As inhibitors of CYP450 enzymes, triazoles can impair metabolism of a coadministered drug, increasing the risk of toxicity. As substrates of the pathway, the concentrations of the triazoles can be substantially affected by concomitant use of medications that inhibit or induce the enzymes, as has been observed for itraconazole and voriconazole.[195,196] **Box 2** lists commonly used classes of medications that have the potential for serious interactions if administered with azoles. Closely examining a patient's medication list is recommended before starting and stopping medications given the high potential for drug–drug interactions. Absorption of the itraconazole oral capsules and the posaconazole oral solution is optimized by gastric acidity (see previous discussion), so proton pump inhibitors and histamine-2 blockers should be avoided.[136–138] Because the triazoles can cause QT prolongation, drug–drug interactions may be encountered by the additive effect of additional QT prolonging agents. Of note, isavuconazole is the only triazole that is not associated with QT prolongation.[85]

ECHINOCANDINS

The echinocandins are a class of semisynthetic lipopeptides composed of cyclic hexapeptides N-linked to a fatty acyl side chain (see **Fig. 1**). The compounds disrupt the fungal cell wall by inhibiting the synthesis of β-1,3 glucan, a fungal cell wall polysaccharide essential for many fungi.[197] For *Candida* spp, this results in fungicidal activity. For *Aspergillus* spp, the echinocandins inhibit cell wall growth primarily at the hyphal tip, producing a fungistatic effect.[198] The 3 echinocandins currently available include caspofungin, micafungin, and anidulafungin.

Spectrum of Activity and Resistance

Caspofungin, micafungin, and anidulafungin demonstrate very similar activities (see **Table 1**). The agents display potent activity against many *Candida* spp, including *C albicans*, *C glabrata*, *C dubliniensis*, *C tropicalis*, and *C krusei*.[91,199,200] For *C parapsilosis* and *C guilliermondii*, MICs are often higher but the echinocandins are often still useful agents for the treatment of these infections clinically.[201] The echinocandins are active against many *Aspergillus* spp, although the activity is fungistatic.[202–204] Additionally, the echinocandins seem to potentiate the activity of triazoles against *Aspergillus* spp in preclinical models.[205,206] The spectrum of activity for the echinocandins does not include *Cryptococcus* spp, endemic dimorphic fungi, Mucorales, *Fusarium* spp, or *Scedosporium* spp.[15,21,74] Resistance to *Candida* spp is relatively low, less than 3%, and is primarily mediated by mutations in 2 conserved regions of the gene-encoding glucan synthase, the echinocandin drug target.[93] Of note, resistance rates for *Candida glabrata* have been increasing and are now reported at rates ranging from 3% to 15%.[207]

Pharmacology

The pharmacokinetic and pharmacodynamic profiles of the echinocandin drugs are quite similar.[10,208–210] The agents are poorly absorbed through the gastrointestinal system and are thus only available in parenteral formulations (see **Table 2**). They can be dosed once daily given their long half-lives (10–26 h).[10,11] Animal studies show the echinocandins demonstrate optimal efficacy following administration of large doses given infrequently.[211–214]

The echinocandins have limited distribution to the central nervous system. Low concentrations are found in the cerebrospinal fluid and eye.[10,11] Therefore, the echinocandins are not ideal agents for infections involving these compartments, such as meningitis or endophthalmitis. The echinocandins are primarily eliminated through nonenzymatic degradation to inactive products.[209] Excretion of the breakdown products is predominantly via the fecal route. Only low concentrations of active drugs are excreted in the urine and caution should be used with treatment of urinary tract infections. Although the echinocandins are not significantly metabolized by the CYP450 enzymes, caspofungin and micafungin undergo hepatic metabolism and dose reduction is recommended for patients with hepatic dysfunction receiving caspofungin.[215]

Clinical Indications

Drugs of the echinocandin class are effective for prevention of invasive fungal infection, empiric treatment of fungal infection, and treatment of candidiasis[155,161–163,165,216–222] (see **Table 2**). Due to their similar activities, caspofungin, micafungin, and anidulafungin are generally used interchangeably.[2] The echinocandins are recommended as first-line agents for the treatment of candidemia and invasive candidiasis based on a meta-analysis of randomized trials showing improved survival with this drug class compared with amphotericin B or triazoles.[155,156,223] The echinocandins also have indications for mucosal (oropharyngeal or esophageal) candidiasis based on trials demonstrating efficacy similar to amphotericin B and fluconazole.[161,162,165,219] However, as parenteral agents, they are not commonly used for this indication.

Although the echinocandins have not been shown to be effective for primary treatment of aspergillosis in a randomized trial, caspofungin has an indication for the treatment of refractory aspergillosis based on salvage therapy investigations.[224,225] Guidelines currently recommend caspofungin or micafungin only as second-line agents.[45] There has been interest in using the echinocandins as adjuvant antifungals for treatment of aspergillosis.[206,226,227] A randomized, controlled trial comparing voriconazole monotherapy and combination therapy with anidulafungin found a trend toward improved outcome in the combination therapy group in a post hoc subgroup analysis. However, this difference did not meet statistical significance to establish superiority.[228] Therefore, there are still only limited data to support the use of combination therapy for the treatment of aspergillosis. Micafungin has approval for prophylaxis of invasive fungal infection based on a randomized trial comparing it to fluconazole in hematopoietic stem cell transplant recipients.[222] It was found to prevent candidiasis and aspergillosis. For patients with neutropenic fever and suspected fungal infection, caspofungin demonstrated therapeutic efficacy with fewer side-effects than amphotericin B.[223] Caspofungin has approval for empiric treatment of fungal infection for this population.

Toxicities

Echinocandins are generally well-tolerated and patients experience very few side effects. The most commonly experienced adverse reactions include gastrointestinal upset, headache, elevation of liver (aminotransferase) tests, or mild infusion reaction.[10,199,200]

Drug–Drug Interactions

Echinocandins demonstrate very few drug–drug interactions because they are not metabolized through the CYP450 enzymatic pathways (see **Box 2**).[10,199,200] Caspofungin has been shown to use the OATP-1B1 transporter, which is also used by other drugs, such as rifampin.[229] Therefore, reduction of caspofungin is recommended in the setting of inducers of this enzyme, including rifampin, phenytoin, or dexamethasone.[210] Mild interactions with the immunosuppressants tacrolimus and cyclosporine are predicted and monitoring of these drug levels is recommendation with coadministration.

REFERENCES

1. McNeil MM, Nash SL, Hajjeh RA, et al. Trends in mortality due to invasive mycotic diseases in the united states, 1980-1997. Clin Infect Dis 2001;33(5): 641–7.
2. Pappas PG, Kauffman CA, Andes D, et al. Clinical practice guidelines for the management of candidiasis: 2009 update by the Infectious Diseases Society of America. Clin Infect Dis 2009;48(5):503–35.
3. Bates DW, Su L, Yu DT, et al. Mortality and costs of acute renal failure associated with amphotericin B therapy. Clin Infect Dis 2001;32(5):686–93.
4. Johnson LB, Kauffman CA. Voriconazole: a new triazole antifungal agent. Clin Infect Dis 2003;36(5):630–7.
5. Nagappan V, Deresinski S. Reviews of anti-infective agents: posaconazole: a broad-spectrum triazole antifungal agent. Clin Infect Dis 2007;45(12):1610–7.
6. Zimmermann T, Yeates RA, Laufen H, et al. Influence of concomitant food intake on the oral absorption of two triazole antifungal agents, itraconazole and fluconazole. Eur J Clin Pharmacol 1994;46(2):147–50.
7. Warn PA, Sharp A, Parmar A, et al. Pharmacokinetics and pharmacodynamics of a novel triazole, isavuconazole: mathematical modeling, importance of tissue concentrations, and impact of immune status on antifungal effect. Antimicrob Agents Chemother 2009;53(8):3453–61.
8. Merck & Co. Inc. Noxafil (posaconazole) [package insert]. Whitehouse Station, NJ: Merck & Co. Inc; 2014.
9. Pascual A, Calandra T, Bolay S, et al. Voriconazole therapeutic drug monitoring in patients with invasive mycoses improves efficacy and safety outcomes. Clin Infect Dis 2008;46(2):201–11.
10. Dodds Ashley ES, Lewis R, Lewis JS, et al. Pharmacology of systemic antifungal agents. Clin Infect Dis 2006;43(S1):S28–39.
11. Okugawa S, Ota Y, Tatsuno K, et al. A case of invasive central nervous system aspergillosis treated with micafungin with monitoring of micafungin concentrations in the cerebrospinal fluid. Scand J Infect Dis 2007;39(4):344–6.
12. Gallis HA, Drew RH, Pickard WW. Amphotericin B: 30 years of clinical experience. Rev Infect Dis 1990;12(2):308–29.
13. Arikan S, Rex JH. Lipid-based antifungal agents: current status. Curr Pharm Des 2001;7(5):393–415.
14. Pfaller MA, Diekema DJ, Messer SA, et al. In vitro activities of voriconazole, posaconazole, and four licensed systemic antifungal agents against Candida species infrequently isolated from blood. J Clin Microbiol 2003;41(1):78–83.
15. Diekema DJ, Messer SA, Hollis RJ, et al. Activities of caspofungin, itraconazole, posaconazole, ravuconazole, voriconazole, and amphotericin B against 448 recent clinical isolates of filamentous fungi. J Clin Microbiol 2003;41(8):3623–6.
16. Pfaller MA, Messer SA, Boyken L, et al. Global trends in the antifungal susceptibility of Cryptococcus neoformans (1990 to 2004). J Clin Microbiol 2005;43(5): 2163–7.
17. Sabatelli F, Patel R, Mann PA, et al. In vitro activities of posaconazole, fluconazole, itraconazole, voriconazole, and amphotericin B against a large collection of clinically important molds and yeasts. Antimicrob Agents Chemother 2006; 50(6):2009–15.

18. Li RK, Ciblak MA, Nordoff N, et al. In vitro activities of voriconazole, itraconazole, and amphotericin B against *Blastomyces dermatitidis, Coccidioides immitis,* and *Histoplasma capsulatum.* Antimicrob Agents Chemother 2000;44(6):1734–6.
19. McGinnis MR, Nordoff N, Li RK, et al. *Sporothrix schenckii* sensitivity to voriconazole, itraconazole and amphotericin B. Med Mycol 2001;39(4):369–71.
20. Meletiadis J, Meis JF, Mouton JW, et al. In vitro activities of new and conventional antifungal agents against clinical *Scedosporium* isolates. Antimicrob Agents Chemother 2002;46(1):62–8.
21. Almyroudis NG, Sutton DA, Fothergill AW, et al. In vitro susceptibilities of 217 clinical isolates of zygomycetes to conventional and new antifungal agents. Antimicrob Agents Chemother 2007;51(7):2587–90.
22. Thompson GR 3rd, Cadena J, Patterson TF. Overview of antifungal agents. Clin Chest Med 2009;30(2):203–15, v.
23. Andes D, Stamsted T, Conklin R. Pharmacodynamics of amphotericin B in a neutropenic-mouse disseminated-candidiasis model. Antimicrob Agents Chemother 2001;45(3):922–6.
24. Andes D, Safdar N, Marchillo K, et al. Pharmacokinetic-pharmacodynamic comparison of amphotericin B (AMB) and two lipid-associated AMB preparations, liposomal AMB and AMB lipid complex, in murine candidiasis models. Antimicrob Agents Chemother 2006;50(2):674–84.
25. Chapman SW, Dismukes WE, Proia LA, et al. Clinical practice guidelines for the management of blastomycosis: 2008 update by the Infectious Diseases Society of America. Clin Infect Dis 2008;46(12):1801–12.
26. Atkinson AJ Jr, Bennett JE. Amphotericin B pharmacokinetics in humans. Antimicrob Agents Chemother 1978;13(2):271–6.
27. Groll AH, Giri N, Petraitis V, et al. Comparative efficacy and distribution of lipid formulations of amphotericin B in experimental *Candida albicans* infection of the central nervous system. J Infect Dis 2000;182(1):274–82.
28. Vogelsinger H, Weiler S, Djanani A, et al. Amphotericin B tissue distribution in autopsy material after treatment with liposomal amphotericin B and amphotericin B colloidal dispersion. J Antimicrob Chemother 2006;57(6):1153–60.
29. Bekersky I, Fielding RM, Dressler DE, et al. Pharmacokinetics, excretion, and mass balance of liposomal amphotericin B (AmBisome) and amphotericin B deoxycholate in humans. Antimicrob Agents Chemother 2002;46(3):828–33.
30. Ostrosky-Zeichner L, Marr KA, Rex JH, et al. Amphotericin B: time for a new "gold standard". Clin Infect Dis 2003;37(3):415–25.
31. Hamill RJ. Amphotericin B formulations: a comparative review of efficacy and toxicity. Drugs 2013;73(9):919–34.
32. Oppenheim BA, Herbrecht R, Kusne S. The safety and efficacy of amphotericin B colloidal dispersion in the treatment of invasive mycoses. Clin Infect Dis 1995; 21(5):1145–53.
33. Walsh TJ, Hiemenz JW, Seibel NL, et al. Amphotericin B lipid complex for invasive fungal infections: analysis of safety and efficacy in 556 cases. Clin Infect Dis 1998;26(6):1383–96.
34. Tollemar J, Andersson S, Ringden O, et al. A retrospective clinical comparison between antifungal treatment with liposomal amphotericin B (AmBisome) and conventional amphotericin B in transplant recipients. Mycoses 1992;35(9–10): 215–20.
35. Linder N, Klinger G, Shalit I, et al. Treatment of Candidaemia in premature infants: comparison of three amphotericin B preparations. J Antimicrob Chemother 2003;52(4):663–7.

36. Casado JL, Quereda C, Oliva J, et al. Candidal meningitis in HIV-infected patients: analysis of 14 cases. Clin Infect Dis 1997;25(3):673–6.
37. Wheat LJ, Freifeld AG, Kleiman MB, et al. Clinical practice guidelines for the management of patients with histoplasmosis: 2007 update by the Infectious Diseases Society of America. Clin Infect Dis 2007;45(7):807–25.
38. Galgiani JN, Ampel NM, Blair JE, et al. Coccidioidomycosis. Clin Infect Dis 2005;41(9):1217–23.
39. Perfect JR, Dismukes WE, Dromer F, et al. Clinical practice guidelines for the management of cryptococcal disease: 2010 update by the Infectious Diseases Society of America. Clin Infect Dis 2010;50(3):291–322.
40. Bennett JE, Dismukes WE, Duma RJ, et al. A comparison of amphotericin B alone and combined with flucytosine in the treatment of cryptococcal meningitis. N Engl J Med 1979;301(3):126–31.
41. Saag MS, Cloud GA, Graybill JR, et al. A comparison of itraconazole versus fluconazole as maintenance therapy for AIDS-associated cryptococcal meningitis. National Institute of Allergy and Infectious Diseases Mycoses Study Group. Clin Infect Dis 1999;28(2):291–6.
42. Spellberg B, Walsh TJ, Kontoyiannis DP, et al. Recent advances in the management of mucormycosis: from bench to bedside. Clin Infect Dis 2009;48(12):1743–51.
43. Kauffman CA, Bustamante B, Chapman SW, et al. Clinical practice guidelines for the management of sporotrichosis: 2007 update by the Infectious Diseases Society of America. Clin Infect Dis 2007;45(10):1255–65.
44. Herbrecht R, Denning DW, Patterson TF, et al. Voriconazole versus amphotericin B for primary therapy of invasive aspergillosis. N Engl J Med 2002;347(6):408–15.
45. Walsh TJ, Anaissie EJ, Denning DW, et al. Treatment of aspergillosis: clinical practice guidelines of the Infectious Diseases Society of America. Clin Infect Dis 2008;46(3):327–60.
46. Pursley TJ, Blomquist IK, Abraham J, et al. Fluconazole-induced congenital anomalies in three infants. Clin Infect Dis 1996;22(2):336–40.
47. Clements JS Jr, Peacock JE Jr. Amphotericin B revisited: reassessment of toxicity. Am J Med 1990;88(5N):22N–7N.
48. Cheng JT, Witty RT, Robinson RR, et al. Amphotericin B nephrotoxicity: increased renal resistance and tubule permeability. Kidney Int 1982;22(6):626–33.
49. Patel R. Antifungal agents. Part I. Amphotericin B preparations and flucytosine. Mayo Clin Proc 1998;73(12):1205–25.
50. Girois SB, Chapuis F, Decullier E, et al. Adverse effects of antifungal therapies in invasive fungal infections: review and meta-analysis. Eur J Clin Microbiol Infect Dis 2005;24(2):119–30.
51. Albengres E, Le Louet H, Tillement JP. Systemic antifungal agents. Drug interactions of clinical significance. Drug Saf 1998;18(2):83–97.
52. Waldorf AR, Polak A. Mechanisms of action of 5-fluorocytosine. Antimicrob Agents Chemother 1983;23(1):79–85.
53. Tassel D, Madoff MA. Treatment of Candida sepsis and Cryptococcus meningitis with 5-fluorocytosine. A new antifungal agent. JAMA 1968;206(4):830–2.
54. Dannaoui E, Meletiadis J, Mouton JW, et al. In vitro susceptibilities of zygomycetes to conventional and new antifungals. J Antimicrob Chemother 2003;51(1):45–52.
55. Sanglard D, Odds FC. Resistance of Candida species to antifungal agents: molecular mechanisms and clinical consequences. Lancet Infect Dis 2002;2(2):73–85.

56. Kontoyiannis DP, Lewis RE. Antifungal drug resistance of pathogenic fungi. Lancet 2002;359(9312):1135–44.
57. Schonebeck J, Polak A, Fernex M, et al. Pharmacokinetic studies on the oral antimycotic agent 5-fluorocytosine in individuals with normal and impaired kidney function. Chemotherapy 1973;18(6):321–36.
58. Vermes A, Guchelaar HJ, Dankert J. Flucytosine: a review of its pharmacology, clinical indications, pharmacokinetics, toxicity and drug interactions. J Antimicrob Chemother 2000;46(2):171–9.
59. Cutler RE, Blair AD, Kelly MR. Flucytosine kinetics in subjects with normal and impaired renal function. Clin Pharmacol Ther 1978;24(3):333–42.
60. Kauffman CA, Frame PT. Bone marrow toxicity associated with 5-fluorocytosine therapy. Antimicrob Agents Chemother 1977;11(2):244–7.
61. Moudgal VV, Sobel JD. Antifungal drugs in pregnancy: a review. Expert Opin Drug Saf 2003;2(5):475–83.
62. Saag MS, Dismukes WE. Azole antifungal agents: emphasis on new triazoles. Antimicrob Agents Chemother 1988;32(1):1–8.
63. Como JA, Dismukes WE. Oral azole drugs as systemic antifungal therapy. N Engl J Med 1994;330(4):263–72.
64. Vanden Bossche H. Biochemical targets for antifungal azole derivatives: hypothesis on the mode of action. Curr Top Med Mycol 1985;1:313–51.
65. Munayyer HK, Mann PA, Chau AS, et al. Posaconazole is a potent inhibitor of sterol 14alpha-demethylation in yeasts and molds. Antimicrob Agents Chemother 2004;48(10):3690–6.
66. Heimark L, Shipkova P, Greene J, et al. Mechanism of azole antifungal activity as determined by liquid chromatographic/mass spectrometric monitoring of ergosterol biosynthesis. J Mass Spectrom 2002;37(3):265–9.
67. Sanati H, Belanger P, Fratti R, et al. A new triazole, voriconazole (UK-109,496), blocks sterol biosynthesis in *Candida albicans* and *Candida krusei*. Antimicrob Agents Chemother 1997;41(11):2492–6.
68. Hitchcock CA, Dickinson K, Brown SB, et al. Interaction of azole antifungal antibiotics with cytochrome P-450-dependent 14 alpha-sterol demethylase purified from *Candida albicans*. Biochem J 1990;266(2):475–80.
69. Pfaller MA, Messer SA, Boyken L, et al. In vitro activities of voriconazole, posaconazole, and fluconazole against 4,169 clinical isolates of *Candida* spp. and *Cryptococcus neoformans* collected during 2001 and 2002 in the ARTEMIS global antifungal surveillance program. Diagn Microbiol Infect Dis 2004;48(3):201–5.
70. Pfaller MA, Messer SA, Hollis RJ, et al. In vitro activities of posaconazole (Sch 56592) compared with those of itraconazole and fluconazole against 3,685 clinical isolates of *Candida* spp. and *Cryptococcus neoformans*. Antimicrob Agents Chemother 2001;45(10):2862–4.
71. Gonzalez GM, Fothergill AW, Sutton DA, et al. In vitro activities of new and established triazoles against opportunistic filamentous and dimorphic fungi. Med Mycol 2005;43(3):281–4.
72. Gonzalez GM, Sutton DA, Thompson E, et al. In vitro activities of approved and investigational antifungal agents against 44 clinical isolates of basidiomycetous fungi. Antimicrob Agents Chemother 2001;45(2):633–5.
73. Sun QN, Fothergill AW, McCarthy DI, et al. In vitro activities of posaconazole, itraconazole, voriconazole, amphotericin B, and fluconazole against 37 clinical isolates of zygomycetes. Antimicrob Agents Chemother 2002;46(5):1581–2.

74. Cuenca-Estrella M, Ruiz-Diez B, Martinez-Suarez JV, et al. Comparative in-vitro activity of voriconazole (UK-109,496) and six other antifungal agents against clinical isolates of *Scedosporium prolificans* and *Scedosporium apiospermum*. J Antimicrob Chemother 1999;43(1):149–51.

75. Pfaller MA, Diekema DJ, Messer SA, et al. In vitro activities of caspofungin compared with those of fluconazole and itraconazole against 3,959 clinical isolates of *Candida* spp., including 157 fluconazole-resistant isolates. Antimicrob Agents Chemother 2003;47(3):1068–71.

76. Pfaller MA, Messer SA, Hollis RJ, et al. In vitro activities of ravuconazole and voriconazole compared with those of four approved systemic antifungal agents against 6,970 clinical isolates of *Candida* spp. Antimicrob Agents Chemother 2002;46(6):1723–7.

77. Alvarado-Ramirez E, Torres-Rodriguez JM. In vitro susceptibility of *Sporothrix schenckii* to six antifungal agents determined using three different methods. Antimicrob Agents Chemother 2007;51(7):2420–3.

78. Pfaller MA, Messer SA, Hollis RJ, et al. In vitro susceptibilities of *Candida* bloodstream isolates to the new triazole antifungal agents BMS-207147, Sch 56592, and voriconazole. Antimicrob Agents Chemother 1998;42(12):3242–4.

79. Pfaller MA, Diekema DJ, Gibbs DL, et al. Results from the ARTEMIS DISK Global Antifungal Surveillance study, 1997 to 2005: an 8.5-year analysis of susceptibilities of *Candida* species and other yeast species to fluconazole and voriconazole determined by CLSI standardized disk diffusion testing. J Clin Microbiol 2007;45(6):1735–45.

80. Pfaller MA, Messer SA, Boyken L, et al. Use of fluconazole as a surrogate marker to predict susceptibility and resistance to voriconazole among 13,338 clinical isolates of *Candida* spp. Tested by clinical and laboratory standards institute-recommended broth microdilution methods. J Clin Microbiol 2007;45(1):70–5.

81. Pfaller MA, Messer SA, Hollis RJ, et al. Antifungal activities of posaconazole, ravuconazole, and voriconazole compared to those of itraconazole and amphotericin B against 239 clinical isolates of *Aspergillus* spp. and other filamentous fungi: report from sentry antimicrobial surveillance program, 2000. Antimicrob Agents Chemother 2002;46(4):1032–7.

82. Guarascio AJ, Slain D. Review of the new delayed-release oral tablet and intravenous dosage forms of posaconazole. Pharmacotherapy 2015;35(2):208–19.

83. Perfect JR, Cox GM, Dodge RK, et al. In vitro and in vivo efficacies of the azole Sch56592 against *Cryptococcus neoformans*. Antimicrob Agents Chemother 1996;40(8):1910–3.

84. Seifert H, Aurbach U, Stefanik D, et al. In vitro activities of isavuconazole and other antifungal agents against *Candida* bloodstream isolates. Antimicrob Agents Chemother 2007;51(5):1818–21.

85. Pettit NN, Carver PL. Isavuconazole: a new option for the management of invasive fungal infections. Ann Pharmacother 2015;49(7):825–42.

86. Perkhofer S, Lechner V, Lass-Florl C, European Committee on Antimicrobial Susceptibility Test. In vitro activity of isavuconazole against *Aspergillus* species and zygomycetes according to the methodology of the European Committee on Antimicrobial Susceptibility Testing. Antimicrob Agents Chemother 2009;53(4):1645–7.

87. Warn PA, Sharp A, Denning DW. In vitro activity of a new triazole BAL4815, the active component of BAL8557 (the water-soluble prodrug), against *Aspergillus* spp. J Antimicrob Chemother 2006;57(1):135–8.

88. Illnait-Zaragozi MT, Martinez GF, Curfs-Breuker I, et al. In vitro activity of the new azole isavuconazole (BAL4815) compared with six other antifungal agents against 162 *Cryptococcus neoformans* isolates from Cuba. Antimicrob Agents Chemother 2008;52(4):1580–2.

89. Gonzalez GM. In vitro activities of isavuconazole against opportunistic filamentous and dimorphic fungi. Med Mycol 2009;47(1):71–6.

90. Lackner M, de Hoog GS, Verweij PE, et al. Species-specific antifungal susceptibility patterns of *Scedosporium* and *Pseudallescheria* species. Antimicrob Agents Chemother 2012;56(5):2635–42.

91. Pfaller MA, Messer SA, Boyken L, et al. Caspofungin activity against clinical isolates of fluconazole-resistant *Candida*. J Clin Microbiol 2003;41(12):5729–31.

92. Pfaller MA, Messer SA, Hollis RJ, et al. Variation in susceptibility of bloodstream isolates of *Candida glabrata* to fluconazole according to patient age and geographic location in the united states in 2001 to 2007. J Clin Microbiol 2009;47(10):3185–90.

93. Perlin DS, Shor E, Zhao Y. Update on antifungal drug resistance. Curr Clin Microbiol Rep 2015;2(2):84–95.

94. van der Linden JW, Arendrup MC, Warris A, et al. Prospective multicenter international surveillance of azole resistance in *Aspergillus fumigatus*. Emerg Infect Dis 2015;21(6):1041–4.

95. Thorpe JE, Baker N, Bromet-Petit M. Effect of oral antacid administration on the pharmacokinetics of oral fluconazole. Antimicrob Agents Chemother 1990;34(10):2032–3.

96. Lazar JD, Wilner KD. Drug interactions with fluconazole. Rev Infect Dis 1990;12(Suppl 3):S327–33.

97. Mian UK, Mayers M, Garg Y, et al. Comparison of fluconazole pharmacokinetics in serum, aqueous humor, vitreous humor, and cerebrospinal fluid following a single dose and at steady state. J Ocul Pharmacol Ther 1998;14(5):459–71.

98. Foulds G, Wajszczuk C, Weidler DJ, et al. Steady state parenteral kinetics of fluconazole in man. Ann N Y Acad Sci 1988;544:427–30.

99. Shiba K, Saito A, Miyahara T. Safety and pharmacokinetics of single oral and intravenous doses of fluconazole in healthy subjects. Clin Ther 1990;12(3):206–15.

100. Cousin L, Berre ML, Launay-Vacher V, et al. Dosing guidelines for fluconazole in patients with renal failure. Nephrol Dial Transplant 2003;18(11):2227–31.

101. Valtonen M, Tiula E, Neuvonen PJ. Effect of continuous venovenous haemofiltration and haemodiafiltration on the elimination of fluconazole in patients with acute renal failure. J Antimicrob Chemother 1997;40(5):695–700.

102. Grant SM, Clissold SP. Fluconazole. A review of its pharmacodynamic and pharmacokinetic properties, and therapeutic potential in superficial and systemic mycoses. Drugs 1990;39(6):877–916.

103. Lange D, Pavao JH, Wu J, et al. Effect of a cola beverage on the bioavailability of itraconazole in the presence of H2 blockers. J Clin Pharmacol 1997;37(6):535–40.

104. Van Peer A, Woestenborghs R, Heykants J, et al. The effects of food and dose on the oral systemic availability of itraconazole in healthy subjects. Eur J Clin Pharmacol 1989;36(4):423–6.

105. Hostetler JS, Hanson LH, Stevens DA. Effect of cyclodextrin on the pharmacology of antifungal oral azoles. Antimicrob Agents Chemother 1992;36(2):477–80.

106. Berenguer J, Ali NM, Allende MC, et al. Itraconazole for experimental pulmonary aspergillosis: comparison with amphotericin B, interaction with cyclosporin A,

and correlation between therapeutic response and itraconazole concentrations in plasma. Antimicrob Agents Chemother 1994;38(6):1303–8.

107. Denning DW, Tucker RM, Hanson LH, et al. Treatment of invasive aspergillosis with itraconazole. Am J Med 1989;86(6 Pt 2):791–800.

108. Denning DW, Tucker RM, Hanson LH, et al. Itraconazole therapy for cryptococcal meningitis and cryptococcosis. Arch Intern Med 1989;149(10): 2301–8.

109. Tucker RM, Denning DW, Arathoon EG, et al. Itraconazole therapy for nonmeningeal coccidioidomycosis: clinical and laboratory observations. J Am Acad Dermatol 1990;23(3 Pt 2):593–601.

110. Hostetler JS, Heykants J, Clemons KV, et al. Discrepancies in bioassay and chromatography determinations explained by metabolism of itraconazole to hydroxyitraconazole: studies of interpatient variations in concentrations. Antimicrob Agents Chemother 1993;37(10):2224–7.

111. Rex JH, Pfaller MA, Galgiani JN, et al. Development of interpretive breakpoints for antifungal susceptibility testing: conceptual framework and analysis of in vitro-in vivo correlation data for fluconazole, itraconazole, and Candida infections. Subcommittee on Antifungal Susceptibility Testing of the National Committee for Clinical Laboratory Standards. Clin Infect Dis 1997;24(2):235–47.

112. Willems L, van der Geest R, de Beule K. Itraconazole oral solution and intravenous formulations: a review of pharmacokinetics and pharmacodynamics. J Clin Pharm Ther 2001;26(3):159–69.

113. Savani DV, Perfect JR, Cobo LM, et al. Penetration of new azole compounds into the eye and efficacy in experimental Candida endophthalmitis. Antimicrob Agents Chemother 1987;31(1):6–10.

114. Haria M, Bryson HM, Goa KL. Itraconazole. A reappraisal of its pharmacological properties and therapeutic use in the management of superficial fungal infections. Drugs 1996;51(4):585–620.

115. De Doncker P, Decroix J, Pierard GE, et al. Antifungal pulse therapy for onychomycosis. A pharmacokinetic and pharmacodynamic investigation of monthly cycles of 1-week pulse therapy with itraconazole. Arch Dermatol 1996;132(1): 34–41.

116. Heykants J, Van Peer A, Van de Velde V, et al. The clinical pharmacokinetics of itraconazole: an overview. Mycoses 1989;32(Suppl 1):67–87.

117. Hardin TC, Graybill JR, Fetchick R, et al. Pharmacokinetics of itraconazole following oral administration to normal volunteers. Antimicrob Agents Chemother 1988;32(9):1310–3.

118. Stevens DA. Itraconazole in cyclodextrin solution. Pharmacotherapy 1999;19(5): 603–11.

119. Boelaert J, Schurgers M, Matthys E, et al. Itraconazole pharmacokinetics in patients with renal dysfunction. Antimicrob Agents Chemother 1988;32(10): 1595–7.

120. Grant SM, Clissold SP. Itraconazole. A review of its pharmacodynamic and pharmacokinetic properties, and therapeutic use in superficial and systemic mycoses. Drugs 1989;37(3):310–44.

121. Purkins L, Wood N, Kleinermans D, et al. Effect of food on the pharmacokinetics of multiple-dose oral voriconazole. Br J Clin Pharmacol 2003;56(Suppl 1):17–23.

122. Theuretzbacher U, Ihle F, Derendorf H. Pharmacokinetic/pharmacodynamic profile of voriconazole. Clin Pharmacokinet 2006;45(7):649–63.

123. Desta Z, Zhao X, Shin JG, et al. Clinical significance of the cytochrome P450 2C19 genetic polymorphism. Clin Pharmacokinet 2002;41(12):913–58.

124. Smith J, Safdar N, Knasinski V, et al. Voriconazole therapeutic drug monitoring. Antimicrob Agents Chemother 2006;50(4):1570–2.
125. Walsh TJ, Karlsson MO, Driscoll T, et al. Pharmacokinetics and safety of intravenous voriconazole in children after single- or multiple-dose administration. Antimicrob Agents Chemother 2004;48(6):2166–72.
126. Trifilio S, Ortiz R, Pennick G, et al. Voriconazole therapeutic drug monitoring in allogeneic hematopoietic stem cell transplant recipients. Bone Marrow Transplant 2005;35(5):509–13.
127. Boyd AE, Modi S, Howard SJ, et al. Adverse reactions to voriconazole. Clin Infect Dis 2004;39(8):1241–4.
128. Andes D, Pascual A, Marchetti O. Antifungal therapeutic drug monitoring: established and emerging indications. Antimicrob Agents Chemother 2009; 53(1):24–34.
129. Smith J, Andes D. Therapeutic drug monitoring of antifungals: pharmacokinetic and pharmacodynamic considerations. Ther Drug Monit 2008;30(2):167–72.
130. Lutsar I, Roffey S, Troke P. Voriconazole concentrations in the cerebrospinal fluid and brain tissue of guinea pigs and immunocompromised patients. Clin Infect Dis 2003;37(5):728–32.
131. Thiel MA, Zinkernagel AS, Burhenne J, et al. Voriconazole concentration in human aqueous humor and plasma during topical or combined topical and systemic administration for fungal keratitis. Antimicrob Agents Chemother 2007; 51(1):239–44.
132. Hariprasad SM, Mieler WF, Holz ER, et al. Determination of vitreous, aqueous, and plasma concentration of orally administered voriconazole in humans. Arch Ophthalmol 2004;122(1):42–7.
133. Alffenaar JW, de Vos T, Uges DR, et al. High voriconazole trough levels in relation to hepatic function: how to adjust the dosage? Br J Clin Pharmacol 2009; 67(2):262–3.
134. Purkins L, Wood N, Greenhalgh K, et al. The pharmacokinetics and safety of intravenous voriconazole - a novel wide-spectrum antifungal agent. Br J Clin Pharmacol 2003;56(Suppl 1):2–9.
135. Courtney R, Wexler D, Radwanski E, et al. Effect of food on the relative bioavailability of two oral formulations of posaconazole in healthy adults. Br J Clin Pharmacol 2004;57(2):218–22.
136. Krishna G, Moton A, Ma L, et al. Pharmacokinetics and absorption of posaconazole oral suspension under various gastric conditions in healthy volunteers. Antimicrob Agents Chemother 2009;53(3):958–66.
137. Courtney R, Radwanski E, Lim J, et al. Pharmacokinetics of posaconazole coadministered with antacid in fasting or nonfasting healthy men. Antimicrob Agents Chemother 2004;48(3):804–8.
138. Alffenaar JW, van Assen S, van der Werf TS, et al. Omeprazole significantly reduces posaconazole serum trough level. Clin Infect Dis 2009;48(6):839.
139. Courtney R, Pai S, Laughlin M, et al. Pharmacokinetics, safety, and tolerability of oral posaconazole administered in single and multiple doses in healthy adults. Antimicrob Agents Chemother 2003;47(9):2788–95.
140. Walsh TJ, Raad I, Patterson TF, et al. Treatment of invasive aspergillosis with posaconazole in patients who are refractory to or intolerant of conventional therapy: an externally controlled trial. Clin Infect Dis 2007;44(1):2–12.
141. Lebeaux D, Lanternier F, Elie C, et al. Therapeutic drug monitoring of posaconazole: a monocentric study with 54 adults. Antimicrob Agents Chemother 2009; 53(12):5224–9.

142. Dolton MJ, Ray JE, Chen SC, et al. Multicenter study of posaconazole therapeutic drug monitoring: exposure-response relationship and factors affecting concentration. Antimicrob Agents Chemother 2012;56(11):5503–10.
143. Ananda-Rajah MR, Grigg A, Slavin MA. Making sense of posaconazole therapeutic drug monitoring: a practical approach. Curr Opin Infect Dis 2012; 25(6):605–11.
144. Ullmann AJ, Lipton JH, Vesole DH, et al. Posaconazole or fluconazole for prophylaxis in severe graft-versus-host disease. N Engl J Med 2007;356(4):335–47.
145. Pitisuttithum P, Negroni R, Graybill JR, et al. Activity of posaconazole in the treatment of central nervous system fungal infections. J Antimicrob Chemother 2005; 56(4):745–55.
146. Riddell JT, Comer GM, Kauffman CA. Treatment of endogenous fungal endophthalmitis: focus on new antifungal agents. Clin Infect Dis 2011;52(5):648–53.
147. Sponsel WE, Graybill JR, Nevarez HL, et al. Ocular and systemic posaconazole(SCH-56592) treatment of invasive *Fusarium solani keratitis* and endophthalmitis. Br J Ophthalmol 2002;86(7):829–30.
148. Krieter P, Flannery B, Musick T, et al. Disposition of posaconazole following single-dose oral administration in healthy subjects. Antimicrob Agents Chemother 2004;48(9):3543–51.
149. Courtney R, Sansone A, Smith W, et al. Posaconazole pharmacokinetics, safety, and tolerability in subjects with varying degrees of chronic renal disease. J Clin Pharmacol 2005;45(2):185–92.
150. Schmitt-Hoffmann A, Roos B, Heep M, et al. Single-ascending-dose pharmacokinetics and safety of the novel broad-spectrum antifungal triazole BAL4815 after intravenous infusions (50, 100, and 200 milligrams) and oral administrations (100, 200, and 400 milligrams) of its prodrug, BAL8557, in healthy volunteers. Antimicrob Agents Chemother 2006;50(1):279–85.
151. Schmitt-Hoffmann A, Roos B, Spickermann J, et al. Effect of mild and moderate liver disease on the pharmacokinetics of isavuconazole after intravenous and oral administration of a single dose of the prodrug BAL8557. Antimicrob Agents Chemother 2009;53(11):4885–90.
152. Anaissie EJ, Darouiche RO, Abi-Said D, et al. Management of invasive candidal infections: results of a prospective, randomized, multicenter study of fluconazole versus amphotericin B and review of the literature. Clin Infect Dis 1996; 23(5):964–72.
153. Rex JH, Bennett JE, Sugar AM, et al. A randomized trial comparing fluconazole with amphotericin B for the treatment of candidemia in patients without neutropenia. Candidemia Study Group and the National Institute. N Engl J Med 1994; 331(20):1325–30.
154. Kullberg BJ, Sobel JD, Ruhnke M, et al. Voriconazole versus a regimen of amphotericin B followed by fluconazole for candidaemia in non-neutropenic patients: a randomised non-inferiority trial. Lancet 2005;366(9495):1435–42.
155. Reboli AC, Rotstein C, Pappas PG, et al. Anidulafungin versus fluconazole for invasive candidiasis. N Engl J Med 2007;356(24):2472–82.
156. Andes DR, Safdar N, Baddley JW, et al. Impact of treatment strategy on outcomes in patients with candidemia and other forms of invasive candidiasis: a patient-level quantitative review of randomized trials. Clin Infect Dis 2012; 54(8):1110–22.
157. Wilcox CM, Darouiche RO, Laine L, et al. A randomized, double-blind comparison of itraconazole oral solution and fluconazole tablets in the treatment of esophageal candidiasis. J Infect Dis 1997;176(1):227–32.

158. Graybill JR, Vazquez J, Darouiche RO, et al. Randomized trial of itraconazole oral solution for oropharyngeal candidiasis in HIV/AIDS patients. Am J Med 1998;104(1):33–9.
159. Phillips P, De Beule K, Frechette G, et al. A double-blind comparison of itraconazole oral solution and fluconazole capsules for the treatment of oropharyngeal candidiasis in patients with AIDS. Clin Infect Dis 1998;26(6): 1368–73.
160. Ally R, Schurmann D, Kreisel W, et al. A randomized, double-blind, double-dummy, multicenter trial of voriconazole and fluconazole in the treatment of esophageal candidiasis in immunocompromised patients. Clin Infect Dis 2001;33(9):1447–54.
161. Villanueva A, Gotuzzo E, Arathoon EG, et al. A randomized double-blind study of caspofungin versus fluconazole for the treatment of esophageal candidiasis. Am J Med 2002;113(4):294–9.
162. de Wet NT, Bester AJ, Viljoen JJ, et al. A randomized, double blind, comparative trial of micafungin (FK463) vs. fluconazole for the treatment of oesophageal candidiasis. Aliment Pharmacol Ther 2005;21(7):899–907.
163. Krause DS, Simjee AE, van Rensburg C, et al. A randomized, double-blind trial of anidulafungin versus fluconazole for the treatment of esophageal candidiasis. Clin Infect Dis 2004;39(6):770–5.
164. Vazquez JA, Skiest DJ, Nieto L, et al. A multicenter randomized trial evaluating posaconazole versus fluconazole for the treatment of oropharyngeal candidiasis in subjects with HIV/AIDS. Clin Infect Dis 2006;42(8):1179–86.
165. de Wet N, Llanos-Cuentas A, Suleiman J, et al. A randomized, double-blind, parallel-group, dose-response study of micafungin compared with fluconazole for the treatment of esophageal candidiasis in HIV-positive patients. Clin Infect Dis 2004;39(6):842–9.
166. Sobel JD, Brooker D, Stein GE, et al. Single oral dose fluconazole compared with conventional clotrimazole topical therapy of *Candida* vaginitis. Fluconazole Vaginitis Study Group. Am J Obstet Gynecol 1995;172(4 Pt 1):1263–8.
167. van Heusden AM, Merkus HM, Euser R, et al. A randomized, comparative study of a single oral dose of fluconazole versus a single topical dose of clotrimazole in the treatment of vaginal candidosis among general practitioners and gynaecologists. Eur J Obstet Gynecol Reprod Biol 1994;55(2):123–7.
168. Osser S, Haglund A, Westrom L. Treatment of Candidal vaginitis. A prospective randomized investigator-blind multicenter study comparing topically applied econazole with oral fluconazole. Acta Obstet Gynecol Scand 1991; 70(1):73–8.
169. Sobel JD, Wiesenfeld HC, Martens M, et al. Maintenance fluconazole therapy for recurrent vulvovaginal candidiasis. N Engl J Med 2004;351(9):876–83.
170. Saag MS, Powderly WG, Cloud GA, et al. Comparison of amphotericin B with fluconazole in the treatment of acute AIDS-associated cryptococcal meningitis. The NIAID Mycoses Study Group and the AIDS Clinical Trials Group. N Engl J Med 1992;326(2):83–9.
171. Powderly WG, Saag MS, Cloud GA, et al. A controlled trial of fluconazole or amphotericin B to prevent relapse of cryptococcal meningitis in patients with the acquired immunodeficiency syndrome. The NIAID AIDS Clinical Trials Group and Mycoses Study Group. N Engl J Med 1992;326(12):793–8.
172. Slavin MA, Osborne B, Adams R, et al. Efficacy and safety of fluconazole prophylaxis for fungal infections after marrow transplantation–a prospective, randomized, double-blind study. J Infect Dis 1995;171(6):1545–52.

173. Bodey GP, Anaissie EJ, Elting LS, et al. Antifungal prophylaxis during remission induction therapy for acute leukemia fluconazole versus intravenous amphotericin B. Cancer 1994;73(8):2099–106.
174. Vardakas KZ, Michalopoulos A, Falagas ME. Fluconazole versus itraconazole for antifungal prophylaxis in neutropenic patients with haematological malignancies: a meta-analysis of randomised-controlled trials. Br J Haematol 2005; 131(1):22–8.
175. Cornely OA, Maertens J, Winston DJ, et al. Posaconazole vs. fluconazole or itraconazole prophylaxis in patients with neutropenia. N Engl J Med 2007;356(4): 348–59.
176. Dismukes WE, Bradsher RW Jr, Cloud GC, et al. Itraconazole therapy for blastomycosis and histoplasmosis. NIAID Mycoses Study Group. Am J Med 1992; 93(5):489–97.
177. Graybill JR, Stevens DA, Galgiani JN, et al. Itraconazole treatment of coccidioidomycosis. NAIAD Mycoses Study Group. Am J Med 1990;89(3):282–90.
178. Restrepo A. Treatment of tropical mycoses. J Am Acad Dermatol 1994;31(3 Pt 2):S91–102.
179. Restrepo A, Robledo J, Gomez I, et al. Itraconazole therapy in lymphangitic and cutaneous sporotrichosis. Arch Dermatol 1986;122(4):413–7.
180. Smith DE, Midgley J, Allan M, et al. Itraconazole versus ketaconazole in the treatment of oral and oesophageal candidosis in patients infected with HIV. AIDS 1991;5(11):1367–71.
181. Pitsouni E, Iavazzo C, Falagas ME. Itraconazole vs fluconazole for the treatment of uncomplicated acute vaginal and vulvovaginal candidiasis in nonpregnant women: a metaanalysis of randomized controlled trials. Am J Obstet Gynecol 2008;198(2):153–60.
182. Nucci M, Biasoli I, Akiti T, et al. A double-blind, randomized, placebo-controlled trial of itraconazole capsules as antifungal prophylaxis for neutropenic patients. Clin Infect Dis 2000;30(2):300–5.
183. Menichetti F, Del Favero A, Martino P, et al. Itraconazole oral solution as prophylaxis for fungal infections in neutropenic patients with hematologic malignancies: a randomized, placebo-controlled, double-blind, multicenter trial. GIMEMA Infection Program. Gruppo Italiano Malattie Ematologiche dell' Adulto. Clin Infect Dis 1999;28(2):250–5.
184. Glasmacher A, Molitor E, Hahn C, et al. Antifungal prophylaxis with itraconazole in neutropenic patients with acute leukemia. Leukemia 1998;12(9): 1338–43.
185. Stevens DA, Lee JY. Analysis of compassionate use itraconazole therapy for invasive aspergillosis by the NIAID Mycoses Study Group criteria. Arch Intern Med 1997;157(16):1857–62.
186. Stevens DA, Schwartz HJ, Lee JY, et al. A randomized trial of itraconazole in allergic bronchopulmonary aspergillosis. N Engl J Med 2000;342(11): 756–62.
187. De Beule K, De Doncker P, Cauwenbergh G, et al. The treatment of aspergillosis and aspergilloma with itraconazole, clinical results of an open international study (1982-1987). Mycoses 1988;31(9):476–85.
188. Perfect JR, Marr KA, Walsh TJ, et al. Voriconazole treatment for less-common, emerging, or refractory fungal infections. Clin Infect Dis 2003;36(9):1122–31.
189. Troke P, Aguirrebengoa K, Arteaga C, et al. Treatment of scedosporiosis with voriconazole: clinical experience with 107 patients. Antimicrob Agents Chemother 2008;52(5):1743–50.

190. Skiest DJ, Vazquez JA, Anstead GM, et al. Posaconazole for the treatment of azole-refractory oropharyngeal and esophageal candidiasis in subjects with HIV infection. Clin Infect Dis 2007;44(4):607–14.
191. Vazquez JA, Skiest DJ, Tissot-Dupont H, et al. Safety and efficacy of posaconazole in the long-term treatment of azole-refractory oropharyngeal and esophageal candidiasis in patients with HIV infection. HIV Clin Trials 2007; 8(2):86–97.
192. Ullmann AJ, Cornely OA, Burchardt A, et al. Pharmacokinetics, safety, and efficacy of posaconazole in patients with persistent febrile neutropenia or refractory invasive fungal infection. Antimicrob Agents Chemother 2006;50(2):658–66.
193. Gubbins PO, Krishna G, Sansone-Parsons A, et al. Pharmacokinetics and safety of oral posaconazole in neutropenic stem cell transplant recipients. Antimicrob Agents Chemother 2006;50(6):1993–9.
194. Lipp HP. Antifungal agents–clinical pharmacokinetics and drug interactions. Mycoses 2008;51(Suppl 1):7–18.
195. Brüggemann RJM, Alffenaar JC, Blijlevens NMA, et al. Pharmacokinetic drug interactions of azoles. Curr Fungal Infect Rep 2008;2(1):20–7.
196. Bruggemann RJ, Alffenaar JW, Blijlevens NM, et al. Clinical relevance of the pharmacokinetic interactions of azole antifungal drugs with other coadministered agents. Clin Infect Dis 2009;48(10):1441–58.
197. Douglas CM, D'Ippolito JA, Shei GJ, et al. Identification of the *fks1* gene of *Candida albicans* as the essential target of 1,3-beta-d-glucan synthase inhibitors. Antimicrob Agents Chemother 1997;41(11):2471–9.
198. Bowman JC, Hicks PS, Kurtz MB, et al. The antifungal echinocandin caspofungin acetate kills growing cells of *Aspergillus fumigatus* in vitro. Antimicrob Agents Chemother 2002;46(9):3001–12.
199. Chandrasekar PH, Sobel JD. Micafungin: a new echinocandin. Clin Infect Dis 2006;42(8):1171–8.
200. Vazquez JA, Sobel JD. Anidulafungin: a novel echinocandin. Clin Infect Dis 2006;43(2):215–22.
201. Barchiesi F, Spreghini E, Tomassetti S, et al. Effects of caspofungin against *Candida guilliermondii* and *Candida parapsilosis*. Antimicrob Agents Chemother 2006;50(8):2719–27.
202. Espinel-Ingroff A. Comparison of in vitro activities of the new triazole Sch56592 and the echinocandins mk-0991 (I-743,872) and ly303366 against opportunistic filamentous and dimorphic fungi and yeasts. J Clin Microbiol 1998;36(10): 2950–6.
203. Nakai T, Uno J, Otomo K, et al. In vitro activity of FK463, a novel lipopeptide antifungal agent, against a variety of clinically important molds. Chemotherapy 2002;48(2):78–81.
204. Messer SA, Kirby JT, Sader HS, et al. Initial results from a longitudinal international surveillance programme for anidulafungin (2003). J Antimicrob Chemother 2004;54(6):1051–6.
205. Kirkpatrick WR, Perea S, Coco BJ, et al. Efficacy of caspofungin alone and in combination with voriconazole in a guinea pig model of invasive aspergillosis. Antimicrob Agents Chemother 2002;46(8):2564–8.
206. Marr KA, Boeckh M, Carter RA, et al. Combination antifungal therapy for invasive aspergillosis. Clin Infect Dis 2004;39(6):797–802.
207. Pfaller MA, Castanheira M, Lockhart SR, et al. Frequency of decreased susceptibility and resistance to echinocandins among fluconazole-resistant bloodstream isolates of *Candida glabrata*. J Clin Microbiol 2012;50(4):1199–203.

208. Hebert MF, Smith HE, Marbury TC, et al. Pharmacokinetics of micafungin in healthy volunteers, volunteers with moderate liver disease, and volunteers with renal dysfunction. J Clin Pharmacol 2005;45(10):1145–52.
209. Eschenauer G, Depestel DD, Carver PL. Comparison of echinocandin antifungals. Ther Clin Risk Manag 2007;3(1):71–97.
210. Kauffman CA, Carver PL. Update on echinocandin antifungals. Semin Respir Crit Care Med 2008;29(2):211–9.
211. Andes D, Diekema DJ, Pfaller MA, et al. In vivo pharmacodynamic characterization of anidulafungin in a neutropenic murine candidiasis model. Antimicrob Agents Chemother 2008;52(2):539–50.
212. Andes D, Marchillo K, Lowther J, et al. In vivo pharmacodynamics of HMR 3270, a glucan synthase inhibitor, in a murine candidiasis model. Antimicrob Agents Chemother 2003;47(4):1187–92.
213. Andes DR, Diekema DJ, Pfaller MA, et al. In vivo pharmacodynamic target investigation for micafungin against Candida albicans and C. Glabrata in a neutropenic murine candidiasis model. Antimicrob Agents Chemother 2008;52(10): 3497–503.
214. Wiederhold NP, Kontoyiannis DP, Chi J, et al. Pharmacodynamics of caspofungin in a murine model of invasive pulmonary aspergillosis: evidence of concentration-dependent activity. J Infect Dis 2004;190(8):1464–71.
215. Wagner C, Graninger W, Presterl E, et al. The echinocandins: comparison of their pharmacokinetics, pharmacodynamics and clinical applications. Pharmacology 2006;78(4):161–77.
216. Kuse ER, Chetchotisakd P, da Cunha CA, et al. Micafungin versus liposomal amphotericin B for Candidaemia and invasive candidosis: a phase III randomised double-blind trial. Lancet 2007;369(9572):1519–27.
217. Ostrosky-Zeichner L, Kontoyiannis D, Raffalli J, et al. International, open-label, noncomparative, clinical trial of micafungin alone and in combination for treatment of newly diagnosed and refractory candidemia. Eur J Clin Microbiol Infect Dis 2005;24(10):654–61.
218. Mora-Duarte J, Betts R, Rotstein C, et al. Comparison of caspofungin and amphotericin B for invasive candidiasis. N Engl J Med 2002;347(25):2020–9.
219. Villanueva A, Arathoon EG, Gotuzzo E, et al. A randomized double-blind study of caspofungin versus amphotericin for the treatment of Candidal esophagitis. Clin Infect Dis 2001;33(9):1529–35.
220. Arathoon EG, Gotuzzo E, Noriega LM, et al. Randomized, double-blind, multicenter study of caspofungin versus amphotericin B for treatment of oropharyngeal and esophageal candidiases. Antimicrob Agents Chemother 2002;46(2):451–7.
221. Kartsonis N, DiNubile MJ, Bartizal K, et al. Efficacy of caspofungin in the treatment of esophageal candidiasis resistant to fluconazole. J Acquir Immune Defic Syndr 2002;31(2):183–7.
222. van Burik JA, Ratanatharathorn V, Stepan DE, et al. Micafungin versus fluconazole for prophylaxis against invasive fungal infections during neutropenia in patients undergoing hematopoietic stem cell transplantation. Clin Infect Dis 2004; 39(10):1407–16.
223. Walsh TJ, Teppler H, Donowitz GR, et al. Caspofungin versus liposomal amphotericin B for empirical antifungal therapy in patients with persistent fever and neutropenia. N Engl J Med 2004;351(14):1391–402.
224. Maertens J, Raad I, Petrikkos G, et al. Efficacy and safety of caspofungin for treatment of invasive aspergillosis in patients refractory to or intolerant of conventional antifungal therapy. Clin Infect Dis 2004;39(11):1563–71.

225. Maertens J, Glasmacher A, Herbrecht R, et al. Multicenter, noncomparative study of caspofungin in combination with other antifungals as salvage therapy in adults with invasive aspergillosis. Cancer 2006;107(12):2888–97.
226. Aliff TB, Maslak PG, Jurcic JG, et al. Refractory *Aspergillus* pneumonia in patients with acute leukemia: successful therapy with combination caspofungin and liposomal amphotericin. Cancer 2003;97(4):1025–32.
227. Kontoyiannis DP, Hachem R, Lewis RE, et al. Efficacy and toxicity of caspofungin in combination with liposomal amphotericin B as primary or salvage treatment of invasive aspergillosis in patients with hematologic malignancies. Cancer 2003;98(2):292–9.
228. Marr KA, Schlamm HT, Herbrecht R, et al. Combination antifungal therapy for invasive aspergillosis: a randomized trial. Ann Intern Med 2015;162(2):81–9.
229. Sandhu P, Lee W, Xu X, et al. Hepatic uptake of the novel antifungal agent caspofungin. Drug Metab Dispos 2005;33(5):676–82.

Basic Genetics and Immunology of Candida Infections

Xiaowen Wang, MD[a,b], Frank L. van de Veerdonk, MD, PhD[a,c],
Mihai G. Netea, MD, PhD[a,c],*

KEYWORDS

- *Candida* • Candidiasis • Genetics • Immunology

KEY POINTS

- Genetic factors play a critical role in the pathogenesis of both mucocutaneous and invasive candida infections.
- Monogenic disorders that impair Th17 deficiency cause chronic mucocutaneous candidiasis.
- Monogenic disorders that are linked to neutrophil deficiencies predispose patients to invasive candidiasis.
- Polymorphisms in genes from the type I interferon pathway increase susceptibility to systemic candidiasis.

INTRODUCTION

Candida species are a genus of yeasts that, under normal circumstances, are nonpathogenic commensal microorganisms in humans. However, they are the predominant opportunistic fungal pathogens, and cause superficial and invasive infection in immunocompromised individuals that is associated with significant morbidity and mortality. Risk factors for candida infections include immunosuppressive therapy, mucosal damage, the presence of indwelling catheters, and prolonged hospitalization.[1] However, mucocutaneous or systemic candidiasis often cannot be explained by just these risk factors, and not all individuals with these risk factors develop candida infections. Therefore, it is thought that genetic factors in addition to these risk factors must play a critical role in the pathogenesis of candida infections.

[a] Department of Internal Medicine, Radboud University Medical Center, Geert Grooteplein Zuid 8, Nijmegen, 6525 GA, The Netherlands; [b] Department of Dermatology, Peking University First Hospital, Xishiku Street 8, Xicheng District, Beijing 10034, China; [c] Radboud Center for Infectious Diseases (RCI), Geert Grooteplein Zuid 8, Nijmegen, 6525 GA, The Netherlands
* Corresponding author. Department of Internal Medicine (463), Radboud University Nijmegen Medical Center, PO Box 9101, Nijmegen 6500 HB, The Netherlands.
E-mail address: mihai.netea@radboudumc.nl

Infect Dis Clin N Am 30 (2016) 85–102
http://dx.doi.org/10.1016/j.idc.2015.10.010
id.theclinics.com

With the development of novel human genetic screening tools, the contribution of genetic factors in the susceptibility to both mucocutaneous and invasive candidiasis has been extensively studied. This work has led to novel insights in the genetic and molecular pathogenesis of candida infections. Among those studies, several genes that impair antifungal immunity have been found to predispose to chronic mucocutaneous candidiasis (CMC) and invasive candidiasis. Meanwhile, common polymorphisms in genes involved in antifungal immunity have also been linked to different types of candida infection, such as recurrent vulvovaginal candidiasis (RVVC) and candidemia. This article summarizes recent findings concerning the genetics and immunology of candida infections, which not only have added to the current understanding of fungal immunology but will also help clinicians to design novel immunotherapeutic approaches.

MONOGENIC INHERITANCE OF CANDIDA INFECTIONS

As its name implies, CMC is characterized by recurrent or persistent infections of the skin, nails, and mucosal membranes with *Candida* species, mainly *Candida albicans*.[2] CMC may present as a distinct clinical entity, in which it is the only or principal manifestation (known as isolated CMC or CMC disease). It may also present as one of the key manifestations of a syndrome in children with primary immunodeficiency (PID) diseases (known as syndromic CMC). CMC can also be observed in addition to increased susceptibility to other infections in patients with acquired or inherited immunodeficiencies.[3] An overview of monogenetic disorders of candida infections is given in **Table 1** and **Fig. 1**.

Isolated Chronic Mucocutaneous Candidiasis

In 2009, autosomal recessive (AR) caspase recruitment domain–containing protein 9 (*CARD9*) deficiencies were discovered to cause isolated CMC.[4] CARD9 is a key adaptor molecule expressed in myeloid cells downstream of the pattern recognition receptors (PRRs) that recognize fungal cell wall components and subsequently activate spleen tyrosine kinase (Syk).[5] After phosphorylation, CARD9 binds B-cell lymphoma 10 (BCL10) and mucosa-associated lymphoid tissue lymphoma translocation gene 1 (MALT1) to form the CBM complex, resulting in nuclear factor kappa B (NF-κB) activation and innate antifungal immunity, thereby triggering the differentiation of naive T cells into T-helper (Th) 17 cells.[6] *CARD9*-deficient patients show reduced tumor necrosis factor (TNF)-α production and circulating interleukin (IL)-17–producing T cells,[4] underscoring the importance of CARD9-dependent pattern recognition signaling in mucocutaneous antifungal host defense.

In 2011, heterozygous gain-of-function (GOF) mutations in signal transducer and activator of transcription 1 (*STAT1*) were shown to result in autosomal dominant (AD) CMC,[7,8] which was confirmed by many other studies as the main hereditary cause of isolated CMC.[3,9–14] STAT1 is the major signaling molecule downstream of interferon (IFN) receptors. Triggered by IFNs, STAT1 translocates to the nucleus and triggers the transcription of IFN-inducible genes, which play a pivotal role in the defense against pathogens.[15] GOF *STAT1* mutations, located in either coiled-coil domain (CCD) or DNA-binding domain (DBD), leads to hyperphosphorylation of STAT1 and accumulation of phosphorylated STAT1 in the nucleus, which may shift the immune response away from a STAT3-mediated induction of Th17 cell generation.[7,8] This shift could be explained by either an increased function of cytokines, such as IL-27 and IFNs that dampen the Th17 response, or less availability of STAT1 molecules to form heterodimers with other STAT molecules, needed to induce optimal Th17 responses.[7] GOF mutation of *STAT1* is also associated with a spectrum of other fungal infections, such as cutaneous fusariosis, disseminated coccidioidomycosis and histoplasmosis, *Penicillium marneffei* infections, and disseminated mucormycosis,[16–19] highlighting the pivotal role of STAT1 in fungal infections. These genetic studies have important clinical implications that contribute to the development of new approaches to treat CMC. Hematopoietic stem cell transplantation (HSCT) has been tried in patients with CMC, but without success.[20] Pilot studies of continuous Granulocyte colony-stimulating factor (G-CSF) therapy and the oral Janus kinase (JAK) family protein tyrosine kinase inhibitor ruxolitinib have been described to successively treat patients with CMC harboring *STAT1* mutations, and these are considered to hold promise as immunotherapies in the future, although treatment with G-CSF has also been reported to fail in 2 patients with *STAT1* GOF mutation.[21–23]

Th17 cells are characterized by their production of IL-17A and IL-17F, which signal through the IL-17RA/RC heterodimer complex, triggering downstream formation of the IL-17R-Act1-TRAF6 complex and leading to NF-κB activation.[24] IL-17A and IL-17F, together with IL-22, promote mucocutaneous antifungal immunity through activating epithelial cells, increasing neutrophils recruitment, and inducing the production of chemokines and antimicrobial peptides.[3] The crucial role of the IL-17 cytokines and IL-17R signaling in antifungal defense is further underscored by the discovery of mutations in these cytokines and their signaling pathway. Partial AD IL-17F deficiency was reported to be the cause of CMC in one family, with mutant IL-17F showing impaired activity.[25] Moreover, complete AR deficiency in IL-17RA, and recently AR deficiency in IL-17RC, were reported in several kindreds of isolated CMC from 2 studies.[25,26] The patients are homozygous for different alleles that abolish the expression of IL-17RA or IL-17RC, which prevents cellular responses of IL-17A and IL-17F signaling.[25,26]

In addition to IL-17 and its receptors, a deficiency in *ACT1*, a key adaptor molecule downstream of IL-17R signaling, has also been reported and the clinical phenotype was characterized by CMC. This missense mutation, located in the SEFIR (SEF/IL17 receptor) domain, impaired the interaction of ACT1 with the IL-17 receptor units, subsequently leading to deficient IL-17 signaling,[27] which again shows the importance of IL-17 in CMC.

Syndromic Chronic Mucocutaneous Candidiasis

Hyper–immunoglobulin (Ig) E syndrome (HIES) is characterized by CMC, increased serum IgE level, eosinophilia, eczema, skeletal abnormalities, and recurrent staphylococcal infections, first described as Job syndrome in 1966.[28] In 2007, loss-of-function mutation in *STAT3* was first discovered to cause AD-HIES.[29,30] Since then, *STAT3* mutations have been identified in more patients with AD-HIES and these mutations now established as the cause of disease in 60% to 70% of patients with HIES.[31] STAT3, another STAT family member, regulates multiple cytokine signaling pathways, including IL-6, IL-21, and IL-23, which are all involved in the development of Th17 cells.[30] In patients with AD-HIES with dominant-negative *STAT3* mutations, peripheral blood cells showed defective IL-6, IL-10, and IL-21 signaling, with impaired induction of RORγt (retinoic acid-related orphan receptor gamma t) messenger RNA, which resulted in greatly diminished Th17 cell differentiation.[29,30,32,33] Impaired Th17 responses are associated with impaired neutrophil chemoattractant factors and epithelial antimicrobial peptides, which in this way increases the susceptibility to candida and staphylococcal infections.[29,30]

Besides the AD trait, HIES was also reported to be AR, with homozygous or compound heterozygous mutations in *DOCK8* (dedicator of cytokinesis 8) as the most

Table 1
Summary of monogenic inheritance of candida infections

Gene	Mode of Inheritance	Disease	Immunologic Phenotype	Refs
Isolated CMC				
STAT1	AD	CMC	Impaired IL-17A and IL-22 production and Th17 differentiation	7,8
CARD9	AR	CMC	Reduced TNF-α production and circulating IL-17 producing T cells	4
IL-17F	AD	CMC	Defective IL-17F bioactivity	25
IL-17RA/C	AR	CMC	Lack of cellular responses to IL-17A and IL-17F	25,26
ACT1	AR	CMC	Impaired IL-17 signaling	27
Syndromic CMC				
STAT3	AD	HIES	Impaired Th17 differentiation and IL-17A and IL-22 production	29,30
DOCK8	AR	HIES	Impaired Th17 differentiation	34
AIRE	AR	APECED	Autoantibodies against IL-17 and IL-22	45
CMC associated PIDs				
TYK2	AR	Increased risk for mycobacterial and viral infections	Reduced Th1 and type I IFN responses	51,53
IL-12RB1	AR	Increased risk for CMC and mycobacterial and salmonella infections	Loss of function of IL-12 and IL-23 receptor, diminished IFN-γ and IL-17	49,50
RORC	AR	Increased risk for candidiasis and mycobacteriosis	Absence of IL-17A/F-producing T cells	54
IL2RA	AR	Candida esophagitis	Reduced number of CD4+ cells	56
MALT1, BCL10, CARD11	AR	Combined immunodeficiencies	Defects of the 3 components of the CBM complex	55

Gene(s)	Inheritance	Disease	Immunological feature	Reference
STAT1	AD	Fatal combined immunodeficiencies	Progressive loss of T- lymphocyte and B-lymphocyte number as well as function	57
NEMO, IKBA, MST1/STK4, CRACM1, and so forth	AR/AD/X linked	Combined immunodeficiencies	T-cell deficiency	58–64
JAK3, RAG1, RAG2, ARTEMIS, and so forth	AR/X linked	Severe combined immunodeficiencies	T-cell deficiency, lymphopenia	65
UNC119, MAGT1, RAG1	AR/AD/X linked	Idiopathic CD4 lymphopenia	Lymphopenia	66–68
Invasive Candida Infections				
CARD9	AR	Candida meningoencephalitis	Reduced Th17 lymphocytes, killing defect of neutrophils	69–71
CYBB, NCF1, NCF2, NCF4, CYBA	X linked/AR	CGD	NADPH oxidase complex deficiency	76
ELA2	AD	Severe congenital neutropenia	Neutropenia	77
HAX1	AR	Severe congenital neutropenia	Neutropenia	78
CD18	AR	Leukocyte adhesion deficiency type 1	Neutrophil adhesion deficiency	79

Abbreviations: AD, autosomal dominant; AIRE, autoimmune regulator; APECED, autoimmune polyendocrinopathy-candidiasis-ectodermal dystrophy; AR, autosomal recessive; BCL10, B-cell lymphoma 10; CARD, caspase recruitment domain-containing protein; CBM, CARD-BCL10-MALT1 complex; CD, cluster of differentiation; CGD, Chronic granulomatous disease; CMC, chronic mucocutaneous candidiasis; DOCK, dedicator of cytokinesis; HIES, Hyper–IgE syndrome; IFN, interferon; IL, interleukin; JAK, Janus kinase; MALT, mucosa-associated lymphoid tissue; NADPH, nicotinamide adenine dinucleotide phosphate; PID, primary immunodeficiency; STAT, signal transducer and activator of transcription; Th, T helper; TNF, tumor necrosis factor; TYK2, tyrosine kinase 2.

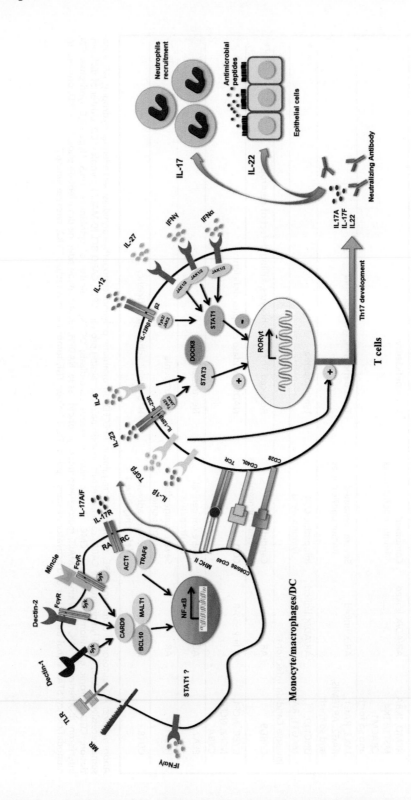

common cause.[34] AR-HIES is a severe entity with a mortality of 48%, characterized as classic AD-HIES, but lack of connective tissue and skeletal disorders, and in addition these patients have a clear increased susceptibility to recurrent viral infections (herpes simplex, varicella zoster, human papilloma and molluscum contagiosum viruses), asthma, severe allergies, and malignancies at a young age.[35–37] DOCK8 is a member of the DOCK180-related family of atypical guanine nucleotide exchange factors, and interacts with Rho GTPases. It has regulatory functions in cell migration, morphology, adhesion, and growth.[38] It is expressed by monocytes, B lymphocytes, and T lymphocytes, and is associated with cytoskeleton formation.[39] DOCK8-deficient patients usually have CD4 and CD8 T-cell lymphopenias, and to a lesser extent decreased natural killer cells and B cells. These patients have mildly to moderately decreased percentages of IL-17–producing cells after activation with anti-CD3 and anti-CD28, although the induction of RORγt expression in naive T cells was intact, suggesting a defect in late differentiation or long-term survival of Th17 cells. These findings could, to some extend, explain an increased susceptibility to CMC.[39] In patients with DOCK8-deficient AR-HIES, several studies suggest HSCT as a curative option that decreases the high mortality associated with this severe immunodeficiency.[40–44]

The syndrome of autoimmune polyendocrinopathy-candidiasis-ectodermal dystrophy (APECED), or autoimmune polyendocrine syndrome 1 (APS-1), is a rare AR syndrome characterized by CMC (which is often the earliest manifestation of the syndrome), multiple autoimmune endocrinopathies, hypoparathyroidism, and adrenal insufficiency. The cause of APECED was found to be mutations in the autoimmune regulator (*AIRE*) gene discovered in 1997.[45] *AIRE* is a transcription factor expressed by medullary thymic epithelial cells, and is responsible for the expression of a wide variety of tissue-specific antigens in the thymus. Nonfunctional *AIRE* in patients leads to impaired central T-cell tolerance, with the generation of autoantibodies. High levels of neutralizing autoantibodies against IL-17A, IL-17F, and/or IL-22 have been

Fig. 1. Crucial pathways involved in the monogenic inheritance of candida infections. After *Candida* is recognized by pathogen recognition receptors in human innate immune cells, the downstream signaling molecule CARD9 (caspase recruitment domain-containing protein 9); forms a complex with BCL-10 (B-cell lymphoma/leukemia 10) and MALT1 (mucosa-associated lymphoid tissue lymphoma translocation protein 1), which drives NF-κB (nuclear factor kappa B) responses. Proinflammatory cytokines, such as interleukin (IL)-1β, IL-6, IL-23, and transforming growth factor beta, are secreted. On binding to receptors on T cells, proinflammatory cytokines signal through STAT3 (signal transducer and activator of transcription 3) and DOCK8 (dedicator of cytokinesis 8), which induces transcription of RORγt (retinoic acid-related orphan receptor gamma t), leading to differentiation of naive T cells toward Th17 (T-helper 17) cells. STAT1 GOF may shift the cellular response from STAT3-mediated Th17 cell activating cytokines toward hyperresponses of Th17 inhibiting cytokines, such as IL-27, interferon (IFN)-γ, and IFN-α. *IL-12Rβ1* and *TYK2* mutations may result in loss of function of IL-12 and IL-23 responses, with diminished IFN-γ and IL-17 production. IL-17 induces secretion of chemokines and colony-stimulating factors, leading to recruitment of neutrophils and enhanced fungal killing, whereas IL-22 induces antimicrobial peptides by epithelial cells. IL-17A and IL-17F signal through the IL-17RA/RC heterodimer complex to trigger NF-κB activation. Neutralizing autoantibodies against IL-17A, IL-17F, and/or IL-22 can directly antagonize IL-17 and IL-22 responses. DC, dendritic cell; FcγR, Fcγ receptor; JAK, Janus kinase; MHC II, major histocompatibility complex class II; MR, mannose receptor; RA, receptor A; Syk, spleen tyrosine kinase; TCR, T-cell receptor; TLR, toll-like receptor; TRAF6, TNF receptor–associated factor 6; TYK2, tyrosine kinase 2.

detected in patients with APECED, which might account for the CMC observed in these patients.[46,47]

Chronic Mucocutaneous Candidiasis Associated with Primary Immunodeficiencies

Mendelian susceptibility to mycobacterial disease (MSMD) is another PID associated with monogenic inheritance, which is characterized by selective susceptibility to atypical mycobacteria. Several genetic causes of MSMD have been reported, mainly with inborn errors of IFN-γ immunity. A subset of patients with MSMD shows susceptibility to both candidiasis and mycobacteria. IL-12Rβ1 deficiency is the most common genetic cause underlying MSMD.[48] The *IL12RB1* gene encodes the first chain of the IL-12 and IL-23 receptors. IL-12 is important for the development of IFN-γ–producing T cells and IFN-γ production, whereas IL-23 is important for the development and maintenance of the Th17 cell population.[49] Therefore, IL-12Rβ1 deficiencies predispose not only to mycobacteria and salmonella infections but also to mild forms of CMC, which have been reported with a frequency of 25% in patients with IL-12Rβ1 deficiency.[50] Tyrosine kinase 2 (Tyk2) is a member of the JAK family, which signals downstream of IL-12 and IL-23, and hence might link to reduced Th1 and type I IFN responses.[51] One case of AR-HIES has been reported to carry a homozygous nonsense mutation in *Tyk2* with mild CMC.[51] However, 8 cases of Tyk2 deficiency without HIES but with mycobacterial and viral infections have been reported recently.[52,53] It is suggested that the core clinical phenotype of Tyk2 deficiency is increased susceptibility to mycobacterial and/or viral infections, caused by impaired responses to IL-12 and IFN-α/β.[53] *RORC*, which encodes RORγ, is the master gene controlling Th17 cell differentiation. Homozygous loss-of-function mutations in *RORC* have been described to cause a PID that is predominantly characterized by an increased susceptibility to mycobacterial infection, and candida infections in some cases.[54]

Patients with combined immunodeficiencies (CID), severe CID (SCID), and idiopathic CD4 lymphopenia may also develop CMC in infancy because of T-cell deficiency, in addition to multiple other infectious and autoimmune diseases. Biallelic loss-of-function mutations in 3 components of the CBM complex, including CARD9, CARD11, BCL10, and MALT1, have recently been linked to CID in 7 patients.[55] A broad range of clinical manifestations of T-lymphocyte and B-lymphocyte defects, including mucosal candidiasis, are described in these patients.[55] CD25, encoded by the *IL2RA* gene, is the alpha subunit of the IL-2 receptor, which is constitutively expressed on T-regulatory cells and involved in the differentiation of effector T cells.[56] In 1995, a patient with a deletion in the *IL2RA* gene was reported to have esophageal candidiasis.[56] Recent studies also found heterozygous mutations of *STAT1* to be associated with progressive CID.[57] Patients show progressive loss of T-lymphocyte and B-lymphocyte numbers and functions, accompanied by increasing autoimmune features and fatal infections, including mucocutaneous candidiasis.[57] Furthermore, other mutations causing CID (*NEMO, IKBA, MST1/STK4, CRACM1*),[58–64] SCID (*JAK3, RAG1, RAG2, ARTEMIS*, and other genes),[65] and idiopathic CD4 lymphopenia (*UNC119, MAGT1, RAG1*)[66–68] were also reported to precipitate CMC and invasive candidiasis as part of the clinical spectrum, showing the crucial role of CD4 T cells in host defense.

Invasive Candida Infections

Unlike in mucocutaneous candidiasis, *Candida* can enter the blood stream and invade deep tissues and organs, causing invasive candidiasis, which has a significant mortality of 26% to 60%.[1] Although most cases of invasive candidiasis are caused by the combination of gene polymorphisms and/or risk factors, mutations in several single genes have been found to be linked to invasive candidiasis.

CARD9 deficiencies predisposing to invasive fungal infections have been reported recently. In 2013, 1 patient with *Candida dubliniensis* meningoencephalitis was reported to have compound heterozygous mutations in *CARD9*, with reduced numbers of Th17 lymphocytes and a selective *C albicans* neutrophil killing defect.[69] In 2014, 1 patient with relapsing *C albicans* meningoencephalitis was discovered to hold homozygous missense mutations in *CARD9*, with normal IL-17 but reduced GM-CSF production, which had a complete clinical remission with GM-CSF therapy.[70] Five more cases with homozygous *CARD9* mutations were reported in 2015, with candida meningoencephalitis.[71] Moreover, idiopathic deep dermatophytosis, subcutaneous phaeohyphomycosis, and invasive exophiala infections have also been reported in AR *CARD9*-deficient patients,[72–75] underscoring the importance of CARD9-dependent pattern recognition signaling in both mucocutaneous and invasive antifungal host defense.

Chronic granulomatous disease (CGD), which is caused by mutations in the genes encoding proteins that form the nicotinamide adenine dinucleotide phosphate (NADPH) oxidase complex, is another typical monogenic disorder linked to high incidence of invasive fungal infection, mostly with invasive aspergillosis but sometimes candidiasis. Mutations in NADPH oxidase complex (X-linked mutations in *CYBB*, and autosomal mutations in *NCF1*, *NCF2*, *NCF4*, *CYBA*) lead to defects in reactive oxygen species production and inability to kill microorganisms.[76] In a study of 368 patients with CGD, *Candida* species were considered as the most common cause of meningitis; the third most common cause of bacteremia, fungemia, and suppurative adenitis; and the fourth cause of death.[76] In addition, invasive candidiasis is also seen in patients with other monogenic disorders such as severe congenital neutropenia (mutations in *ELA2* and *HAX1*),[77,78] and leukocyte adhesion deficiency type 1 (mutation in *CD18*).[79] These diseases highlight the importance of sufficient numbers of phagocytic cells and the ability of granulocytes to reach the site of infection in preventing invasive candidiasis.

POLYGENIC INHERITANCE OF CANDIDA INFECTIONS

Despite the monogenic disorders of candida infections described earlier, most of these infections cannot be explained by monogenic disorders, but are more likely to be a consequence of both the well-known classic risk factors and polygenic inheritance leading to increased susceptibility. Several studies have investigated the role of genetic factors in patients at risk to develop candida infections, and linked single-nucleotide polymorphisms (SNPs) to the increased risk for both mucosal and invasive candida infections. An overview of polygenetic inheritance of candida infections is shown in **Table 2**.

Several studies that investigated genetic susceptibility to CMC, RVVC, and intra-abdominal candidiasis (IAC) have suggested a role for polymorphisms in certain PRRs and cytokines. A homozygous *dectin-1* Y238X polymorphism was first described in a family to cause RVVC and onychomycosis, with diminished capacity of beta-glucan recognition and Th17 responses.[80] This early stop codon SNP has further been shown to be associated with increased *Candida* colonization in a cohort of patients with HSCT,[81] but not with systemic candidiasis, in a case-control study of patients with candidemia.[82] *TLR3* polymorphisms have also been shown to influence susceptibility to CMC because of decreased IFN-γ production.[83,84] Polymorphisms in mannose-binding lectin (MBL), a soluble PRR, have

Table 2
Summary of polygenic inheritance of candida infections

Gene	SNP	rs Number	Disease	Immunologic Phenotype	Refs
Dectin-1	Y238X	rs16910526	Candida colonization, RVVC, onychomycosis	Cytokine responses deficiency of beta-glucan recognition	80,81
PTPN22	R620W	rs2476601	CMC and microbial infections	Unknown	92
TLR3	L412F	rs3775291	CMC and bacterial and CMV infections	Decreased IFN-γ levels	83,84
DEFB1	44C/G	rs1800972	Candida carriage and Candida colonization	Unknown	89,93
NLPR3	Variable number of tandem repeats in intron 4	—	RVVC	Impaired IL-1β production	88
IL-4	589T/C	rs2243250	RVVC	Increased vaginal IL-4, reduced NO and MBL levels	91
	589T/C, 33T/C, 1098G/T	rs2243250, rs2070874, rs243248	Chronic disseminated candidiasis	Unknown	90
MBL2	Codon 54 Allele B	—	RVVC	Reduced vaginal MBL levels	85,86
	R52C, G54D, G57E,	rs5030737, rs1800450, rs1800451	Intra-abdominal candidiasis	Reduced MBL levels	87
TNFA	308G/A	rs1800629	Intra-abdominal candidiasis	Unknown	89
IL-10	1082A/G	rs1800896	Persistent candidemia	Higher Candida-induced IL-10 production	97

Gene	Variant	SNP	Association	Description	Ref
IL-12B	2724ins/del	rs41292470	Persisting candidemia	Lower Candida-induced IFN-γ production	97
TLR1	R80T, N248S, S602I	rs5743611, rs4833095, rs5743618	Candidemia	Decreased production of IL-1β, IL-6, and IL-8 after stimulation	94
TLR2	R753Q	rs5743708	Candidemia	Decreased levels of IFN-γ and IL-8	95
TLR4	D299G, T399I	rs4986790, rs4986791	Candidemia and Candida colonization	Increased IL-10 production	94,96
CCL8	—	1kg_17_29697448	Candidemia	Defective type I IFN pathway	99
STAT1	—	rs16833172	Candidemia	Defective type I IFN pathway	99
SP110	—	rs3769845	Candidemia	Defective type I IFN pathway	99
PSMB8	—	rs3198005	Candidemia	Defective type I IFN pathway	99
CD58	—	rs17035850, rs12025416	Candidemia	Decreased capacity of macrophages to kill Candida	100
LCE4A/C1orf68	—	rs4845320	Candidemia	Impaired epithelial barrier function	100
TAGAP	—	rs3127214	Candidemia	KO mice incapable of clearing Candida from organs	100
MDA5(IFIH1)	—	rs1990760 and rs3747517	Candidemia and CMC	Lower levels of MDA5, altered cytokine response to C albicans	98

Abbreviations: CMV, cytomegalovirus; KO, knockout; MBL, mannose-binding lectin; MDA 5, Melanoma Differentiation-Associated protein 5; TLR, Toll-like receptor; TNFA, tumor necrosis factor-alpha.

been linked to RVVC and IAC in 3 studies.[85–87] Moreover, polymorphisms in the *NLRP3* gene that encodes a subunit of the inflammasome have been associated with increased risk of RVVC.[88] Polymorphisms in key cytokine genes such as *TNF* have been associated with an increased risk of IAC and *Candida* colonization in high-risk surgical patients in intensive care units (ICUs),[89] and polymorphisms in IL-4 are associated with both chronic disseminated candidiasis[90] and RVVC.[91] Polymorphisms in the gene encoding the protein PTPN22, which is involved in T-cell and B-cell receptor signaling, was associated with an increased risk of CMC in 1 study.[92] Polymorphism in *DEFB1* coding for beta defensin-1, which acts as an antimicrobial peptide contributing to anti-*Candida* epithelial immunity, was associated with *Candida* colonization[93] and increased susceptibility to candida infections in ICU surgical patients.[89]

Given the high mortality of candidemia in hospitalized patients, an increasing number of studies have tried to identify genetic polymorphisms that might contribute to the cause and severity of candidemia. Three SNPs in *TLR1* that influence the proinflammatory cytokines in response to Toll-like receptor (TLR) 1/TLR2 agonists have been shown to increase susceptibility to candidemia.[94] In another cohort of ICU patients in Germany, polymorphisms in *TLR2* were found in 5.2% of ICU patients with septic shock, with altered cytokine release (increased TNF-α but reduced IFN-γ and IL-8 levels) in response to *Candida*.[95] TLR4 D299G and T399I polymorphisms have initially been suggested to increase the risk for candidemia in nonneutropenic patients,[96] but a larger study did not support this observation.[94] In addition, polymorphisms in the cytokine genes *IL-10* and *IL-12B* resulting in low production of proinflammatory cytokines were associated with persistent candidemia in a cohort study of 338 patients with candidemia.[97]

One characteristic of invasive disease caused by *Candida* is the formation of hyphae. Macrophages that are exposed to yeasts that form hyphae show a different transcription profile than when they are exposed to *Candida* mutants that cannot form hyphae. This difference involved genes associated with the Retinoic-acid-inducible gene-I-like signaling cascade. When this pathway was explored in 227 patients with candidemia, SNPs in the *MDA5* (*IFIH1*) gene, which encodes a cytosolic receptor for viral double-stranded RNA, were associated with increased risk to develop candidemia.[98] Based on immunologic studies in knockout mice and humans, polymorphisms in MDA5 were shown to produce an altered cytokine response to *C albicans*.[98] By integrating transcriptional analysis and functional genomics, Smeekens and colleagues[99] identified the type I IFN pathway as *Candida*-specific host defense mechanisms in humans. Polymorphisms in genes from the type I IFN pathway, including *CCL8*, *STAT1*, *SP110*, and *PSMB8*, modulated *Candida*-induced cytokine production and were correlated with increased susceptibility to systemic candidiasis.[99] By using genome-wide association studies with 118,989 SNPs across 186 loci in a large candidemia cohort, Kumar and colleagues[100] recently identified 3 novel genetic risk factors associated with candidemia, including SNPs located in *CD58*, *LCE4A-C1orf68*, and *TAGAP*. These data provided novel insights into these proteins and their role in invasive fungal infection. CD58 was shown to be important for controlling *Candida* growth when phagocytosed by macrophages, whereas TAGAP-deficient mice showed higher mortality in a model with invasive candidiasis and the TAGAP deficiency was associated with decreased TNF production. Therefore, the use of novel genetic techniques and a system biology approach has the capacity to identify novel insights in pathogenesis, such as the identification of the type 1 IFN pathway, which is crucial for viral host defense but now has also been linked to candida infection.

SUMMARY

In recent years, genetic susceptibility to candida infections has been extensively explored, which has led to novel insights into the pathogenesis of candidiasis. Next-generation sequencing in particular has contributed to the identification of monogenetic disorders associated with candida infections. This approach has identified key pathways in the host defense against candida infections, such as the importance of an optimal IL-17 signaling pathway in preventing mucocutaneous candidiasis, and the unexpected role of the type 1 IFN pathway in invasive fungal infection. These studies not only contribute to new insights but will prove to be an essential element to guide the development of future immunotherapeutic strategies.

REFERENCES

1. Das I, Nightingale P, Patel M, et al. Epidemiology, clinical characteristics, and outcome of candidemia: Experience in a tertiary referral center in the UK. Int J Infect Dis 2011;15(11):e759–63.
2. Lilic D. New perspectives on the immunology of chronic mucocutaneous candidiasis. Curr Opin Infect Dis 2002;15(2):143–7.
3. Puel A, Cypowyj S, Marodi L, et al. Inborn errors of human IL-17 immunity underlie chronic mucocutaneous candidiasis. Curr Opin Allergy Clin Immunol 2012; 12(6):616–22.
4. Glocker EO, Hennigs A, Nabavi M, et al. A homozygous CARD9 mutation in a family with susceptibility to fungal infections. N Engl J Med 2009;361(18):1727–35.
5. Romani L. Immunity to fungal infections. Nat Rev Immunol 2011;11(4):275–88.
6. Drummond RA, Saijo S, Iwakura Y, et al. The role of Syk/CARD9 coupled C-type lectins in antifungal immunity. Eur J Immunol 2011;41(2):276–81.
7. Liu L, Okada S, Kong XF, et al. Gain-of-function human STAT1 mutations impair IL-17 immunity and underlie chronic mucocutaneous candidiasis. J Exp Med 2011;208(8):1635–48.
8. van de Veerdonk FL, Plantinga TS, Hoischen A, et al. STAT1 mutations in autosomal dominant chronic mucocutaneous candidiasis. N Engl J Med 2011; 365(1):54–61.
9. Smeekens SP, Plantinga TS, van de Veerdonk FL, et al. STAT1 hyperphosphorylation and defective IL12R/IL23R signaling underlie defective immunity in autosomal dominant chronic mucocutaneous candidiasis. PLoS One 2011;6(12): e29248.
10. Hori T, Ohnishi H, Teramoto T, et al. Autosomal-dominant chronic mucocutaneous candidiasis with STAT1-mutation can be complicated with chronic active hepatitis and hypothyroidism. J Clin Immunol 2012;32(6):1213–20.
11. Takezaki S, Yamada M, Kato M, et al. Chronic mucocutaneous candidiasis caused by a gain-of-function mutation in the STAT1 DNA-binding domain. J Immunol 2012; 189(3):1521–6.
12. Soltesz B, Toth B, Shabashova N, et al. New and recurrent gain-of-function STAT1 mutations in patients with chronic mucocutaneous candidiasis from eastern and central Europe. J Med Genet 2013;50(9):567–78.
13. Mizoguchi Y, Tsumura M, Okada S, et al. Simple diagnosis of STAT1 gain-of-function alleles in patients with chronic mucocutaneous candidiasis. J Leukoc Biol 2014;95(4):667–76.
14. Yamazaki Y, Yamada M, Kawai T, et al. Two novel gain-of-function mutations of STAT1 responsible for chronic mucocutaneous candidiasis disease: Impaired

production of IL-17a and IL-22, and the presence of anti-IL-17F autoantibody. J Immunol 2014;193(10):4880–7.

15. Najjar I, Fagard R. STAT1 and pathogens, not a friendly relationship. Biochimie 2010;92(5):425–44.

16. Sampaio EP, Hsu AP, Pechacek J, et al. Signal transducer and activator of transcription 1 (STAT1) gain-of-function mutations and disseminated coccidioidomycosis and histoplasmosis. J Allergy Clin Immunol 2013;131(6):1624–34.

17. Wang X, Lin Z, Gao L, et al. Exome sequencing reveals a signal transducer and activator of transcription 1 (STAT1) mutation in a child with recalcitrant cutaneous fusariosis. J Allergy Clin Immunol 2013;131(4):1242–3.

18. Kumar N, Hanks ME, Chandrasekaran P, et al. Gain-of-function signal transducer and activator of transcription 1 (STAT1) mutation-related primary immunodeficiency is associated with disseminated mucormycosis. J Allergy Clin Immunol 2014;134(1):236–9.

19. Lee PP, Mao H, Yang W, et al. *Penicillium marneffei* infection and impaired IFN-gamma immunity in humans with autosomal-dominant gain-of-phosphorylation STAT1 mutations. J Allergy Clin Immunol 2014;133(3):894–6.e5.

20. Aldave JC, Cachay E, Nunez L, et al. A 1-year-old girl with a gain-of-function STAT1 mutation treated with hematopoietic stem cell transplantation. J Clin Immunol 2013;33(8):1273–5.

21. Wildbaum G, Shahar E, Katz R, et al. Continuous G-CSF therapy for isolated chronic mucocutaneous candidiasis: Complete clinical remission with restoration of IL-17 secretion. J Allergy Clin Immunol 2013;132(3):761–4.

22. Higgins E, Al Shehri T, McAleer MA, et al. Use of ruxolitinib to successfully treat chronic mucocutaneous candidiasis caused by gain-of-function signal transducer and activator of transcription 1 (STAT1) mutation. J Allergy Clin Immunol 2015;135(2):551–3.

23. van de Veerdonk FL, Koenen HJ, van der Velden WJ, et al. Immunotherapy with G-CSF in patients with chronic mucocutaneous candidiasis. Immunol Lett 2015; 167(1):54–6.

24. Gu C, Wu L, Li X. Il-17 family: Cytokines, receptors and signaling. Cytokine 2013; 64(2):477–85.

25. Puel A, Cypowyj S, Bustamante J, et al. Chronic mucocutaneous candidiasis in humans with inborn errors of interleukin-17 immunity. Science 2011;332(6025):65–8.

26. Ling Y, Cypowyj S, Aytekin C, et al. Inherited IL-17RC deficiency in patients with chronic mucocutaneous candidiasis. J Exp Med 2015;212(5):619–31.

27. Boisson B, Wang C, Pedergnana V, et al. An ACT1 mutation selectively abolishes interleukin-17 responses in humans with chronic mucocutaneous candidiasis. Immunity 2013;39(4):676–86.

28. Davis SD, Schaller J, Wedgwood RJ. Job's syndrome. Recurrent, "cold", staphylococcal abscesses. Lancet 1966;1(7445):1013–5.

29. Holland SM, DeLeo FR, Elloumi HZ, et al. STAT3 mutations in the hyper-IgE syndrome. N Engl J Med 2007;357(16):1608–19.

30. Minegishi Y, Saito M, Tsuchiya S, et al. Dominant-negative mutations in the DNA-binding domain of STAT3 cause hyper-IgE syndrome. Nature 2007;448(7157): 1058–62.

31. Farmand S, Sundin M. Hyper-IgE syndromes: Recent advances in pathogenesis, diagnostics and clinical care. Curr Opin Hematol 2015;22(1):12–22.

32. Saito M, Nagasawa M, Takada H, et al. Defective IL-10 signaling in hyper-IgE syndrome results in impaired generation of tolerogenic dendritic cells and induced regulatory T cells. J Exp Med 2011;208(2):235–49.

33. Ma CS, Avery DT, Chan A, et al. Functional STAT3 deficiency compromises the generation of human T follicular helper cells. Blood 2012;119(17):3997–4008.

34. Engelhardt KR, McGhee S, Winkler S, et al. Large deletions and point mutations involving the dedicator of cytokinesis 8 (DOCK8) in the autosomal-recessive form of hyper-IgE syndrome. J Allergy Clin Immunol 2009;124(6):1289–302.e4.

35. Sabry A, Hauk PJ, Jing H, et al. Vaccine strain varicella-zoster virus-induced central nervous system vasculopathy as the presenting feature of DOCK8 deficiency. J Allergy Clin Immunol 2014;133(4):1225–7.

36. Aydin SE, Kilic SS, Aytekin C, et al. DOCK8 deficiency: Clinical and immunological phenotype and treatment options - a review of 136 patients. J Clin Immunol 2015;35(2):189–98.

37. Engelhardt KR, Gertz ME, Keles S, et al. The extended clinical phenotype of 64 patients with dedicator of cytokinesis 8 deficiency. J Allergy Clin Immunol 2015; 136(2):402–12.

38. Zhang Q, Davis JC, Lamborn IT, et al. Combined immunodeficiency associated with DOCK8 mutations. N Engl J Med 2009;361(21):2046–55.

39. Su HC. Dedicator of cytokinesis 8 (DOCK8) deficiency. Curr Opin Allergy Clin Immunol 2010;10(6):515–20.

40. Bittner TC, Pannicke U, Renner ED, et al. Successful long-term correction of autosomal recessive hyper-IgE syndrome due to DOCK8 deficiency by hematopoietic stem cell transplantation. Klin Padiatr 2010;222(6):351–5.

41. McDonald DR, Massaad MJ, Johnston A, et al. Successful engraftment of donor marrow after allogeneic hematopoietic cell transplantation in autosomal-recessive hyper-IgE syndrome caused by dedicator of cytokinesis 8 deficiency. J Allergy Clin Immunol 2010;126(6):1304–5.e3.

42. Gatz SA, Benninghoff U, Schutz C, et al. Curative treatment of autosomal-recessive hyper-IgE syndrome by hematopoietic cell transplantation. Bone Marrow Transplant 2011;46(4):552–6.

43. Metin A, Tavil B, Azik F, et al. Successful bone marrow transplantation for DOCK8 deficient hyper IgE syndrome. Pediatr Transplant 2012;16(4):398–9.

44. Kawaguch K, Matsubara K, Uchida Y, et al. Successful treatment with allogenic hematopoietic stem cell transplantation of a severe congenital neutropenia patient harboring a novel ELANE mutation. Rinsho Ketsueki 2014;55(11):2294–9.

45. Finnish-German AC. An autoimmune disease, APECED, caused by mutations in a novel gene featuring two PHD-type zinc-finger domains. Nat Genet 1997; 17(4):399–403.

46. Puel A, Doffinger R, Natividad A, et al. Autoantibodies against IL-17A, IL-17F, and IL-22 in patients with chronic mucocutaneous candidiasis and autoimmune polyendocrine syndrome type I. J Exp Med 2010;207(2):291–7.

47. Kisand K, Boe Wolff AS, Podkrajsek KT, et al. Chronic mucocutaneous candidiasis in APECED or thymoma patients correlates with autoimmunity to Th17-associated cytokines. J Exp Med 2010;207(2):299–308.

48. Fieschi C, Dupuis S, Catherinot E, et al. Low penetrance, broad resistance, and favorable outcome of interleukin 12 receptor beta1 deficiency: Medical and immunological implications. J Exp Med 2003;197(4):527–35.

49. Ouederni M, Sanal O, Ikinciogullari A, et al. Clinical features of candidiasis in patients with inherited interleukin 12 receptor beta1 deficiency. Clin Infect Dis 2014;58(2):204–13.

50. de Beaucoudrey L, Samarina A, Bustamante J, et al. Revisiting human IL-12Rbeta1 deficiency: A survey of 141 patients from 30 countries. Medicine 2010;89(6): 381–402.

51. Minegishi Y, Saito M, Morio T, et al. Human tyrosine kinase 2 deficiency reveals its requisite roles in multiple cytokine signals involved in innate and acquired immunity. Immunity 2006;25(5):745–55.
52. Kilic SS, Hacimustafaoglu M, Boisson-Dupuis S, et al. A patient with tyrosine kinase 2 deficiency without hyper-IgE syndrome. J Pediatr 2012;160(6): 1055–7.
53. Kreins AY, Ciancanelli MJ, Okada S, et al. Human TYK2 deficiency: Mycobacterial and viral infections without hyper-IgE syndrome. J Exp Med 2015;212(10): 1641–62.
54. Okada S, Markle JG, Deenick EK, et al. Immunodeficiencies. Impairment of immunity to *Candida* and *Mycobacterium* in humans with bi-allelic RORC mutations. Science 2015;349(6248):606–13.
55. Perez de Diego R, Sanchez-Ramon S, Lopez-Collazo E, et al. Genetic errors of the human caspase recruitment domain-B-cell lymphoma 10-mucosa-associated lymphoid tissue lymphoma-translocation gene 1 (CBM) complex: Molecular, immunologic, and clinical heterogeneity. J Allergy Clin Immunol 2015. [Epub ahead of print].
56. Sakaguchi S, Sakaguchi N, Asano M, et al. Immunologic self-tolerance maintained by activated T cells expressing IL-2 receptor alpha-chains (CD25). Breakdown of a single mechanism of self-tolerance causes various autoimmune diseases. J Immunol 1995;155(3):1151–64.
57. Sharfe N, Nahum A, Newell A, et al. Fatal combined immunodeficiency associated with heterozygous mutation in STAT1. J Allergy Clin Immunol 2014;133(3): 807–17.
58. Feske S, Gwack Y, Prakriya M, et al. A mutation in Orai1 causes immune deficiency by abrogating CRAC channel function. Nature 2006;441(7090):179–85.
59. Morgan NV, Goddard S, Cardno TS, et al. Mutation in the TCRα subunit constant gene (TRAC) leads to a human immunodeficiency disorder characterized by a lack of TCRαβ+ T cells. J Clin Invest 2011;121(2):695–702.
60. Ouederni M, Vincent QB, Frange P, et al. Major histocompatibility complex class II expression deficiency caused by a RFXANK founder mutation: A survey of 35 patients. Blood 2011;118(19):5108–18.
61. Picard C, Casanova JL, Puel A. Infectious diseases in patients with IRAK-4, Myd88, NEMO, or IkappaBalpha deficiency. Clin Microbiol Rev 2011;24(3): 490–7.
62. Abdollahpour H, Appaswamy G, Kotlarz D, et al. The phenotype of human STK4 deficiency. Blood 2012;119(15):3450–7.
63. Nehme NT, Pachlopnik Schmid J, Debeurme F, et al. MST1 mutations in autosomal recessive primary immunodeficiency characterized by defective naive T-cell survival. Blood 2012;119(15):3458–68.
64. Schimke LF, Rieber N, Rylaarsdam S, et al. A novel gain-of-function IKBA mutation underlies ectodermal dysplasia with immunodeficiency and polyendocrinopathy. J Clin Immunol 2013;33(6):1088–99.
65. Puck JM. Neonatal screening for severe combined immunodeficiency. Curr Opin Pediatr 2011;23(6):667–73.
66. Kuijpers TW, Ijspeert H, van Leeuwen EM, et al. Idiopathic CD4+ T lymphopenia without autoimmunity or granulomatous disease in the slipstream of RAG mutations. Blood 2011;117(22):5892–6.
67. Li FY, Chaigne-Delalande B, Kanellopoulou C, et al. Second messenger role for Mg2+ revealed by human T-cell immunodeficiency. Nature 2011;475(7357): 471–6.

68. Gorska MM, Alam R. A mutation in the human uncoordinated 119 gene impairs TCR signaling and is associated with CD4 lymphopenia. Blood 2012;119(6):1399–406.
69. Drewniak A, Gazendam RP, Tool AT, et al. Invasive fungal infection and impaired neutrophil killing in human CARD9 deficiency. Blood 2013;121(13):2385–92.
70. Gavino C, Cotter A, Lichtenstein D, et al. CARD9 deficiency and spontaneous central nervous system candidiasis: Complete clinical remission with GM-CSF therapy. Clin Infect Dis 2014;59(1):81–4.
71. Lanternier F, Mahdaviani SA, Barbati E, et al. Inherited CARD9 deficiency in otherwise healthy children and adults with *Candida* species-induced meningo-encephalitis, colitis, or both. J Allergy Clin Immunol 2015;135(6):1558–68.e2.
72. Lanternier F, Barbati E, Meinzer U, et al. Inherited CARD9 deficiency in 2 unrelated patients with invasive *Exophiala* infection. J Infect Dis 2015;211(8):1241–50.
73. Lanternier F, Pathan S, Vincent QB, et al. Deep dermatophytosis and inherited CARD9 deficiency. N Engl J Med 2013;369(18):1704–14.
74. Wang X, Wang W, Lin Z, et al. CARD9 mutations linked to subcutaneous phaeohyphomycosis and Th17 cell deficiencies. J Allergy Clin Immunol 2014;133(3):905–8.e3.
75. Jachiet M, Lanternier F, Rybojad M, et al. Posaconazole treatment of extensive skin and nail dermatophytosis due to autosomal recessive deficiency of CARD9. JAMA Dermatol 2015;151(2):192–4.
76. Winkelstein JA, Marino MC, Johnston RB Jr, et al. Chronic granulomatous disease. Report on a national registry of 368 patients. Medicine 2000;79(3):155–69.
77. Dale DC, Person RE, Bolyard AA, et al. Mutations in the gene encoding neutrophil elastase in congenital and cyclic neutropenia. Blood 2000;96(7):2317–22.
78. Klein C, Grudzien M, Appaswamy G, et al. HAX1 deficiency causes autosomal recessive severe congenital neutropenia (Kostmann disease). Nat Genet 2007;39(1):86–92.
79. Fischer A, Lisowska-Grospierre B, Anderson DC, et al. Leukocyte adhesion deficiency: Molecular basis and functional consequences. Immunodefic Rev 1988;1(1):39–54.
80. Ferwerda B, Ferwerda G, Plantinga TS, et al. Human dectin-1 deficiency and mucocutaneous fungal infections. N Engl J Med 2009;361(18):1760–7.
81. Plantinga TS, van der Velden WJ, Ferwerda B, et al. Early stop polymorphism in human dectin-1 is associated with increased *Candida* colonization in hematopoietic stem cell transplant recipients. Clin Infect Dis 2009;49(5):724–32.
82. Rosentul DC, Plantinga TS, Oosting M, et al. Genetic variation in the dectin-1/CARD9 recognition pathway and susceptibility to candidemia. J Infect Dis 2011;204(7):1138–45.
83. Nahum A, Dadi H, Bates A, et al. The I412f variant of toll-like receptor 3 (TLR3) is associated with cutaneous candidiasis, increased susceptibility to cytomegalovirus, and autoimmunity. J Allergy Clin Immunol 2011;127(2):528–31.
84. Nahum A, Dadi H, Bates A, et al. The biological significance of TLR3 variant, L412F, in conferring susceptibility to cutaneous candidiasis, CMV and autoimmunity. Autoimmun Rev 2012;11(5):341–7.
85. Babula O, Lazdane G, Kroica J, et al. Relation between recurrent vulvovaginal candidiasis, vaginal concentrations of mannose-binding lectin, and a mannose-binding lectin gene polymorphism in Latvian women. Clin Infect Dis 2003;37(5):733–7.
86. Giraldo PC, Babula O, Goncalves AK, et al. Mannose-binding lectin gene polymorphism, vulvovaginal candidiasis, and bacterial vaginosis. Obstet Gynecol 2007;109(5):1123–8.

87. van Till JW, Modderman PW, de Boer M, et al. Mannose-binding lectin deficiency facilitates abdominal *Candida* infections in patients with secondary peritonitis. Clin Vaccine Immunol 2008;15(1):65–70.
88. Lev-Sagie A, Prus D, Linhares IM, et al. Polymorphism in a gene coding for the inflammasome component NALP3 and recurrent vulvovaginal candidiasis in women with vulvar vestibulitis syndrome. Am J Obstet Gynecol 2009;200(3):303.e1–6.
89. Wojtowicz A, Tissot F, Lamoth F, et al. Polymorphisms in tumor necrosis factor-alpha increase susceptibility to intra-abdominal *Candida* infection in high-risk surgical ICU patients. Crit Care Med 2014;42(4):e304–8.
90. Choi EH, Foster CB, Taylor JG, et al. Association between chronic disseminated candidiasis in adult acute leukemia and common IL4 promoter haplotypes. J Infect Dis 2003;187(7):1153–6.
91. Babula O, Lazdane G, Kroica J, et al. Frequency of interleukin-4 (IL-4) -589 gene polymorphism and vaginal concentrations of IL-4, nitric oxide, and mannose-binding lectin in women with recurrent vulvovaginal candidiasis. Clin Infect Dis 2005;40(9):1258–62.
92. Nahum A, Bates A, Sharfe N, et al. Association of the lymphoid protein tyrosine phosphatase, R620W variant, with chronic mucocutaneous candidiasis. J Allergy Clin Immunol 2008;122(6):1220–2.
93. Jurevic RJ, Bai M, Chadwick RB, et al. Single-nucleotide polymorphisms (SNPS) in human beta-defensin 1: High-throughput SNP assays and association with *Candida* carriage in type I diabetics and nondiabetic controls. J Clin Microbiol 2003;41(1):90–6.
94. Plantinga TS, Johnson MD, Scott WK, et al. Toll-like receptor 1 polymorphisms increase susceptibility to candidemia. J Infect Dis 2012;205(6):934–43.
95. Woehrle T, Du W, Goetz A, et al. Pathogen specific cytokine release reveals an effect of TLR2 Arg753Gln during *Candida* sepsis in humans. Cytokine 2008;41(3):322–9.
96. Van der Graaf CA, Netea MG, Morre SA, et al. Toll-like receptor 4 Asp299Gly/Thr399Ile polymorphisms are a risk factor for *Candida* bloodstream infection. Eur Cytokine Netw 2006;17(1):29–34.
97. Johnson MD, Plantinga TS, van de Vosse E, et al. Cytokine gene polymorphisms and the outcome of invasive candidiasis: A prospective cohort study. Clin Infect Dis 2012;54(4):502–10.
98. Jaeger M, van der Lee R, Cheng SC, et al. The RIG-I-like helicase receptor mda5 (IFIH1) is involved in the host defense against *Candida* infections. Eur J Clin Microbiol Infect Dis 2015;34(5):963–74.
99. Smeekens SP, Ng A, Kumar V, et al. Functional genomics identifies type I interferon pathway as central for host defense against *Candida albicans*. Nat Commun 2013;4:1342.
100. Kumar V, Cheng SC, Johnson MD, et al. Immunochip SNP array identifies novel genetic variants conferring susceptibility to candidaemia. Nat Commun 2014;5:4675.

Invasive Candidiasis

Todd P. McCarty, MD, Peter G. Pappas, MD*

KEYWORDS

- *Candida* • Invasive candidiasis • Antifungals • Bloodstream infection
- Fungal infection

KEY POINTS

- *Candida* is a leading cause of hospital-acquired bloodstream infections, in particular in patients admitted to intensive care units.
- Non–culture-based molecular diagnostic assays have the potential to improve time to treatment, thereby improving morbidity and mortality.
- Echinocandins are the treatment of choice for most cases of invasive candidiasis.
- Targeted antifungal prophylaxis decreases rates of invasive candidiasis and may influence mortality.

INTRODUCTION

Invasive infection due to *Candida* species is a condition associated with medical progress. It is a common health care–associated infection and is widely recognized as a major cause of infection-related morbidity and mortality. There are at least 15 distinct *Candida* species that cause human disease, but more than 95% of invasive disease is caused by the 5 most common pathogens: *C albicans*, *C glabrata*, *C tropicalis*, *C parapsilosis*, and *C krusei*. Serious infections due to these organisms are generally referred to as invasive candidiasis (IC). Mucosal *Candida* infections, including those involving the oropharynx, esophagus, and vagina, are not part of this review. Rather, the focus of this review is on the epidemiology, pathogenesis, diagnosis, clinical manifestations, and management of IC.

EPIDEMIOLOGY

Candidemia ranks as the third or fourth most common cause of health care–associated bloodstream infection (BSI) and is a leading cause of BSIs in the intensive care unit (ICU). A recent multicenter point-prevalence survey identified *Candida* spp as the most common health care–associated bloodstream pathogen.[1] At least 50% of episodes of candidemia occur in an ICU setting, reflecting the complexity of illness usually associated with

University of Alabama at Birmingham, 1900 University Boulevard, 229 THT, Birmingham, AL 35294-0006, USA
* Corresponding author.
E-mail address: pappas@uab.edu

Infect Dis Clin N Am 30 (2016) 103–124
http://dx.doi.org/10.1016/j.idc.2015.10.013
0891-5520/16/$ – see front matter © 2016 Elsevier Inc. All rights reserved.

id.theclinics.com

this infection. There are well-recognized risk factors associated with IC that apply to all hospitalized persons but especially to those in an ICU. Premature low-birth-weight neonates are at extraordinary high risk of candidemia, and the highest incidence of candidemia occurs in the neonatal ICU. The most common risk factors include the presence of an indwelling central venous catheter (CVC), exposure to broad-spectrum antibacterial agents, prolonged ICU stay with or without assisted ventilation (greater than 3 days), recent major surgery, necrotizing pancreatitis, any type of hemodialysis, and immunosuppression.[2,3] A more complete list of risk factors for IC is depicted in **Table 1**.

Community-acquired candidemia is a relatively new observation in the Unites States and other developed countries, reflecting the increasing utilization of parenteral outpatient antimicrobial therapy through a permanent or semipermanent venous access device (eg, Hickman catheter, peripherally inserted cannulated catheter).[4] This phenomenon has led to the observation that as many as 20% to 30% of patients with candidemia are categorized as health care associated and community acquired.

Species distribution is important in all forms of candidiasis; there is considerable geographic, center-to-center, and unit-to-unit variability in the prevalence of pathogenic *Candida* species.[5–9] Indeed, candidiasis is not one but rather several diseases, with each *Candida* species presenting its own unique characteristics with respect to tissue tropism, propensity to cause invasive disease, virulence, and antifungal susceptibility. A working knowledge of the local epidemiology and rates of antifungal resistance is critical in making informed clinical and therapeutic decisions while awaiting culture and susceptibility data.

In the United States, *C albicans* accounts for approximately 50% of bloodstream *Candida* isolates. *C glabrata* is the second most common bloodstream pathogen, representing up to 25% to 30% in some series.[10] *C glabrata* is more common among patients aged greater than 60 years and in solid organ transplants. This pathogen is uncommon in the neonatal ICU (NICU).[5] *C tropicalis* and *C parapsilosis* generally represent 10% to 15% of isolates, depending on the region and the study population. For example, in Latin America, *C parapsilosis* and *C tropicalis* are both more common in adults than *C glabrata*.[9] *C tropicalis* is recognized commonly in India, Latin America, and other tropical and subtropical regions. *C krusei* is the least common of the 5 major species and is a prominent pathogen among patients with hematologic malignancies and others who have received prolonged azole prophylaxis.

Table 1
Risk factors for IC

Immunocompromised	Nonimmunocompromised	Neonates
In addition to →	Broad-spectrum antibiotics	← In addition to
Granulocytopenia	Any type of renal dialysis	Gestational age
Stem cell transplant	Central venous catheter	Low APGAR
Mucositis	IV drug use	Length of NICU stay
Graft vs host disease	Severity of illness	H_2 blockers
Type of chemotherapy	Total parenteral nutrition	Shock
Organ transplants	GI perforation or surgery	Intubation
	Candida colonization	GI disease
	Diabetes	Congenital malformations
	Length of stay in ICU	
	Pancreatitis	
	Sepsis	

Abbreviations: GI, gastrointestinal; GVHD, graft-versus-host disease; IV, intravenous; NICU, neonatal ICU.

PATHOGENESIS

Candida species are normal human flora and are typically found in the gastrointestinal tract and are common colonizers of the genitourinary tract and skin. The pathogenesis of IC generally results from a combination of increased fungal burden with an alteration of the skin and mucous membranes as a means of keeping pathogens external. In particular, *Candida* is adept at surface adherence and the formation of biofilms both on body surfaces as well as prosthetic devices, including urinary catheters and intra-vascular devices.[11] *Candida* species are able to convert from the yeast phase to the hyphal phase on adherence to a surface.[12] Additionally, the formation of biofilms leads to upregulation of azole-resistance mechanisms as well as the development of persister cells with even higher levels of antifungal resistance.[13–16]

All arms of the immune system are involved in the response to candidal infections. Lymphocytes are crucial to the development of cell-mediated immunity to *Candida* species and the prevention of mucosal disease. In particular, deficiencies in the T-helper 17 cell line impair the mucosal immune response to *C albicans* leading to an increase in colonization and disease.[17] Monocytes and neutrophils damage and destroy pseudohyphae and blastospores. Consequently, patients with significant neutrophil dysfunction or leukopenia have a strong propensity toward the development of candidemia and other forms of IC. Complement and immunoglobulins are required for optimal opsonization and intracellular killing of the organism, and deficiency of either of these components can be associated with more complicated or refractory disease. Regardless of the importance of these underlying conditions in the pathogenesis of candidiasis, iatrogenic factors, such as antibiotic exposure, instrumentation, and immunosuppression, are the most important influences on the genesis and outcomes among patients with IC.

DIAGNOSIS

The gold standard of diagnosis in IC is culture, in particular culture from sterile sites, such as blood, peritoneal fluid, and pleural fluid. However, blood cultures are insensitive and identify only approximately 50% of all patients with IC based on data from several autopsy studies.[18] Most (95%) blood cultures that are ultimately positive for *Candida* species become positive within 96 hours, but time to positivity is species dependent; for example, *C glabrata* grows much more slowly than *C albicans*. Other factors that influence the sensitivity of blood culture include the volume of blood, antifungal drug exposure, and the specific blood culture technique. The reliance on blood culture remains a significant obstacle to making clinical decisions regarding early intervention with antifungal therapy. The development of reliable nonculture assays is critical to providing the opportunity for earlier intervention with more targeted antifungal therapy among large numbers of at-risk patients.[18]

Data from several retrospective studies suggest that early and effective treatment confers a survival benefit from *Candida* sepsis.[19,20] Moreover, early identification to the species level facilitates therapeutic decision making based on the likelihood of fluconazole susceptibility or resistance and allows for informed alterations in therapy while awaiting formal antifungal sensitivity data. Thus, the development of rapid, non–culture-based technologies is a high priority in the effort to influence the management and improve outcomes for patients with IC.

Currently there are 4 Food and Drug Administration (FDA)–approved technologies that may help to bridge this gap: matrix-assisted laser desorption/ionization time-of-flight (MALDI-TOF), peptide nucleic acid fluorescent in situ hybridization (PNA-FISH), the β-D glucan (Fungitell, Associates of Cape Cod, Inc, East Falmouth, MA) assay, and the T2Candida assay (T2 Biosystems, Lexington, MA).

MALDI-TOF is a postculture technique that uses mass spectroscopy and requires pure growth of an organism on artificial media; therefore, it has no influence on time to diagnosis of candidemia. MALDI-TOF can provide species identification within 10 to 15 minutes once an organism is isolated on artificial media. This identification is generally 1.0 to 1.5 days sooner than conventional methods, with the most dramatic difference noted for nonalbicans *Candida* species.[21–23]

PNA-FISH can be performed directly on a positive blood culture result rather than waiting for the growth of pure colonies.[24] The test exists as commercially available multi-species kits, with a positive result narrowing the identification to a paired result (*C albicans/tropicalis* vs *C glabrata/krusei* vs *C parapsilosis*), not to the level of single species specificity.[25] Although this assay provides prompt species identification, diagnosis is reliant on a positive culture.

β-D-glucan (BDG) is a cell wall constituent of *Candida* spp, *Aspergillus* spp, *Pneumocystis jiroveci*, selected dematiaceous fungi, and several other fungi. In this respect, it is a pan-fungal diagnostic test. The assay has performance characteristics that are reasonably well defined among patients with IC. Using a cutoff value of 80 pg/mL in patients with proven IC, in meta-analyses of BDG studies, the pooled sensitivity and specificity for diagnosing IC were 75% to 80% and 80%, respectively.[26–28] Its performance is optimized by requiring 2 successive positive assays to define a true-positive result. True-positive results are not specific for IC; for this reason, among patient populations who are also at risk for invasive mold infections, such as hematopoietic cell transplant recipients, BDG offers a theoretic advantage over other assays. Its use has been limited by its nonspecificity, expense, and the tedious nature of performing the test.

The T2Candida assay is a polymerase chain reaction (PCR)–based assay that uses magnetic resonance detection to identify the presence of *Candida* organisms in whole blood. The assay provides the same paired species level result as does PNA-FISH.[29] The key difference is that the assay is performed on whole blood, ideally collected in parallel with routine or fungal blood cultures, allowing the rapid diagnosis of candidemia with additional species level information. Once the specimen has been processed, results are available in as soon as 3 to 4 hours. The largest prospective study of this assay demonstrated excellent positive and negative predictive values of 91.7% and 99.6%, respectively.[30] To date, there are too few data from the real world use of the assay in practice; but it has significant promise as a rapid, sensitive, and specific non–culture-based assay for the early diagnosis of candidemia. The overall performance of the assay in noncandidemic IC is unknown at this time.

Other non–FDA-approved tests include several commercially available PCR assays. A major limitation of PCR studies is the lack of standardized methodologies and multicenter validation of assay performance. Compared with cultures, PCR assays of various blood fractions have been shown to shorten the time to diagnosis of IC and initiation of antifungal therapy.[31,32] The pooled sensitivity and specificity of PCR for suspected IC in a recent meta-analysis were 95% and 92%, respectively.[31] In probable IC, the sensitivity of PCR and blood cultures was 85% and 38%, respectively.

In Europe, a whole-blood, multiplex real-time PCR (SeptiFast [Roche, Basel, Switzerland]) that detects 19 bacteria and 6 fungi (*C albicans, C glabrata, C parapsilosis, C tropicalis, C krusei*, and *Aspergillus fumigatus*) has been investigated in several studies of sepsis and neutropenic fever. In one study among candidemic patients, the sensitivity of the test was 94%.[33]

ANTIFUNGAL SUSCEPTIBILITY TESTING

Once an organism has been isolated, an important step in characterizing the organism is antifungal susceptibility testing. Efforts to develop standardized, reproducible, and relevant susceptibility testing methods for fungi have resulted in the development of the Clinical and Laboratory Standards Institute (CLSI) M27-A3 and the European Committee on Antimicrobial Susceptibility Testing methodologies for susceptibility testing of yeasts.[34] Interpretive break points for susceptibility take into account the minimum inhibitory concentration (MIC) as well as pharmacokinetic/pharmacodynamic data and animal model data. Break points have been established for most antifungals for the 5 most common *Candida* species (**Table 2**).[35–38] In many instances, clinical break points have decreased from those used previously. For *C glabrata*, there are no break points established for itraconazole, posaconazole, or voriconazole.

Table 2
Clinical break points for antifungal agents against common *Candida* species

| Organism | Antifungal Agent | Clinical Break Point (mcg/mL)[a] | | | |
		S	SDD	I	R
C albicans	Fluconazole	≤2	4	—	≥8
	Itraconazole	≤0.12	0.25–0.5	—	≥1
	Voriconazole	≤0.12	—	0.25–0.5	≥1
	Posaconazole	—	—	—	—
	Anidulafungin	<0.25	—	0.5	≥1
	Caspofungin	≤0.25	—	0.5	≥1
	Micafungin	≤0.25	—	0.5	≥1
C glabrata	Fluconazole	—	32	—	≥64
	Itraconazole	—	—	—	—
	Voriconazole	—	—	—	—
	Posaconazole	—	—	—	—
	Anidulafungin	≤0.12	—	0.25	≥0.5
	Caspofungin	≤0.12	—	0.25	≥0.5
	Micafungin	≤0.06	—	0.12	≥0.25
C parapsilosis	Fluconazole	≤2	4	—	≥8
	Itraconazole	—	—	—	—
	Voriconazole	≤0.12	—	0.25–0.5	≥1
	Posaconazole	—	—	—	—
	Anidulafungin	≤2	—	4	≥8
	Caspofungin	≤2	—	4	≥8
	Micafungin	≤2	—	4	≥8
C tropicalis	Fluconazole	≤2	4	—	≥8
	Itraconazole	—	—	—	—
	Voriconazole	≤0.12	—	0.25–0.5	≥1
	Posaconazole	—	—	—	—
	Anidulafungin	≤0.25	—	0.5	≥1
	Caspofungin	≤0.25	—	0.5	≥1
	Micafungin	≤0.25	—	0.5	≥1
C krusei	Fluconazole	—	—	—	—
	Itraconazole	—	—	—	—
	Voriconazole	≤0.5	—	1	≥2
	Posaconazole	—	—	—	—
	Anidulafungin	≤0.25	—	0.5	≥1
	Caspofungin	≤0.25	—	0.5	≥1
	Micafungin	≤0.25	—	0.5	≥1

Abbreviations: I, intermediate; R, resistant; S, susceptible; SDD, susceptible dose dependent.
  [a] Clinical break points adopted by the CLSI. Where no values are entered, there are insufficient data to establish clinical break points.

The susceptibility of *Candida* to the currently available antifungal agents is generally predictable if the species of the infecting isolate is known. Antifungal resistance in *C albicans* remains uncommon.[39] Recent surveillance studies suggest triazole resistance among *C glabrata* isolates has become common enough that it is difficult to rely on these agents for therapy without susceptibility testing.[9,40,41] A similar trend has begun to emerge for a smaller proportion of *C glabrata* isolates and the echinocandins.[40,42,43]

The value of susceptibility testing for other *Candida* species is less clear, although resistance among *C tropicalis* and *C parapsilosis* is increasingly reported from institutions that use antifungal agents extensively.[44,45] Because of these trends, susceptibility testing is generally recommended to guide the management of candidemia and IC.[46]

CLINICAL MANIFESTATIONS

IC is most commonly manifest as candidemia, but it can occur at virtually any anatomic site. A few syndromes compose most cases. A review of these most common syndromes in addition to less common but classic clinical manifestations follows.

Candidemia

BSI with *Candida* is the most commonly recognized form of IC, accounting for more than half of all IC cases. A positive blood culture result for *Candida* should be thoroughly investigated because of the high risk of morbidity and mortality. All-cause mortality rates are high across the age spectrum, especially associated with *Candida* sepsis, ranging from 5% to 71%.[47–53] However, most experts agree that the attributable mortality associated with candidemia is 15% to 20% in adults. Among the many clinical manifestations of IC, candidemia has been given the most attention in epidemiologic surveys and clinical trials because of its frequency, the ease of defining the disorder, and the relative ease of identifying patients for inclusion into clinical trials.[5–9,48,54–56]

CVCs and other intravascular devices are commonly implicated in candidemia; but other sources must be considered, especially among neutropenic patients in whom the gastrointestinal tract is a common source. Most experts agree that thoughtful patient-specific management of CVCs is critical in the overall management of candidemia.[57] Several researchers have demonstrated that mortality is closely linked to the timing of therapy and/or source control.[19,20,57–60] That is, earlier intervention with appropriate antifungal therapy and removal of a contaminated CVC or drainage of infected material is generally associated with better overall outcomes.[19,20,57–60]

Neonatal Candidiasis

Candida spp are the third most common pathogen associated with BSI in NICUs in the United States,[61] although the incidence has decreased dramatically over the past decade.[62–64] Neonatal candidiasis is associated with significant risk of death, neurodevelopmental impairment in extremely low-birth-weight infants who weigh 1000 g or less, and increased health care costs.[65–70] These infants are at high risk to have central nervous system (CNS) involvement as a complication of candidemia.[71,72] *C albicans* and *C parapsilosis* account for 80% to 90% of neonatal IC.[64,73]

Neonatal candidiasis differs from invasive disease in older patients in that neonates are more likely to present with nonspecific or subtle signs and symptoms of infection. Meningitis is seen frequently in association with candidemia, but approximately half of neonates with *Candida* meningitis do not have a positive blood culture.[71] CNS involvement should be assumed to be present in the neonate who has candidemia and signs and symptoms suggesting meningoencephalitis because cerebrospinal fluid (CSF) findings of *Candida* infection may be unreliable. Neurodevelopmental impairment is common in survivors; thus, careful long-term follow-up is critical.[65,67,68,70]

Acute Disseminated Candidiasis

Acute disseminated candidiasis is a life-threatening manifestation of this infection and occurs almost exclusively among patients with neutropenia who have undergone cytotoxic chemotherapy for a hematologic malignancy. Most of these patients are acutely ill, have positive blood cultures, and a characteristic diffuse, discrete hemorrhagic and papular rash consistent with small vessel vasculitis. Multiple organs may be involved; an autopsy study has demonstrated that the lungs are the most common target for metastatic infection, followed by the gastrointestinal tract, kidneys, liver, and spleen.[74]

Endovascular Infection

The chief manifestations of endovascular *Candida* infection are infective endocarditis (IE) and infection involving implantable intracardiac devices. The incidence of *Candida* endocarditis has increased concurrently with the general increase in *Candida* infections. Endocarditis should be suspected when blood cultures are persistently positive, when a patient with candidemia has persistent fever despite appropriate treatment, or when a new heart murmur, heart failure, or embolic phenomena occur in the setting of candidemia.[75] Most cases occur following cardiac valvular surgery; but other risk factors include injection drug use, cancer chemotherapy, prolonged presence of CVCs, and prior bacterial endocarditis. The signs, symptoms, and complications are generally similar to those of bacterial endocarditis, except for the frequent occurrence of large emboli to major vessels. A prospective cohort of endocarditis via the International Collaboration on Endocarditis examined the epidemiology and treatment impact of *Candida* IE and noted 59% mortality at 1 year.[76] Almost three-quarters of cases were attributed to *C parapsilosis* and *C albicans*, and approximately 50% were associated with a prosthetic valve.

There are a few case reports and a single retrospective review of *Candida* infections of pacemakers and cardiac defibrillators.[77-82] The entire device should be removed and antifungal therapy given for 4 to 6 weeks depending on whether the infection involves the wires in addition to the generator pocket.[77,79-82] Medical therapy alone is usually inadequate.[78] There are also isolated case reports of *Candida* infections involving ventricular assist devices.[83-86]

Osteomyelitis and Arthritis

Vertebral osteomyelitis, with or without discitis, is an increasingly common disorder that is usually associated with unrecognized or untreated candidemia. This disorder has been described with many of the pathogenic *Candida* species, and symptoms usually manifest several weeks to months after an episode of candidemia. The intervertebral disk and vertebral bodies are the preferred sites of involvement, with patients presenting with chronic progressively severe local back pain, usually without concomitant fever, weight loss, or other constitutional symptoms. As with other forms are vertebral osteomyelitis and discitis, there is a risk of nerve root compression syndromes including complete loss of function.

Candida bone infections can occur at a wide variety of other sites, usually as a consequence of BSI and less commonly through direct inoculation.[87] The sternum and ribs constitute a large proportion of cases.[87,88] Systemic manifestations of infection were uncommon in non-neutropenic patients, with local complaints of pain, erythema, and swelling present in nearly all patients.[87]

Candida prosthetic joint infections occur rarely as an intraoperative event or as a consequence of candidemia in patients with a preexisting prosthetic joint. Hips and knees are the most common sites of involvement. Clinical signs and symptoms are usually very indolent.

Endophthalmitis

Most cases of *Candida* endophthalmitis are endogenous, that is, as a consequence of candidemia. Endogenous infections can be manifested as isolated chorioretinitis or as chorioretinitis with extension into the vitreous, leading to vitritis.[89–92] Estimates of ocular involvement associated with candidemia have ranged as high as 37%; but more recent data suggest that this is a much less common complication, with estimates less than 20%.[93,94] *C albicans* accounts for approximately 90% of cases of endogenous endophthalmitis, but most *Candida* species have been reported.

Chronic Disseminated Candidiasis (Hepatosplenic Candidiasis)

Chronic disseminated candidiasis is seen almost exclusively among patients who have undergone myeloablative chemotherapy associated with neutropenia. On recovery from neutropenia, patients with this disorder develop low-grade fever; right upper quadrant pain, often associated with a palpable and tender liver; splenomegaly; and an elevated serum alkaline phosphatase. Imaging studies (MRI, computed tomography [CT], or abdominal ultrasound) reveal multiple focal abnormalities in the liver, spleen, kidneys, and, rarely, the lungs.[95] Parenchymal lesions develop following neutrophil recovery, suggesting that an adequate host inflammatory response is a prerequisite to the development of radiographically visible lesions, which are rarely seen during the period of neutropenia. Among patients with a history of documented candidemia, the diagnosis can be inferred from the clinical laboratory and radiographic findings. In the absence of documented candidemia, a CT-directed liver biopsy for histopathology and culture is generally recommended to establish a diagnosis.[43,95,96] Yield from blood and tissue culture tends to be poor; histopathology is generally more helpful for diagnosis.

Other

Candida has been reported as the etiologic agent of infection in virtually every visceral organ and body cavity; however, these remain relatively rare manifestations of disease. *Candida* species may cause meningitis, septic arthritis, tenosynovitis, isolated involvement of the kidney, the intra-abdominal cavity, and, rarely, pneumonia. These less common manifestations of IC are not discussed here in detail. The diagnosis of these forms of visceral candidiasis is usually based on the isolation of *Candida* species from sterilely obtained specimens. There remains little debate over whether *Candida* is a true pathogen in the peritoneum; there are clearly distinct populations whereby *Candida* contributes to poor outcomes.[97,98] *Candida* pneumonia is a rare disorder that is seen almost exclusively among severely immunocompromised patients; the isolation of *Candida* from respiratory secretions should be viewed with great skepticism unless accompanied by histopathologic evidence confirming invasive disease. Meningitis usually occurs as a complication of candidemia; but it should be considered in patients with prosthetic devices in the CNS, such as intraventricular shunts.[99,100]

TREATMENT
General Principles of Therapy

Treatment of IC is largely based on data derived from controlled clinical trials among patients with candidemia and other forms of IC. There have been no prospective studies that evaluate the treatment of less common forms of IC. Insights into the appropriate management of these patients are derived almost entirely from anecdotal experience and retrospective case series. A synopsis of the treatment recommendations based on the 2016 Infectious Diseases Society of America's guidelines for the treatment of candidiasis is included in **Table 3**.[46]

The management of IC has evolved significantly over the last 30 years, but the general principles of therapy remain the same. There are several important considerations in choosing initial antifungal therapy among patients with proven or suspected IC: What is the presumed source of Candida infection, and is it an easily removable or drainable source? What is the severity of illness? What are the comorbidities and underlying disorders? What are the dominant Candida species in this unit/location? What are the susceptibility patterns of Candida species in this particular health care setting? Is there a recent history of antifungal exposure? Is there clinical evidence to suggest involvement of the CNS, cardiac valves, liver, spleen, eyes, and/or kidneys? Is there a patient history of intolerance to specific antifungal agent?

Regardless of the choice of initial therapy for IC, specific lengths of therapy are now recommended depending on the site of involvement and, in the case of candidemia, the rapidity of clearance of Candida from the bloodstream. For patients with documented candidemia, 14 days of effective antifungal therapy following the first negative blood culture is recommended. A dilated funduscopic examination during the first week of antifungal therapy in non-neutropenic patients is recommended for all patients with documented candidemia to exclude occult ocular involvement. For neutropenic patients, this procedure should be delayed until neutrophil recovery, as the characteristic findings of ocular candidiasis are often delayed.

Echinocandins

The echinocandins (caspofungin, anidulafungin, and micafungin) demonstrate significant fungicidal activity against most Candida species; each of these agents has demonstrated success in approximately 70% to 75% of patients in randomized, comparative clinical trials.[101–106] These agents are only available as parenteral preparations.[107–109] Despite this limitation, documented superb efficacy, few drug interactions, excellent patient tolerance, and concerns about fluconazole resistance have led clinicians to favor the echinocandins as initial therapy for most adult patients with candidemia. These agents are sufficiently similar to be considered interchangeable.[105,110] The MICs of the echinocandins are low for most Candida species, including C glabrata and C krusei.[36,111,112] However, recent reports have described treatment failure associated with resistant strains of C glabrata.[43,113,114] C parapsilosis demonstrates innately higher MICs to the echinocandins compared with other Candida species, but recent data suggest this may be clinically insignificant.

Each of these agents has been studied for the treatment of IC,[102–105] and each has demonstrated efficacy in these situations. A combined analysis of 7 of the largest randomized clinical trials comparing the treatment of candidemia and IC and involving almost 2000 patients found that initial therapy with an echinocandin was a significant predictor of survival.[57]

All echinocandins have minimal adverse effects. Echinocandins achieve therapeutic concentrations in all infection sites with the exception of the eye, CNS, and urine.[115]

Table 3
Treatment of candidemia and other forms of IC therapy

Condition	Primary	Alternative	Duration	Comments
Candidemia				
Non-neutropenic adults	Caspo 70 mg loading then 50 mg/d; Mica 100 mg/d; or Anid 200 mg loading, then 100 mg/d	Flu 800 mg/d loading, then 400 mg/d	14 d after last positive blood culture and resolution of signs and symptoms	Remove all intravascular catheters, if possible.
Neonates	AmB 1.0 mg/kg/d IV; or Flu 12 mg/kg/d IV	LFAmB 3–5 mg/kg/d	14–21 d after resolution of signs and symptoms and negative repeat blood cultures	Occult CNS and other organ involvement must be ruled out. Use LFAmB with caution if urinary involvement suspected.
Neutropenia	Caspo 70 mg loading, then 50 mg/d; Mica 100 mg/d; or Anid 200 mg loading, then 100 mg/d	LFAmB 3–5 mg/kg/d or Flu 800 mg loading, then 400 mg/d	14 d after last positive blood culture and resolution of signs and symptoms and resolved neutropenia	Removal of all intravascular catheters is controversial in neutropenic patients; gastrointestinal source is common.
Chronic disseminated candidiasis	LFAmB, 3–5 mg/kg/d; or Caspo 70 mg loading, then 50 mg/d; or Mica 100 mg/d; or Anid 200 mg loading, then 100 mg/d	Flu, 6 mg/kg/d	3–6 mo and resolution or calcification of radiologic lesions	Flu may be given after 1–2 wk of LFAmB or an echinocandin if clinically stable or improved; steroids may be beneficial in those with persistent fever.

Condition				Comments
Endocarditis	LFAmB 3–5 mg/kg/d ± 5-FC 25 mg/kg po qid; or Caspo 150 mg/d; Mica 150 mg/d; Anid 200 mg/d	Flu 6–12 mg/kg/d IV/po	At least 6 wk after valve replacement	Valve replacement is almost always necessary; long-term suppression with Flu has been successful among selected patients who cannot undergo valve replacement. Consider step down to Vori or Posa for susceptible, Flu-resistant isolates.
Osteoarticular	Flu 400 mg/d or Caspo 50 mg/d; Mica 100 mg/d or Anid 100 md/d	LFAmB 3–5 mg/kg/d	6–12 mo +/– surgery	Step down therapy to Flu after at least 2 wk induction with an echinocandin or LFAmB.
Endophthalmitis	Flu 800 mg loading, then 400 mg/d; or Vori 400 mg × 2 loading, then 300 mg bid; or LFAmB 3–5 mg/kg/d	Intravitreal AmB 5–10 mcg or Vori 100 mcg	4–6 wk at least after surgery	Vitrectomy is usually performed when vitreitis is present.
Cystitis	Flu 200 mg/d; or 5-FC 25 mg/kg qid for Flu-resistant isolates	AmB 0.3–0.6 mg/kg/d	1–2 wk	Echinocandins have minimal role in cystitis. For upper tract disease, treat as for candidemia.

Abbreviations: AmB, amphotericin B; Anid, anidulafungin; Caspo, caspofungin; 5-FC, 5-fluorocytosine; Flu, fluconazole; IV, intravenously; LFAmB, lipid formulation of amphotericin B; Mica, micafungin; Posa, posaconazole; Vori, voriconazole.

None of the echinocandins require dosage adjustment for renal insufficiency or dialysis. The usual intravenous dosing regimens for IC are as follows: caspofungin, loading dose 70 mg then 50 mg daily; anidulafungin, loading dose 200 mg then 100 mg daily; and micafungin, 100 mg daily (no loading dose needed).

The emergence of echinocandin-resistant *Candida* isolates, especially *C glabrata*, has been clearly documented; this finding seems to be associated with worse clinical outcomes.[7,9,42,116–119] Fluconazole resistance is a frequent finding among echinocandin-resistant isolates,[6,48] further limiting therapeutic choices.

Triazoles

Fluconazole, itraconazole, voriconazole, posaconazole, and a new expanded spectrum triazole, isavuconazole, demonstrate similar in vitro activity against most *Candida* species.[35,36,111,112,120,121] Each of the azoles has less activity against *C glabrata* and *C krusei* than against other *Candida* species. All of the azole antifungals inhibit cytochrome P450 enzymes.[122] In earlier clinical trials, fluconazole demonstrated efficacy comparable with that of amphotericin B (AmB) deoxycholate for the treatment of candidemia.[123,124] Fluconazole is readily absorbed, with oral bioavailability resulting in concentrations equal to approximately 90% of those achieved by intravenous administration.[125] Among the triazoles, fluconazole has the greatest penetration into the CSF and vitreous, achieving concentrations of more than 70% of those in serum.[115,126–128] For this reason, it is often used in the treatment of CNS and intraocular *Candida* infections. Fluconazole achieves urine concentrations that are 10 to 20 times the concentrations in serum, thus, is the preferred treatment option for symptomatic cystitis.[115] For patients with IC, fluconazole should be administered with an average loading dose of 800 mg (12 mg/kg), followed by an average daily dose of 400 mg (6 mg/kg). A higher dose level (800 mg daily, 12 mg/kg) has been suggested for therapy for susceptible *C glabrata* infections, but this has not been validated in clinical trials.

Voriconazole is effective for IC,[129,130] but its role in the routine management of this disorder is limited. Its clinical use is generally limited to step-down oral therapy in patients with infection due to *C krusei* and fluconazole-resistant, voriconazole-susceptible *C glabrata*. It is available in oral and intravenous formulations. Following 2 loading dosages of 6 mg/kg every 12 hours, a maintenance dosage of 3 mg/kg every 12 hours is recommended. Voriconazole does not accumulate in active form in the urine and, thus, should not be used for urinary candidiasis.

Other currently available azoles offer little benefit in the management of IC. Itraconazole is only available in oral formulations. It has not been well studied for IC and is generally reserved for patients with mucosal/esophageal candidiasis who have failed fluconazole.[131] Posaconazole does not have an indication for primary therapy for IC. It demonstrates in vitro activity against *Candida* species that is similar to that of voriconazole, but clinical data are inadequate to make recommendations for the treatment of IC. Isavuconazole is a recently approved expanded spectrum triazole antifungal with excellent in vitro activity versus *Candida* spp. A recently completed international trial comparing treatment with isavuconazole or an echinocandin for IC did not meet predetermined criteria for noninferiority (Astellas US, personal communication, L Kovanda, MS, 2015); thus, it is unlikely to play an important role in management of IC.

The major role for fluconazole in the current management of IC is for step-down therapy once patients have become clinically stable following successful induction with an echinocandin. This transition usually occurs within 5 to 7 days of echinocandin therapy but is variable depending on patient response and clinician preference. Several recent open-label, noncomparative studies have examined outcomes when this strategy was used in candidemic patients. There has been no observed difference in outcomes among patients who received only an echinocandin compared with those who were switched to an oral azole.[114,132,133] From these data and other clinical trials,[102,103,105,124,130] step-down therapy to fluconazole or voriconazole is reasonable for patients who have improved clinically and have susceptible organism.

Amphotericin B Formulations

Most published experience with AmB for the treatment of IC is with the deoxycholate preparation (AmB-d). Two lipid formulations of AmB (LFAmB) have been developed and are generally available: AmB lipid complex (ABLC) and liposomal AmB. These agents possess the same spectrum of activity versus *Candida* spp as AmB-d, but daily dosing regimens and toxicity profiles differ for each agent. For most forms of IC, the typical intravenous dosage for AmB-d is 0.5 to 0.7 mg/kg daily; but dosages as high as 1 mg/kg daily may be considered for IC caused by less susceptible species, such as *C glabrata* and *C krusei*. The usual dosage for LFAmB is 3 to 5 mg/kg daily. LFAmB all have considerably less nephrotoxicity[134,135] and generally fewer infusion-related reactions than AmB-d. There are no data suggesting superior clinical efficacy of LFAmB versus AmB-d in the treatment of IC. Data demonstrating that AmB-d–induced nephrotoxicity is associated with a 6.6-fold increase in mortality have led many clinicians to use LFAmB in proven or suspected IC, especially in the ICU.[136]

EMPIRICAL THERAPY

Empirical therapy for IC in the ICU is a complex issue, and it constitutes one of the most common uses of antifungal compounds. Current strategies for initiating empirical antifungal therapy include an evaluation of risk factors and use of surrogate markers. Empirical antifungal therapy is considered in critically ill patients with risk factors for IC and no other known cause of clinical deterioration. An echinocandin is appropriate in hemodynamically unstable patients, those previously exposed to an azole, and in those colonized with azole-resistant *Candida* species.[46] There are no data guiding the appropriate duration of empirical antifungal therapy among patients who have a clinical response, but it should probably not differ from the treatment of documented candidemia. Conversely, therapy can be stopped after several days in the absence of clinical response if cultures and surrogate markers are negative.[46]

Very few clinical studies have evaluated the efficacy of empirical antifungal therapy in the ICU. In a randomized clinical trial of ICU patients at risk for IC and with unexplained fever, empirical fluconazole (800 mg daily for 14 days) was not associated with better outcomes when compared with placebo.[137] A recent study comparing caspofungin with placebo among ICU patients with signs of infection, *Candida* colonization, and clinical risk factors for IC was stopped prematurely because of poor patient accrual, confirming the difficulty in conducting these trials.

PREVENTION

For ICUs that show very high rates of IC, in excess of the expected rates of less than 5% of patients, antifungal prophylaxis may be warranted in selected patients who are at highest risk.[138] Two randomized placebo-controlled trials have shown a reduction in the incidence of IC in single units or single hospitals when fluconazole prophylaxis was used broadly in the ICU.[139,140] In a smaller study, fluconazole prophylaxis was shown to decrease *Candida* intra-abdominal infections in high-risk patients in the surgical ICU.[141] A recent multicenter placebo-controlled, blinded clinical trial of caspofungin prophylaxis targeting only those ICU patients who met specific criteria for high risk showed a trend toward reduction of IC.[142]

Several meta-analyses have demonstrated that fluconazole prophylaxis is associated with a reduction in IC,[143,144] but only one has shown a reduction in mortality from IC.[144] A Cochrane analysis confirms the importance of targeted prophylaxis in high-risk patients.[145]

REFERENCES

1. Magill SS, Edwards JR, Bamberg W, et al. Multistate point-prevalence survey of health care-associated infections. N Engl J Med 2014;370(13):1198–208.
2. Pittet D, Monod M, Suter PM, et al. Candida colonization and subsequent infections in critically ill surgical patients. Ann Surg 1994;220(6):751–8.
3. Blumberg HM, Jarvis WR, Soucie JM, et al. Risk factors for candidal bloodstream infections in surgical intensive care unit patients: the NEMIS prospective multicenter study. The National Epidemiology of Mycosis Survey. Clin Infect Dis 2001;33(2):177–86.
4. Cleveland AA, Harrison LH, Farley MM, et al. Declining incidence of candidemia and the shifting epidemiology of Candida resistance in two US metropolitan areas, 2008-2013: results from population-based surveillance. PLoS One 2015;10(3):e0120452.
5. Pfaller M, Neofytos D, Diekema D, et al. Epidemiology and outcomes of candidemia in 3648 patients: data from the Prospective Antifungal Therapy (PATH Alliance(R)) registry, 2004-2008. Diagn Microbiol Infect Dis 2012;74(4):323–31.
6. Diekema D, Arbefeville S, Boyken L, et al. The changing epidemiology of healthcare-associated candidemia over three decades. Diagn Microbiol Infect Dis 2012;73(1):45–8.
7. Pfaller MA, Messer SA, Moet GJ, et al. Candida bloodstream infections: comparison of species distribution and resistance to echinocandin and azole antifungal agents in Intensive Care Unit (ICU) and non-ICU settings in the SENTRY Antimicrobial Surveillance Program (2008-2009). Int J Antimicrob Agents 2011;38(1):65–9.
8. Pfaller MA, Moet GJ, Messer SA, et al. Candida bloodstream infections: comparison of species distributions and antifungal resistance patterns in community-onset and nosocomial isolates in the SENTRY Antimicrobial Surveillance Program, 2008-2009. Antimicrob Agents Chemother 2011;55(2):561–6.
9. Pfaller MA, Moet GJ, Messer SA, et al. Geographic variations in species distribution and echinocandin and azole antifungal resistance rates among Candida bloodstream infection isolates: report from the SENTRY Antimicrobial Surveillance Program (2008 to 2009). J Clin Microbiol 2011;49(1):396–9.
10. Matsumoto E, Boyken L, Tendolkar S, et al. Candidemia surveillance in Iowa: emergence of echinocandin resistance. Diagn Microbiol Infect Dis 2014;79(2): 205–8.
11. Mayer FL, Wilson D, Hube B. Candida albicans pathogenicity mechanisms. Virulence 2013;4(2):119–28.
12. Saville SP, Lazzell AL, Chaturvedi AK, et al. Use of a genetically engineered strain to evaluate the pathogenic potential of yeast cell and filamentous forms during Candida albicans systemic infection in immunodeficient mice. Infect Immun 2008;76(1):97–102.
13. LaFleur MD, Kumamoto CA, Lewis K. Candida albicans biofilms produce antifungal-tolerant persister cells. Antimicrob Agents Chemother 2006;50(11): 3839–46.
14. Ramage G, Rajendran R, Sherry L, et al. Fungal biofilm resistance. Int J Microbiol 2012;2012:528521.

15. Al-Fattani MA, Douglas LJ. Penetration of Candida biofilms by antifungal agents. Antimicrob Agents Chemother 2004;48(9):3291–7.
16. Shin JH, Kee SJ, Shin MG, et al. Biofilm production by isolates of Candida species recovered from nonneutropenic patients: comparison of blood-stream isolates with isolates from other sources. J Clin Microbiol 2002; 40(4):1244–8.
17. Gow NA, van de Veerdonk FL, Brown AJ, et al. Candida albicans morphogenesis and host defence: discriminating invasion from colonization. Nat Rev Microbiol 2012;10(2):112–22.
18. Clancy CJ, Nguyen MH. Finding the "missing 50%" of invasive candidiasis: how nonculture diagnostics will improve understanding of disease spectrum and transform patient care. Clin Infect Dis 2013;56(9):1284–92.
19. Garey KW, Rege M, Pai MP, et al. Time to initiation of fluconazole therapy impacts mortality in patients with candidemia: a multi-institutional study. Clin Infect Dis 2006;43(1):25–31.
20. Morrell M, Fraser VJ, Kollef MH. Delaying the empiric treatment of candida bloodstream infection until positive blood culture results are obtained: a potential risk factor for hospital mortality. Antimicrob Agents Chemother 2005;49(9): 3640–5.
21. Lacroix C, Gicquel A, Sendid B, et al. Evaluation of two matrix-assisted laser desorption ionization-time of flight mass spectrometry (MALDI-TOF MS) systems for the identification of Candida species. Clin Microbiol Infect 2014; 20(2):153–8.
22. Tan KE, Ellis BC, Lee R, et al. Prospective evaluation of a matrix-assisted laser desorption ionization-time of flight mass spectrometry system in a hospital clinical microbiology laboratory for identification of bacteria and yeasts: a bench-by-bench study for assessing the impact on time to identification and cost-effectiveness. J Clin Microbiol 2012;50(10):3301–8.
23. Marklein G, Josten M, Klanke U, et al. Matrix-assisted laser desorption ionization-time of flight mass spectrometry for fast and reliable identification of clinical yeast isolates. J Clin Microbiol 2009;47(9):2912–7.
24. Wilson DA, Joyce MJ, Hall LS, et al. Multicenter evaluation of a Candida albicans peptide nucleic acid fluorescent in situ hybridization probe for characterization of yeast isolates from blood cultures. J Clin Microbiol 2005;43(6): 2909–12.
25. Hall L, Le Febre KM, Deml SM, et al. Evaluation of the Yeast Traffic Light PNA FISH probes for identification of Candida species from positive blood cultures. J Clin Microbiol 2012;50(4):1446–8.
26. Karageorgopoulos DE, Vouloumanou EK, Ntziora F, et al. beta-D-glucan assay for the diagnosis of invasive fungal infections: a meta-analysis. Clin Infect Dis 2011;52(6):750–70.
27. Lu Y, Chen YQ, Guo YL, et al. Diagnosis of invasive fungal disease using serum $(1{\rightarrow}3)$-beta-D-glucan: a bivariate meta-analysis. Intern Med 2011;50(22): 2783–91.
28. Onishi A, Sugiyama D, Kogata Y, et al. Diagnostic accuracy of serum 1,3-beta-D-glucan for pneumocystis jiroveci pneumonia, invasive candidiasis, and invasive aspergillosis: systematic review and meta-analysis. J Clin Microbiol 2012; 50(1):7–15.
29. Neely LA, Audeh M, Phung NA, et al. T2 magnetic resonance enables nanoparticle-mediated rapid detection of candidemia in whole blood. Sci Transl Med 2013;5(182):182ra154.

30. Mylonakis E, Clancy CJ, Ostrosky-Zeichner L, et al. T2 magnetic resonance assay for the rapid diagnosis of candidemia in whole blood: a clinical trial. Clin Infect Dis 2015;60(6):892–9.
31. Avni T, Leibovici L, Paul M. PCR diagnosis of invasive candidiasis: systematic review and meta-analysis. J Clin Microbiol 2011;49(2):665–70.
32. McMullan R, Metwally L, Coyle PV, et al. A prospective clinical trial of a real-time polymerase chain reaction assay for the diagnosis of candidemia in nonneutropenic, critically ill adults. Clin Infect Dis 2008;46(6):890–6.
33. Lucignano B, Ranno S, Liesenfeld O, et al. Multiplex PCR allows rapid and accurate diagnosis of bloodstream infections in newborns and children with suspected sepsis. J Clin Microbiol 2011;49(6):2252–8.
34. Clinical and Laboratory Standards Institute, Reference method for broth dilution antifungal susceptibility testing of yeasts (monograph). 3rd informational supplement. 2008.
35. Pfaller MA, Andes D, Arendrup MC, et al. Clinical breakpoints for voriconazole and Candida spp. revisited: review of microbiologic, molecular, pharmacodynamic, and clinical data as they pertain to the development of species-specific interpretive criteria. Diagn Microbiol Infect Dis 2011;70(3):330–43.
36. Pfaller MA, Castanheira M, Diekema DJ, et al. Triazole and echinocandin MIC distributions with epidemiological cutoff values for differentiation of wild-type strains from non-wild-type strains of six uncommon species of Candida. J Clin Microbiol 2011;49(11):3800–4.
37. Pfaller MA, Espinel-Ingroff A, Canton E, et al. Wild-type MIC distributions and epidemiological cutoff values for amphotericin B, flucytosine, and itraconazole and Candida spp. as determined by CLSI broth microdilution. J Clin Microbiol 2012;50(6):2040–6.
38. Pfaller MA, Diekema DJ, Andes D, et al. Clinical breakpoints for the echinocandins and Candida revisited: integration of molecular, clinical, and microbiological data to arrive at species-specific interpretive criteria. Drug Resist Updat 2011;14(3):164–76.
39. Pfaller MA, Diekema DJ, Sheehan DJ. Interpretive breakpoints for fluconazole and Candida revisited: a blueprint for the future of antifungal susceptibility testing. Clin Microbiol Rev 2006;19(2):435–47.
40. Pfaller MA, Castanheira M, Lockhart SR, et al. Frequency of decreased susceptibility and resistance to echinocandins among fluconazole-resistant bloodstream isolates of Candida glabrata. J Clin Microbiol 2012;50(4): 1199–203.
41. Pfaller MA, Castanheira M, Messer SA, et al. Variation in Candida spp. distribution and antifungal resistance rates among bloodstream infection isolates by patient age: report from the SENTRY Antimicrobial Surveillance Program (2008-2009). Diagn Microbiol Infect Dis 2010;68(3):278–83.
42. Alexander BD, Johnson MD, Pfeiffer CD, et al. Increasing echinocandin resistance in Candida glabrata: clinical failure correlates with presence of FKS mutations and elevated minimum inhibitory concentrations. Clin Infect Dis 2013; 56(12):1724–32.
43. Dannaoui E, Desnos-Ollivier M, Garcia-Hermoso D, et al. Candida spp. with acquired echinocandin resistance, France, 2004-2010. Emerg Infect Dis 2012; 18(1):86–90.
44. Ben-Ami R, Olshtain-Pops K, Krieger M, et al. Antibiotic exposure as a risk factor for fluconazole-resistant Candida bloodstream infection. Antimicrob Agents Chemother 2012;56(5):2518–23.

45. Oxman DA, Chow JK, Frendl G, et al. Candidaemia associated with decreased in vitro fluconazole susceptibility: is Candida speciation predictive of the susceptibility pattern? J Antimicrob Chemother 2010;65(7):1460–5.

46. Pappas PG, Kauffman CA, Andes D, et al. Clinical practice guideline for the management of candidiasis: 2015 update by the Infectious Diseases Society of America. Clin Infect Dis 2015, in press.

47. Bassetti M, Righi E, Ansaldi F, et al. A multicenter study of septic shock due to candidemia: outcomes and predictors of mortality. Intensive Care Med 2014; 40(6):839–45.

48. Pappas PG, Rex JH, Lee J, et al. A prospective observational study of candidemia: epidemiology, therapy, and influences on mortality in hospitalized adult and pediatric patients. Clin Infect Dis 2003;37(5):634–43.

49. Zaoutis TE, Argon J, Chu J, et al. The epidemiology and attributable outcomes of candidemia in adults and children hospitalized in the United States: a propensity analysis. Clin Infect Dis 2005;41(9):1232–9.

50. Pien BC, Sundaram P, Raoof N, et al. The clinical and prognostic importance of positive blood cultures in adults. Am J Med 2010;123(9):819–28.

51. Horn DL, Ostrosky-Zeichner L, Morris MI, et al. Factors related to survival and treatment success in invasive candidiasis or candidemia: a pooled analysis of two large, prospective, micafungin trials. Eur J Clin Microbiol Infect Dis 2010; 29(2):223–9.

52. Hassan I, Powell G, Sidhu M, et al. Excess mortality, length of stay and cost attributable to candidaemia. J Infect 2009;59(5):360–5.

53. Falagas ME, Apostolou KE, Pappas VD. Attributable mortality of candidemia: a systematic review of matched cohort and case-control studies. Eur J Clin Microbiol Infect Dis 2006;25(7):419–25.

54. Wisplinghoff H, Bischoff T, Tallent SM, et al. Nosocomial bloodstream infections in US hospitals: analysis of 24,179 cases from a prospective nationwide surveillance study. Clin Infect Dis 2004;39(3):309–17.

55. Gudlaugsson O, Gillespie S, Lee K, et al. Attributable mortality of nosocomial candidemia, revisited. Clin Infect Dis 2003;37(9):1172–7.

56. Morgan J, Meltzer MI, Plikaytis BD, et al. Excess mortality, hospital stay, and cost due to candidemia: a case-control study using data from population-based candidemia surveillance. Infect Control Hosp Epidemiol 2005;26(6): 540–7.

57. Andes DR, Safdar N, Baddley JW, et al. Impact of treatment strategy on outcomes in patients with candidemia and other forms of invasive candidiasis: a patient-level quantitative review of randomized trials. Clin Infect Dis 2012; 54(8):1110–22.

58. Kollef M, Micek S, Hampton N, et al. Septic shock attributed to Candida infection: importance of empiric therapy and source control. Clin Infect Dis 2012; 54(12):1739–46.

59. Grim SA, Berger K, Teng C, et al. Timing of susceptibility-based antifungal drug administration in patients with Candida bloodstream infection: correlation with outcomes. J Antimicrob Chemother 2012;67(3):707–14.

60. Ostrosky-Zeichner L, Kullberg BJ, Bow EJ, et al. Early treatment of candidemia in adults: a review. Med Mycol 2011;49(2):113–20.

61. Hocevar SN, Edwards JR, Horan TC, et al. Device-associated infections among neonatal intensive care unit patients: incidence and associated pathogens reported to the National Healthcare Safety Network, 2006-2008. Infect Control Hosp Epidemiol 2012;33(12):1200–6.

62. Aliaga S, Clark RH, Laughon M, et al. Changes in the incidence of candidiasis in neonatal intensive care units. Pediatrics 2014;133(2):236–42.
63. Fisher BT, Ross RK, Localio AR, et al. Decreasing rates of invasive candidiasis in pediatric hospitals across the United States. Clin Infect Dis 2014;58(1):74–7.
64. Chitnis AS, Magill SS, Edwards JR, et al. Trends in Candida central line-associated bloodstream infections among NICUs, 1999-2009. Pediatrics 2012; 130(1):e46–52.
65. Benjamin DK Jr, Stoll BJ, Fanaroff AA, et al. Neonatal candidiasis among extremely low birth weight infants: risk factors, mortality rates, and neurodevelopmental outcomes at 18 to 22 months. Pediatrics 2006;117(1):84–92.
66. Zaoutis TE, Heydon K, Localio R, et al. Outcomes attributable to neonatal candidiasis. Clin Infect Dis 2007;44(9):1187–93.
67. Wynn JL, Tan S, Gantz MG, et al. Outcomes following candiduria in extremely low birth weight infants. Clin Infect Dis 2012;54(3):331–9.
68. Stoll BJ, Hansen NI, Adams-Chapman I, et al. Neurodevelopmental and growth impairment among extremely low-birth-weight infants with neonatal infection. JAMA 2004;292(19):2357–65.
69. Smith PB, Morgan J, Benjamin JD, et al. Excess costs of hospital care associated with neonatal candidemia. Pediatr Infect Dis J 2007;26(3):197–200.
70. Benjamin DK Jr, Smith PB, Arrieta A, et al. Safety and pharmacokinetics of repeat-dose micafungin in young infants. Clin Pharmacol Ther 2010;87(1):93–9.
71. Cohen-Wolkowiez M, Smith PB, Mangum B, et al. Neonatal Candida meningitis: significance of cerebrospinal fluid parameters and blood cultures. J Perinatol 2007;27(2):97–100.
72. Fernandez M, Moylett EH, Noyola DE, et al. Candidal meningitis in neonates: a 10-year review. Clin Infect Dis 2000;31(2):458–63.
73. Steinbach WJ, Roilides E, Berman D, et al. Results from a prospective, international, epidemiologic study of invasive candidiasis in children and neonates. Pediatr Infect Dis J 2012;31(12):1252–7.
74. Lewis RE, Cahyame-Zuniga L, Leventakos K, et al. Epidemiology and sites of involvement of invasive fungal infections in patients with haematological malignancies: a 20-year autopsy study. Mycoses 2013;56(6):638–45.
75. Card L, Lofland D. Candidal endocarditis presenting with bilateral lower limb ischemia. Clin Lab Sci 2012;25(3):130–4.
76. Arnold CJ, Johnson M, Bayer AS, et al. Candida infective endocarditis: an observational cohort study with a focus on therapy. Antimicrob Agents Chemother 2015;59(4):2365–73.
77. Joly V, Belmatoug N, Leperre A, et al. Pacemaker endocarditis due to Candida albicans: case report and review. Clin Infect Dis 1997;25(6):1359–62.
78. Roger PM, Boissy C, Gari-Toussaint M, et al. Medical treatment of a pacemaker endocarditis due to Candida albicans and to Candida glabrata. J Infect 2000; 41(2):176–8.
79. Tascini C, Bongiorni MG, Tagliaferri E, et al. Micafungin for Candida albicans pacemaker-associated endocarditis: a case report and review of the literature. Mycopathologia 2013;175(1–2):129–34.
80. Brown LA, Baddley JW, Sanchez JE, et al. Implantable cardioverter-defibrillator endocarditis secondary to Candida albicans. Am J Med Sci 2001;322(3):160–2.
81. Hindupur S, Muslin AJ. Septic shock induced from an implantable cardioverter-defibrillator lead-associated Candida albicans vegetation. J Interv Card Electrophysiol 2005;14(1):55–9.

82. Halawa A, Henry PD, Sarubbi FA. Candida endocarditis associated with cardiac rhythm management devices: review with current treatment guidelines. Mycoses 2011;54(4):e168–74.
83. Bagdasarian NG, Malani AN, Pagani FD, et al. Fungemia associated with left ventricular assist device support. J Cardiovasc Surg 2009;24(6):763–5.
84. Shoham S, Shaffer R, Sweet L, et al. Candidemia in patients with ventricular assist devices. Clin Infect Dis 2007;44(2):e9–12.
85. Aslam S, Hernandez M, Thornby J, et al. Risk factors and outcomes of fungal ventricular-assist device infections. Clin Infect Dis 2010;50(5):664–71.
86. Cabrera AG, Khan MS, Morales DL, et al. Infectious complications and outcomes in children supported with left ventricular assist devices. J Heart Lung Transplant 2013;32(5):518–24.
87. Gamaletsou MN, Kontoyiannis DP, Sipsas NV, et al. Candida osteomyelitis: analysis of 207 pediatric and adult cases (1970-2011). Clin Infect Dis 2012;55(10):1338–51.
88. Slenker AK, Keith SW, Horn DL. Two hundred and eleven cases of Candida osteomyelitis: 17 case reports and a review of the literature. Diagn Microbiol Infect Dis 2012;73(1):89–93.
89. Binder MI, Chua J, Kaiser PK, et al. Endogenous endophthalmitis: an 18-year review of culture-positive cases at a tertiary care center. Medicine (Baltimore) 2003;82(2):97–105.
90. Lingappan A, Wykoff CC, Albini TA, et al. Endogenous fungal endophthalmitis: causative organisms, management strategies, and visual acuity outcomes. Am J Ophthalmol 2012;153(1):162–6.
91. Shah CP, McKey J, Spirn MJ, et al. Ocular candidiasis: a review. Br J Ophthalmol 2008;92(4):466–8.
92. Khan FA, Slain D, Khakoo RA. Candida endophthalmitis: focus on current and future antifungal treatment options. Pharmacotherapy 2007;27(12):1711–21.
93. Oude Lashof AM, Rothova A, Sobel JD, et al. Ocular manifestations of candidemia. Clin Infect Dis 2011;53(3):262–8.
94. Brooks RG. Prospective study of Candida endophthalmitis in hospitalized patients with candidemia. Arch Intern Med 1989;149(10):2226–8.
95. Rammaert B, Desjardins A, Lortholary O. New insights into hepatosplenic candidosis, a manifestation of chronic disseminated candidosis. Mycoses 2012; 55(3):e74–84.
96. Sallah S, Semelka RC, Wehbie R, et al. Hepatosplenic candidiasis in patients with acute leukaemia. Br J Haematol 1999;106(3):697–701.
97. Montravers P, Dupont H, Gauzit R, et al. Candida as a risk factor for mortality in peritonitis. Crit Care Med 2006;34(3):646–52.
98. Rex JH. Candida in the peritoneum: passenger or pathogen? Crit Care Med 2006;34(3):902–3.
99. O'Brien D, Stevens NT, Lim CH, et al. Candida infection of the central nervous system following neurosurgery: a 12-year review. Acta Neurochir 2011;153(6): 1347–50.
100. Bagheri F, Cervellione KL, Maruf M, et al. Candida parapsilosis meningitis associated with shunt infection in an adult male. Clin Neurol Neurosurg 2010;112(3): 248–51.
101. Krause DS, Simjee AE, van Rensburg C, et al. A randomized, double-blind trial of anidulafungin versus fluconazole for the treatment of esophageal candidiasis. Clin Infect Dis 2004;39(6):770–5.
102. Mora-Duarte J, Betts R, Rotstein C, et al. Comparison of caspofungin and amphotericin B for invasive candidiasis. N Engl J Med 2002;347(25):2020–9.

103. Kuse ER, Chetchotisakd P, da Cunha CA, et al. Micafungin versus liposomal amphotericin B for candidaemia and invasive candidosis: a phase III randomised double-blind trial. Lancet 2007;369(9572):1519–27.
104. Reboli AC, Shorr AF, Rotstein C, et al. Anidulafungin compared with fluconazole for treatment of candidemia and other forms of invasive candidiasis caused by Candida albicans: a multivariate analysis of factors associated with improved outcome. BMC Infect Dis 2011;11:261.
105. Pappas PG, Rotstein CM, Betts RF, et al. Micafungin versus caspofungin for treatment of candidemia and other forms of invasive candidiasis. Clin Infect Dis 2007;45(7):883–93.
106. Betts RF, Nucci M, Talwar D, et al. A multicenter, double-blind trial of a high-dose caspofungin treatment regimen versus a standard caspofungin treatment regimen for adult patients with invasive candidiasis. Clin Infect Dis 2009; 48(12):1676–84.
107. Chandrasekar PH, Sobel JD. Micafungin: a new echinocandin. Clin Infect Dis 2006;42(8):1171–8.
108. Deresinski SC, Stevens DA. Caspofungin. Clin Infect Dis 2003;36(11):1445–57.
109. Vazquez JA, Sobel JD. Anidulafungin: a novel echinocandin. Clin Infect Dis 2006;43(2):215–22.
110. Kohno S, Izumikawa K, Yoshida M, et al. A double-blind comparative study of the safety and efficacy of caspofungin versus micafungin in the treatment of candidiasis and aspergillosis. Eur J Clin Microbiol Infect Dis 2013;32(3):387–97.
111. Pfaller MA, Boyken L, Hollis RJ, et al. In vitro susceptibility of invasive isolates of Candida spp. to anidulafungin, caspofungin, and micafungin: six years of global surveillance. J Clin Microbiol 2008;46(1):150–6.
112. Pfaller MA, Boyken L, Hollis RJ, et al. Wild-type MIC distributions and epidemiological cutoff values for the echinocandins and Candida spp. J Clin Microbiol 2010;48(1):52–6.
113. Shields RK, Nguyen MH, Press EG, et al. Anidulafungin and micafungin MIC breakpoints are superior to that of caspofungin for identifying FKS mutant Candida glabrata strains and echinocandin resistance. Antimicrob Agents Chemother 2013;57(12):6361–5.
114. Vazquez J, Reboli AC, Pappas PG, et al. Evaluation of an early step-down strategy from intravenous anidulafungin to oral azole therapy for the treatment of candidemia and other forms of invasive candidiasis: results from an open-label trial. BMC Infect Dis 2014;14:97.
115. Dodds Ashley ES, Lewis R, Lewis JS, et al. Pharmacology of systemic antifungal agents. Clin Infect Dis 2006;43:S28–39.
116. Lewis JS 2nd, Wiederhold NP, Wickes BL, et al. Rapid emergence of echinocandin resistance in Candida glabrata resulting in clinical and microbiologic failure. Antimicrob Agents Chemother 2013;57(9):4559–61.
117. Castanheira M, Woosley LN, Messer SA, et al. Frequency of FKS mutations among Candida glabrata isolates from a 10-year global collection of bloodstream infection isolates. Antimicrob Agents Chemother 2014;58(1):577–80.
118. Shields RK, Nguyen MH, Press EG, et al. Caspofungin MICs correlate with treatment outcomes among patients with Candida glabrata invasive candidiasis and prior echinocandin exposure. Antimicrob Agents Chemother 2013;57(8): 3528–35.
119. Beyda ND, Lewis RE, Garey KW. Echinocandin resistance in Candida species: mechanisms of reduced susceptibility and therapeutic approaches. Ann Pharmacother 2012;46(7–8):1086–96.

120. Pfaller MA, Andes D, Diekema DJ, et al. Wild-type MIC distributions, epidemiological cutoff values and species-specific clinical breakpoints for fluconazole and Candida: time for harmonization of CLSI and EUCAST broth microdilution methods. Drug Resist Updat 2010;13(6):180–95.

121. Pfaller MA, Castanheira M, Messer SA, et al. Echinocandin and triazole antifungal susceptibility profiles for Candida spp., Cryptococcus neoformans, and Aspergillus fumigatus: application of new CLSI clinical breakpoints and epidemiologic cutoff values to characterize resistance in the SENTRY Antimicrobial Surveillance Program (2009). Diagn Microbiol Infect Dis 2011;69(1): 45–50.

122. Bruggemann RJ, Alffenaar JW, Blijlevens NM, et al. Clinical relevance of the pharmacokinetic interactions of azole antifungal drugs with other coadministered agents. Clin Infect Dis 2009;48(10):1441–58.

123. Rex JH, Bennett JE, Sugar AM, et al. A randomized trial comparing fluconazole with amphotericin B for the treatment of candidemia in patients without neutropenia. Candidemia Study Group and the National Institute. N Engl J Med 1994; 331(20):1325–30.

124. Rex JH, Pappas PG, Karchmer AW, et al. A randomized and blinded multicenter trial of high-dose fluconazole plus placebo versus fluconazole plus amphotericin B as therapy for candidemia and its consequences in nonneutropenic subjects. Clin Infect Dis 2003;36(10):1221–8.

125. Zimmermann T, Yeates RA, Laufen H, et al. Influence of concomitant food intake on the oral absorption of two triazole antifungal agents, itraconazole and fluconazole. Eur J Clin Pharmacol 1994;46(2):147–50.

126. Thaler F, Bernard B, Tod M, et al. Fluconazole penetration in cerebral parenchyma in humans at steady state. Antimicrob Agents Chemother 1995;39(5): 1154–6.

127. Tod M, Lortholary O, Padoin And C. Intravitreous penetration of fluconazole during endophthalmitis. Clin Microbiol Infect 1997;3(3):379A.

128. Tucker RM, Williams PL, Arathoon EG, et al. Pharmacokinetics of fluconazole in cerebrospinal fluid and serum in human coccidioidal meningitis. Antimicrob Agents Chemother 1988;32(3):369–73.

129. Ally R, Schurmann D, Kreisel W, et al. A randomized, double-blind, double-dummy, multicenter trial of voriconazole and fluconazole in the treatment of esophageal candidiasis in immunocompromised patients. Clin Infect Dis 2001;33(9):1447–54.

130. Kullberg BJ, Sobel JD, Ruhnke M, et al. Voriconazole versus a regimen of amphotericin B followed by fluconazole for candidaemia in non-neutropenic patients: a randomised non-inferiority trial. Lancet 2005;366(9495):1435–42.

131. Eichel M, Just-Nubling G, Helm EB, et al. [Itraconazole suspension in the treatment of HIV-infected patients with fluconazole-resistant oropharyngeal candidiasis and esophagitis]. Mycoses 1996;39(Suppl 1):102–6.

132. Nucci M, Colombo AL, Petti M, et al. An open-label study of anidulafungin for the treatment of candidaemia/invasive candidiasis in Latin America. Mycoses 2014; 57(1):12–8.

133. Mootsikapun P, Hsueh PR, Talwar D, et al. Intravenous anidulafungin followed optionally by oral voriconazole for the treatment of candidemia in Asian patients: results from an open-label phase III trial. BMC Infect Dis 2013;13:219.

134. Safdar A, Ma J, Saliba F, et al. Drug-induced nephrotoxicity caused by amphotericin B lipid complex and liposomal amphotericin B: a review and meta-analysis. Medicine (Baltimore) 2010;89(4):236–44.

135. Walsh TJ, Hiemenz JW, Seibel NL, et al. Amphotericin B lipid complex for invasive fungal infections: analysis of safety and efficacy in 556 cases. Clin Infect Dis 1998;26(6):1383–96.
136. Bates DW, Su L, Yu DT, et al. Mortality and costs of acute renal failure associated with amphotericin B therapy. Clin Infect Dis 2001;32(5):686–93.
137. Schuster MG, Edwards JE Jr, Sobel JD, et al. Empirical fluconazole versus placebo for intensive care unit patients: a randomized trial. Ann Intern Med 2008; 149(2):83–90.
138. Ostrosky-Zeichner L. Prophylaxis or preemptive therapy of invasive candidiasis in the intensive care unit? Crit Care Med 2004;32(12):2552–3.
139. Pelz RK, Hendrix CW, Swoboda SM, et al. Double-blind placebo controlled trial of prophylactic fluconazole to prevent Candida infcetions in critically ill surgical patients. Ann Surg 2001;233:542–8.
140. Garbino J, Lew DP, Romand JA, et al. Prevention of severe Candida infections in nonneutropenic, high-risk, critically ill patients: a randomized, double-blind, placebo-controlled trial in patients treated by selective digestive decontamination. Intensive Care Med 2002;28(12):1708–17.
141. Eggimann P, Francioli P, Bille J, et al. Fluconazole prophylaxis prevents intraabdominal candidiasis in high-risk surgical patients. Crit Care Med 1999; 27(6):1066–72.
142. Ostrosky-Zeichner L, Shoham S, Vazquez J, et al. MSG-01: A randomized, double-blind, placebo-controlled trial of caspofungin prophylaxis followed by preemptive therapy for invasive candidiasis in high-risk adults in the critical care setting. Clin Infect Dis 2014;58(9):1219–26.
143. Vardakas KZ, Samonis G, Michalopoulos A, et al. Antifungal prophylaxis with azoles in high-risk, surgical intensive care unit patients: a meta-analysis of randomized, placebo-controlled trials. Crit Care Med 2006;34(4):1216–24.
144. Cruciani M, de Lalla F, Mengoli C. Prophylaxis of Candida infections in adult trauma and surgical intensive care patients: a systematic review and meta-analysis. Intensive Care Med 2005;31(11):1479–87.
145. Playford E, Webster A, Sorrell T. Antifungal agents for preventing fungal infections in non-neutropenic critically ill patients. Cochrane Database Syst Rev 2001;(1):CD004920.

Invasive Aspergillosis

Current Strategies for Diagnosis and Management

Jose Cadena, MD[a], George R. Thompson III, MD[b],
Thomas F. Patterson, MD[a],*

KEYWORDS

- Aspergillosis • Invasive pulmonary aspergillosis • Resistance
- Chronic cavitary aspergillosis • Aspergilloma

KEY POINTS

- Invasive aspergillosis remains a major cause of morbidity and mortality in immunosuppressed hosts.
- Laboratory confirmation of invasive aspergillosis remains a priority to help direct therapy and to evaluate for possible antifungal resistance.
- Voriconazole remains the recommended therapy for patients with invasive aspergillosis.
- New antifungal agents including new drugs like isavuconazole and new formulations of posaconazole offer the potential for improved outcome in patients with invasive aspergillosis.
- The role of combination therapy remains controversial but can be considered in high risk patients like those with hematological malignancy and severe disease.
- Prophylaxis may improve outcome in highest risk patients.

INTRODUCTION

The spectrum of aspergillosis encompasses a broad range of clinical entities, from noninvasive forms, such as allergic bronchopulmonary aspergillosis (ABPA) and chronic pulmonary aspergillosis syndromes, to invasive pulmonary aspergillosis (IPA) with possible widespread dissemination (**Fig. 1**).[1,2]

[a] Division of Infectious Diseases, Department of Medicine, The University of Texas Health Science Center and South Texas Veterans Health Care System, 7703 Floyd Curl Drive, San Antonio, TX 78229-3900, USA; [b] Division of Infectious Diseases, Department of Internal Medicine, University of California - Davis, 1 Shields Avenue, Tupper Hall, Room 3146, Davis, CA, USA
* Corresponding author. Division of Infectious Diseases, Department of Medicine, University of Texas Health Science Center San Antonio, 7703 Floyd Curl Drive, MSC 7881, San Antonio, TX 78229-3900.
E-mail address: patterson@uthscsa.edu

Infect Dis Clin N Am 30 (2016) 125–142
http://dx.doi.org/10.1016/j.idc.2015.10.015
0891-5520/16/$ — see front matter Published by Elsevier Inc.

id.theclinics.com

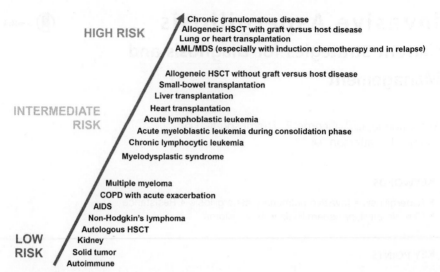

Fig. 1. Spectrum of risk for IA. (*Data from* Pagano L, Akova M, Dimopoulos G, et al. Risk assessment and prognostic factors for mould-related diseases in immunocompromised patients. J Antimicrob Chemother 2011;66(Suppl 1):i5–14.)

Although most frequently affecting the lungs, aspergillosis can develop within virtually any organ system and disseminated disease is particularly common among patients with prolonged granulocytopenia following chemotherapy.

Despite advances in the diagnosis and treatment of invasive aspergillosis (IA), mortality rates remain high, especially in the immunosuppressed host. During the past decade, triazole resistance has emerged in some regions of the world and is particularly concerning for management given the limited options to treat azole-resistant infections and the possibility that this may led to failure of prophylaxis in immunocompromised hosts. Cryptic species of *Aspergillus*, strains that are difficult to identify morphologically, have also become increasingly important given the higher azole antifungal minimum inhibitory concentrations (MICs) of some of these species, the difficulty in differentiating these organisms on phenotypic appearance alone, and the uncertain clinical outcomes and therapeutic challenges they represent.

Despite these challenges, new diagnostic methods and antifungal agents have emerged in attempts to further reduce mortality from IPA. These newer agents possess potential advantages compared with existing agents, such as improved bioavailability (posaconazole tablets) and reduced toxicity (isavuconazole). These additions to the therapeutic armamentarium have been welcomed and provide clinicians with additional options during treatment.

MYCOLOGY AND EPIDEMIOLOGY

There are more than 250 species of *Aspergillus*, with several subgenera and multiple sections (previously known as groups).[3,4] The most common species isolated in cases of invasive disease are *A fumigatus*, followed by *A flavus*, *A terreus*, and *A niger* (**Table 1**).[5] Additional species have also been implicated in infection of severely immunocompromised patients. In most cases, identification to the genus level is not difficult; however, when poorly sporulating isolates are observed, identification even to the species complex level may be challenging.[6] Most species of *Aspergillus* reproduce

Table 1
Frequency of *Aspergillus* spp received in a fungal reference laboratory

A fumigatus	57%
A flavus	12%
A niger	10%
A terreus	12%
Others	9%
A nidulans	2%
A calidoustus	2%
A sydowii	2%
A versicolor	2%

From Sutton DA, Fothergill AW, Rinaldi MG. *Aspergillus* in vitro antifungal susceptibility data: new millennium trends. In: Abstracts of advances against aspergillosis. San Francisco (CA), September 9–11, 2004. [abstract: 16].

asexually but some species may have a teleomorph (sexual) form. Despite the identification of anamorph or teleomorph stages, the term *Aspergillus* is most commonly used under the convention of one fungus, one name.[7–9]

Investigators have found cryptic *Aspergillus* species that are morphologically indistinguishable from the main *Aspergillus* sections. However, many of these species have been shown to possess elevated triazole MICs.[10] Identification of these organisms is based on molecular methods such as sequencing of the internal transcriber spacer region, beta-tubulin, calmodulin, and actin genes.[11] The description of cryptic species began with *A lentulus*, which was found to be a subset of *A fumigatus* with poor sporulation and elevated triazole MICs. After this, *Neosartorya pseudofischeri* was identified, followed by the discovery of *A udagawae*, *A viridinutans*, *A fumigatiaffinis*, and *A novofumigatus* in the section *Fumigati*. Other examples of cryptic aspergillosis include *A alliaceous* (section *Flavi*), *A carneau* and *A alabamensis* (section *Terrei*); *A tubingensis*, *A awamori*, and *A acidus* (section *Nigri*); and *A calidoustus*, *A insuetus*, and *A kevei* (section *Usti*), among many others. The lack of a standardized identification process has led to challenges in definitive identification of these organisms and interlaboratory differences. The relevance of proper identification in treatment selection and outcomes remains a topic of debate because most clinical trials have not identified isolates with this degree of scrutiny and most subjects enrolled in clinical trials have only probable disease with a clinical picture, radiographic findings, and blood test or bronchoalveolar lavage (BAL) result (eg, galactomannan [GM]) suggesting IA without recovery of an actual isolate for definitive identification.

Studies from transplant patients in which detailed identification was performed found that up to 10% of isolates causing disease may belong to the these cryptic species and, although they exhibit elevated triazole MICs in vitro, there are not sufficient data to suggest a difference in outcomes.[10]

IA continues to increase and recent data from the Path Alliance Registry (from 2004 to 2007) have shown IA is the most common fungal infection in hematopoietic stem cell transplant (HSCT) recipients.[12] The continued increase, despite the use of anti-mold prophylaxis, may be secondary to the growing number of immunosuppressed patients, the use of more aggressive chemotherapy protocols, more aggressive immunosuppressive practices in solid organ transplant recipients, and perhaps greater physician awareness and the use of increasingly sensitive diagnostic tests.

Aspergillus spp are found in the environment and are unavoidable. Organisms can be found in water, food, air, and soil and thus have a clear environmental niche. Regional differences in precipitation, humidity, and temperature play a role in the environmental burden of *Aspergillus* and earlier reports have found a correlation between the incidence of infection and geoclimatic patterns.[13]

Patients undergoing HSCT are at the greatest risk of IA, in particular IPA and sinus disease. Risk factors in this population include prolonged neutropenia, defects in cell-mediated immunity, and prolonged immunosuppressive therapy for graft-versus-host disease (GVHD). Individual patient risk varies depending on the type of stem cell transplant (SCT), ranging from 0.5% to 3.9% among allogeneic transplant recipients with lower rates in those receiving autologous SCT.[14] Improvements in hematology and stem cell transplantation techniques have led to decreasing durations and frequency of neutropenia, and the use of granulocyte colony stimulating factors may further decrease the periods of higher risk for IPA. These changes have resulted in the shifting of IA to a bimodal temporal distribution. The highest risk continues to be in early transplantation (<20 days) and a second peak in incidence is observed greater than 100 days after transplant (due to the use of corticosteroids and other medications in the treatment of GVHD). IA risk also increases with repeated courses of chemotherapy or long-term relative neutropenia in conditions such as myeloproliferative syndromes.[15]

IA is also common among patients undergoing solid organ transplantation (SOT), in particular, lung transplant recipients, with an incidence of up to 10% to 15% in past studies.[16,17] The risk of IA varies depending on the organ transplanted, the degree of immunosuppression, metabolic factors, and infection with immunomodulatory viruses (eg, cytomegalovirus).[14]

The increased risk of IA among lung transplant recipients is due to colonization with *Aspergillus* in either the native or transplanted lung, reduced mucociliary clearance, and continued exposure of the transplanted tissue to the external environment.[18] Most cases of IA in lung transplant recipients occur within 6 months of transplantation but some cases may occur at a later date.[14]

More recently, critically ill patients without traditional risk factors have been identified as an at-risk population.[19,20] Chronic obstructive pulmonary disease is one of the most common predisposing conditions due to the high rate of *Aspergillus* spp airway colonization in these patients. In addition, decompensated liver disease or cirrhosis, acquired immunodeficiency syndrome (AIDS), corticosteroid therapy for management of acute respiratory distress syndrome, impaired mucociliary clearance after resolution of pneumonia (viral or bacterial), immune deficiency following prolonged illness, and autoimmune disease have also been identified as significant risk factors.[21,22]

IA can occur in other immunosuppressed hosts outside the intensive care unit, including AIDS patients, patients with primary immunodeficiency, or those receiving immunosuppressive medications such as tumor necrosis factor-α blockers.[5,23,24]

HOST SUSCEPTIBILITY

Inhaled conidia pose an invasive threat and trigger both innate and adaptive immune responses. Conidia interact with leukocytes and epithelial cells within the respiratory tract and, following hyphal invasion, with endothelial cells. Neutrophils have little inflammatory response toward *Aspergillus* spp until germination is observed. Conidia (but not hyphae), bind the host soluble receptor pentraxin-3 via GM and this reaction increases the uptake by alveolar macrophages, dendritic cells, and drives the Th1 immune response. Other aspects of innate immunity, including the toll-like receptors (TLRs) 2 and 4 are also necessary for immune recognition of conidia.

Once germination occurs, *Aspergillus* cell wall composition is altered, and β-(1–3)-glucan is exposed, resulting in dectin-1 signaling in a stage-specific manner. This mechanism may have developed to restrict the host inflammatory response by ignoring nongerminating or resting conidia.

Following phagocytosis by alveolar macrophages, nicotinamide adenine dinucleotide phosphate (NADPH)-dependent killing occurs. Therefore, defects of this pathway, such as those that occur in chronic granulomatous disease, impair fungal killing and result in continued fungal growth and infection within the host.

These processes also require a coordinated T-cell response as illustrated by the prolonged period of risk in allogeneic HSCT patients during receipt of high-dose corticosteroid therapy. The mechanism by which these T-cell responses benefit the host is incompletely understood. Previous studies have shown hyphal damage is significantly higher when the organism is in vitro with T cells, antigen-presenting cells (APCs), and neutrophils than it is with neutrophils alone or with either T cells or APCs. These findings support the ability of *Aspergillus*-responsive T cells to enhance neutrophil function.

Host genomic factors that may predispose patients to IA or poor outcomes have been investigated. Y238X, an early stop codon within the dectin-1 gene, does seem to be a moderate risk factor for the development of IA.[25] However, in HSCT recipients, this polymorphism does not alter the course of infection. Polymorphisms within TLR4 and pentraxin-3 in transplant donors have also been shown to predispose to IA in the recipient.[26] Additional studies are ongoing and further elucidation of genomic risk factors may drive therapeutic decision-making in the future.

CLINICAL MANIFESTATIONS

The clinical presentation of aspergillosis is diverse and depends on both the site of involvement and the ability of the host to generate a robust and coordinated immune response. The upper airways, trachea, bronchi, lung parenchyma, and contiguous structures are those most frequently involved; however, dissemination or infection may occur in any organ system. Clinical syndromes may be classified into allergic manifestations of aspergillosis, noninvasive saprophytic infections, semi-invasive syndromes, and invasive disease.

NONINVASIVE DISEASE
Aspergilloma

An aspergilloma, or *Aspergillus* fungus ball, forms inside a pre-existing pulmonary cavity caused by emphysema, malignancy, or pulmonary tuberculosis. It can be seen on imaging as a freely moveable solid mass within a cavity. Clinical manifestations range from asymptomatic and incidentally discovered radiographic findings to life-threating hemoptysis requiring emergent intervention. Symptomatic aspergilloma can be managed with surgical resection; however, in many patients, underlying structural lung disease and low pulmonary reserve preclude operative intervention; a combination of embolization and antifungal therapy are required to achieve disease stabilization in this subset of patients.[27]

Allergic Bronchopulmonary Aspergillosis

ABPA is a clinical syndrome caused by hypersensitivity to *Aspergillus* spp and is characterized by the presence of chronic immune activation, pulmonary infiltrates, and asthma. Bronchiectasis may also develop in time. Criteria for diagnosis include the presence of bronchial asthma, immediate skin reactivity to *A fumigatus*, elevated serum immunoglobulin (Ig)-E titers, pulmonary infiltrates, central bronchiectasis, eosinophilia, and anti-IgG precipitins against *Aspergillus*. However, none of the findings are pathognomonic of this clinical syndrome. High-resolution computed tomography (CT) of the chest may show characteristic central bronchiectasis but radiological patterns vary and, late in the disease process, fibrosis and cavities are common. Patients are frequently initiated on combination corticosteroids and itraconazole following diagnosis in an attempt to rapidly improve patient symptoms. However, earlier studies have illustrated the corticosteroid-sparing effects of itraconazole during treatment of ABPA and, following initial improvement, frequent attempts to reduce and/or remove corticosteroid therapy should be undertaken. There are limited data with the use of other azoles and alternative therapies such as omalizumab. Patients who fail therapy or exhibit intolerance to itraconazole can frequently be successfully managed with other triazoles such as voriconazole or posaconazole.[28]

Chronic Forms of Pulmonary Aspergillosis

Semi-invasive forms of aspergillosis are likely to represent a continuum with invasive disease. The most common clinical syndrome is chronic cavitary pulmonary aspergillosis, which is characterized by the presence of cavitary lung lesions, chronic respiratory symptoms, and *Aspergillus* spp serum-precipitating antibodies.[29–31] There can be direct invasion of *Aspergillus* spp into the surrounding lung parenchyma and progressive damage with worsening pulmonary symptoms, enlargement of the cavity, and a subsequent decline in lung reserve.[31] Mortality at 1 year can exceed 50%. The initiation of antifungal therapy reduces mortality to 50% at 5 years.[27,32]

INVASIVE DISEASE
Invasive Pulmonary Aspergillosis

Traditionally, most patients with IPA were noted to present 10 to 21 days following HSCT in the setting of profound granulocytopenia.[33] However, recent reports have shown a shift in epidemiology, with less than one-third of patients being neutropenic at the time of IPA diagnosis.[34]

Clinical manifestations of IPA include cough, fever, chest pain or pleuritic pain, dyspnea, and hemoptysis. In neutropenic hosts, symptoms may be more subtle given their relative inability to mount an appropriate inflammatory response. In this patient population, fever may be absent and other symptoms, such as hemoptysis and pleuritic chest pain, secondary to angioinvasion may be more prominent.[35]

The classic radiological finding associated with IPA is the halo sign, which is an area of low attenuation surrounding a pulmonary nodule. However, imaging findings in high-risk patients are usually nonspecific and indistinguishable from other pulmonary infections. Imaging may show diffuse pulmonary infiltrates, pleural-based densities, cavitary lesions, and/or less commonly pleural effusions.[36] Initial findings on CT scan may be followed by an incremental increase in the volume of the lesions in the first 7 days; this increase correlates with bone marrow recovery and immune reconstitution.[37] These radiographic abnormalities may continue to evolve and later cavitate, leading to the air crescent sign.[38] These changes are common and can occur even with early and effective antifungal therapy.[39]

Histopathological features of *Aspergillus* are useful to confirm the diagnosis, although it is frequently not possible to obtain tissue for analysis due to underlying host factors precluding invasive diagnostic testing, such as thrombocytopenia or hemodynamic instability. When tissue is obtained, angioinvasion is typical of disease. Morphologic features suggestive of IPA are the presence of dichotomous branching hyphae. However, these morphologic findings are also observed with infection from other hyaline molds and cultures are required for definitive identification.

The mortality of IPA remains high but some investigators have reported up to a 50% reduction in mortality with prompt initiation of effective antifungal therapy.[40,41]

Tracheobronchial Aspergillosis

The significance of *Aspergillus* spp in respiratory cultures is variable and may range from colonization to infection.[42,43] Tracheobronchial aspergillosis (TA) is defined as infection entirely or almost entirely confined to the tracheobronchial tree. The most common underlying conditions reported in the literature among patients with TA are solid organ transplant (44%, in particular, lung transplant), hematological malignancy (21%), neutropenia (18%), and chronic obstructive pulmonary disease (15%). Most patients who develop TA were receiving long-term corticosteroids or chemotherapy.[44] Clinical features of TA include cough, chest pain, fever, and hemoptysis, all nonspecific symptoms that may lead to a delay in diagnosis. Typical findings on bronchoscopy include pseudomembranes and ulcerative lesions. Bronchoscopy is usually required for diagnosis due to the poor sensitivity and specificity of sputum cultures. In lung transplant patients, TA of the anastomotic site may led to dehiscence.[43]

TA is managed with systemic antifungals, similar to IPA. Voriconazole is the agent of choice and systemic liposomal amphotericin B (L-AMB), or other mold-active triazoles, can be used as alternatives. Some experts use inhaled AMB in addition to the systemic azoles, particularly in lung transplant patients.

Extrapulmonary Involvement

Aspergillosis rhinosinusitis

Sinus aspergillosis may present as a fungus ball of the sinus cavity, allergic sinusitis, granulomatous rhinosinusitis, or as invasive sinus disease. Invasive fungal sinusitis can be acute with a fulminant and rapid clinical course, such as in the immunosuppressed population or, less commonly, in patients without identifiable immune defects, as a chronic granulomatous form with progression through the sinus mucosa, underlying tissue, and bone. This latter form is seen primarily in the Middle East for reasons that are unclear but may relate to host immunogenetic factors.[45]

Acute invasive sinusitis occurs primarily in immunocompromised patients and is characterized by pain, facial swelling, purulent rhinorrhea, and nasal obstruction. It is usually localized to one sinus and can compromise surrounding cranial nerves due to direct invasion. Tissue is required to confirm the diagnosis and, pathologically, angioinvasion, ischemic tissue necrosis, and bone necrosis are observed. CT imaging shows thickening of the sinus and nasal cavity mucosa and later can show bone and tissue destruction. MRI has an increased sensitivity for assessment of tissue invasion and is the preferred modality for initial evaluation and follow-up.[46,47]

Management of invasive sinus aspergillosis usually requires surgical debridement, reduction of immunosuppression, when feasible, and antifungal therapy (similar to IPA). Sinus aspergillomas require removal of the fungus ball and appropriate sinus drainage. Voriconazole is the antifungal of choice; however, in cases in which zygomycosis is a consideration, initial therapy with a lipid AMB formulation is appropriate pending definitive diagnosis.

Ocular Aspergillosis

Aspergillosis of the eye can present as dacryocystitis, periorbital cellulitis, endophthalmitis, vitritis, or may be secondary to contiguous extension from invasive sinusitis or dissemination from a primary pulmonary site. Keratitis also is a common ocular manifestation following local exposure.

Endophthalmitis usually presents with impaired vision, a painful eye, and debris within the anterior chamber. Management usually requires intraocular AMB, with partial vitrectomy. Voriconazole is the treatment of choice for most other ocular manifestations although natamycin is commonly used for A keratitis.[1,48]

Aspergillus osteomyelitis

A osteomyelitis is a rare entity. It is most often seen in patients with significant immunosuppression, including chronic granulomatous disease, hematological malignancies, SOT, HIV infection, steroid therapy, or prior or concurrent pulmonary aspergillosis. Infections following penetrating trauma or as a complication of recent surgery or procedure have also been reported. The most common locations reported in the literature include the spine (49%), skull base, paranasal sinuses and jaw (18%), ribs (9%), and long bones (9%), but it may affect any site. Patients usually present with nonspecific systemic symptoms and localized pain and erythema as well as loss of function of the affected bone or joint.[49] Therapy usually involves surgical debridement and systemic antifungal therapy.

Central Nervous System Aspergillosis

Central nervous system (CNS) aspergillosis usually occurs in patients with neutropenia. Most patients have previous or concurrent IPA or invasive sinus infection. The clinical presentation usually includes fever (57%), neurologic deficits (35%), seizures (28%), mental status changes (21%), and headache (14%). Cerebrospinal fluid analysis is not typically useful for diagnosis because most CNS aspergillosis manifests as a mass lesion instead of meningitis. Management includes systemic therapy with voriconazole and a previous report has suggested improved outcomes in patients who undergo surgical intervention.

DIAGNOSIS

Aspergillus spp grow well on standard media, although the use of fungal-specific media may increase the recovery of the organism. It is not always easy to delineate the clinical significance of positive cultures from nonsterile sites and interpretation in the context of individualized risk factors, symptoms, and radiological findings is required. Furthermore, antifungal therapy may decrease the yield of cultures.[50,51]

Definitive diagnosis requires tissue biopsy with direct visualization of the branching septate hyphae on microscopic examination and/or recovery of the organism. Obtaining tissue may be challenging in thrombocytopenia or in hosts with coagulation disorders; it may not be possible in patients with high oxygen requirements.

Given the challenges of obtaining tissue and the variable yield of cultures, nonculture-based diagnostics have been developed and remain an active focus of research efforts. Antigen detection of GM, a component of the Aspergillus cell wall, is the most frequently used methodology. The sensitivity of testing is variable and depends on the host (44%–90%). For example, the sensitivity in patients with hematologic malignancy is higher than in those with lesser degrees of immunosuppression, and patients on antifungal therapy may have falsely negative GM results.[52,53] Conversely, false-positive results have historically been reported in patients receiving piperacillin-tazobactam and amoxicillin-clavulanate, and among patients with histoplasmosis or blastomycosis, although recent reports have shown no cross reactions with piperacillin-tazobactam.[54] The use of serial enzyme immunoassay (EIA) testing for screening high-risk patients (such as those with hematological malignancy) is reserved for those not on antimold prophylaxis because the sensitivity of the assay is significantly reduced in those patients.[55] Use of the Platelia EIA (BioRad, Hercules, CA) is recommended in symptomatic patients suspected of having IPA; it can also be used on BAL fluid, even for patients receiving antimold therapy.[56]

Serum GM determination also provides prognostic information with declining values associated with improvements in patient outcomes.[57] BAL testing exhibits increased sensitivity compared with serum testing.[58] The sensitivity of GM testing in BAL fluid is, however, reduced in patients receiving prophylactic or empiric antifungal therapy. The positive predictive value is also decreased among patients receiving effective antifungal prophylaxis, in whom most positive tests represent false positives, and only 12% of positive results representing true disease.

Serum $(1 \rightarrow 3)$-β-D-glucan (another component of the fungal cell wall) determination also may be helpful, although this marker is not specific for *Aspergillus* and its presence may indicate various other invasive fungal infections.[59] The negative predictive value of $(1 \rightarrow 3)$-β-D-glucan has generated interest in its use as a screening test in high-risk patients.[60]

Recently, a point-of-care lateral flow device for the detection of GM was introduced into the diagnostic armamentarium for IA. This test has a sensitivity that has been reported close to 100%, a specificity of approximately 80%, and a negative predictive value among patients with proven IA. This sensitivity was still high (around 82%) when probable cases were included. However, the sensitivity is reduced in patients already receiving antifungal therapy, similar to the aforementioned tests.

To date, polymerase chain reaction (PCR) testing has not been widely adopted due to a lack of standardization. However, data continue to emerge suggesting the usefulness of combined PCR and GM testing. When comparing blood samples, antigen testing using GM has been shown to exhibit a greater specificity than PCR. Conversely, when BAL samples are examined, PCR seems to have a higher specificity ($\sim$93%) than GM testing of the same sample (85%), with similar sensitivity. Several clinical trials using the combination of GM and PCR have shown a sensitivity of 98% when used in concert. The use of empiric antifungal therapy can be reduced in patients with negative results with no worsening of patient mortality, with recent data using a combined approach suggesting an improved outcome.[61] Data on the use of PCR based methods to make the diagnosis of IA have been recently reviewed.[62]

The emergence of antifungal resistance in *Aspergillus* spp has also led to the development of additional nucleic acid based assays (AsperGenius, PathoNostics B.V., Netherlands) capable of identifying resistance mutations known to confer antifungal resistance, although they are not yet available in the United States. Sensitivity has been reported as 78% and specificity 100%.[63] Additional tests, using multilocus sequence typing (MLST) sequence alignment generated by multiplex reaction from patient sputum samples with possible or probable IA, have also been developed and have shown promising results.[64]

TREATMENT

The antifungal armamentarium has expanded, during the past decades, from AMB deoxycholate to L-AMB preparations, and from itraconazole to voriconazole, posaconazole (initially a liquid suspension formulation, followed by oral tablets and an intravenous [IV] preparation), and more recently isavuconazole (available in IV and oral formulations).[65]

Triazoles

The triazoles exert their antifungal effects by inhibiting the cytochrome P450 (CYP)-dependent 14-α-demethylase, blocking the conversion of lanosterol to ergosterol.

This results in the inhibition of fungal cell growth and replication. The variable affinity of azoles to the 14-α-demethylase accounts for their respective differences in activity against different organisms. Azoles may also cause inhibition of several CYP-dependent human enzymes, leading to clinically relevant adverse events and the potential for drug-drug interactions.

Voriconazole

Voriconazole, a second-generation triazole, is available in oral and IV formulations and remains the treatment of choice for IA.[66] A prospective randomized trial showed the superiority of voriconazole over AMB deoxycholate.[67] Subsequent publications and clinical experience in a variety of clinical forms have provided additional data regarding the efficacy of voriconazole.[1]

Adverse events during voriconazole therapy include liver function test abnormalities (15% of patients), gastrointestinal toxicities (nausea, vomiting, diarrhea), and skin rashes. Other, less common, adverse events include hallucinations, visual abnormalities (associated with higher serum concentrations, transient and reversible), and fluorosis or cutaneous malignancy with long-term administration.[68]

Treatment with voriconazole requires the administration of a loading dose of 6 mg/kg IV every 12 hours for 2 doses, followed by 4 mg/kg every 12 hours. Oral therapy in adults is usually 200 mg twice a day after the loading dose. However, it can be optimized by administering 4 mg/kg/dose twice daily and using therapeutic drug monitoring.[1] Pediatric patients require higher doses of voriconazole and a maintenance dosage of 7 mg/kg twice a day is recommended. Loading dose in the pediatric population has not been well studied.[1]

Dosing in adults is not predictable due to a variety of factors, including gender, age, liver disease, and potential genetic polymorphisms in CYP2C19. There is some evidence that therapeutic drug monitoring (TDM) in patients with aspergillosis may lead to improved patient outcomes and reduce toxicity.[69] TDM is recommended when available, with a goal trough of between 1 and 5.5 μg/mL.[70] The IV formulation contains a cyclodextrin vehicle that can accumulate in patients with renal impairment, although no adverse events have been demonstrated and this remains largely a theoretic concern.[71,72]

Posaconazole

Posaconazole is a triazole with a similar structure to itraconazole. It is highly active in vitro against *Aspergillus* spp. When it was initially developed, it was only available in a suspension and administered in divided doses 2 to 4 times per day with a meal or oral supplement to increase absorption. Steady state could not be reached for up to 7 days, making its use during primary therapy problematic. Posaconazole is metabolized in the liver through glucuronidation and can have drug interactions involving CYP450 3A4 isoenzymes.

Posaconazole prophylaxis has been used in high-risk patients undergoing bone marrow transplant with graft versus host disease and in patients with acute myelogenous leukemia and myelodysplastic syndrome.[73,74] Some experts may recommend TDM for posaconazole when using the solution for prophylaxis because lower levels have been associated with a higher rate of invasive fungal infections.[75] Newer formulations of posaconazole, including an oral delayed-release tablet and an IV formulation, have since been developed. The tablet contains a pH-sensitive polymer and is administered as 300 mg twice daily for 2 doses, then 300 mg daily. The tablet is superior to the oral suspension in oral bioavailability and target drug levels are readily attained in most patients. The role of TDM during administration of the tablet or IV formulations has not been determined and higher drug levels have not been definitively associated with toxicity to date.

Itraconazole

Itraconazole is an azole available in oral capsules. Absorption of the capsules is erratic and thus is not recommended for severely ill patients. Side effects include nausea, vomiting, hypertriglyceridemia, hypokalemia, and hepatotoxicity.[76] It can also have negative inotropic effects, and should be used with caution in patients with heart failure or a reduced ejection fraction. Itraconazole is administered as 200 mg orally twice a day with meals. Itraconazole is primarily used in noninvasive or chronic forms of aspergillosis, or following intolerance or toxicity to other triazoles.[77] When used for IA, TDM is recommended.

Isavuconazole

Isavuconazole has potent activity against *Aspergillus* spp in vitro, including some isolates with decreased susceptibility to other triazoles.[78] It was initially compared with voriconazole for the treatment of IA and was shown to be noninferior and to have 17% fewer side effects than voriconazole.[79] It is administered orally as 200 mg tablets 3 times daily for 6 doses, followed by 200 mg daily thereafter. The IV formulation does not contain cyclodextrin as a solubilizing agent. It is available in oral and IV preparations as the prodrug isavuconazonium sulfate and, following administration, plasma esterases cleave the prodrug into the active form isavuconazole. Isavuconazole has excellent oral bioavailability (98%), is greater than 99% protein bound, and has a prolonged half-life of 100 to 130 hours. Isavuconazole does act as both a substrate and inhibitor of CYP3A4, P-glycoprotein, and organic cation transporter 2; therefore, drug-drug interactions may occur. Common side effects include nausea, vomiting, and diarrhea; however, drug discontinuation in preclinical studies was uncommon. Similar to other triazoles, hepatic toxicity may occur and monitoring of liver function tests during therapy is recommended.[80]

Echinocandins

The echinocandins inhibit the synthesis of 1,3-β-D-glucan, via inhibition of the glucan synthase enzyme. Caspofungin, micafungin, and anidulafungin are currently available in IV formulations only. They are well tolerated, have limited drug-drug interactions, and adverse events are uncommon.[81] Echinocandins inhibit the growth of *Aspergillus* spp but they are fungistatic, rather than fungicidal. A pharmacodynamic parameter may limit its efficacy in immunocompromised hosts. Caspofungin has been approved for salvage therapy in IPA but efficacy is only 33% when used in severely immunocompromised patients.[82] The use of micafungin has been studied in chronic pulmonary aspergillosis and as salvage therapy, with a 44% survival rate in the latter group.[83–86] Based on lack of data in primary therapy, echinocandins are not recommended as first-line agents and are reserved for the salvage setting or in combination with another antifungal class. See later discussion on the role of combination therapy with a triazole and an echinocandin.

Amphotericin B

AMB is a polyene that is fungicidal and appears to act by forming large extramembranous aggregates that extract ergosterol from lipid bilayers, resulting in cell death and leading to the formation of ion channels, which has been historically thought to be the primary mechanism of action associated with destruction of the fungi.[87] AMB deoxycholate was the first-line therapeutic agent for IA for decades, with the exception of *A terreus*, which is inherently resistant. However, due to toxicity and poor outcomes among immunosuppressed patients, and the superiority of voriconazole in a random-ized clinical trial, AMB deoxycholate has been relegated for those intolerant or refrac-tory to first-line agents.[5,88,89]

Lipid formulations of AMB are less nephrotoxic, are preferred to AMB deoxycholate, and are recommend for use as an alternative first-line agent when voriconazole is not tolerated or is contraindicated. AMB lipid complex is used in doses of 5 mg/kg/d IV daily. L-AMB is used in doses of 3 to 5 mg/kg/d. Higher doses of L-AMB (10 mg/kg) have been shown not to be more effective than lower doses in the treatment of IA but were associated with increased toxicity.[90]

Combination Therapy

Despite the availability of voriconazole for therapy for IA, mortality remains high and attempts to further improve outcomes are ongoing. In vitro, animal models, and retrospective data have suggested a benefit of combined triazole and echinocandin therapy. A recent study designed specifically to evaluate combination therapy ran-domized subjects to voriconazole alone or voriconazole plus anidulafungin. The pri-mary endpoint was met in 19.5% of the subjects in the combination group and 27.8% of the subjects in the voriconazole group; however, the difference was not statistically significant ($P = .087$).[91] There was no difference in adverse outcomes be-tween groups. A subset analysis of those subjects diagnosed by a positive GM did show a statistically improved outcome ($P<.05$) with reduced mortality in those sub-jects receiving combination therapy compared with those receiving voriconazole monotherapy (15.7% vs 27.3%). Thus, initial combination therapy is not routinely rec-ommended but may still be considered in high-risk patients, such as those with he-matologic malignancy and severe disease, although the benefit has not been definitively proven.

ANTIFUNGAL RESISTANCE

Aspergillus spp with decreased susceptibility to azoles have been reported and their prevalence is increasing, particularly within the United Kingdom and the Netherlands (increasing from 1.7% to 6%). In the United States, triazole resistance is about 4%.

In a recent study of 21 centers in 18 countries, between 2009 to 2011, a total of 3788 isolates were analyzed (77% of these were A fumigatus species complex). Resistance was observed in 3.2% of the isolates assessed but resistance was highly variable and largely correlated with different regions (range 0%–26% among the centers). Among all subjects with IA, azole-resistance was documented in 5.1%.[92]

Azole resistance in clinical Aspergillus isolates has been linked to mutations in the CYP51A gene, which encodes the Cyp51A enzyme (responsible for a step in the ergosterol biosynthesis), and the development of tandem repeats in the promoter re-gion for this same gene (the most common being a lysine to histidine substitution at codon 98; TR34/L98H).

Given the lack of data regarding the correlation between MIC and patient outcomes, the Clinical Laboratory Standards Institute (CLSI) has abstained from establishing break-points for Aspergillus and other molds. In Europe, the European Union Committee on Antimicrobial Susceptibility Testing (EUCAST) has recently established susceptibility breakpoints for itraconazole, posaconazole, and voriconazole for Aspergillus spp.

The development of resistance, including recovery of resistant isolates from the environment, has been met with significant concern and is likely related to the use of fungicides in numerous agricultural practices and commercial products (eg, environmental fungicides and outdoor paint to prevent wood rot).

Management of patients with azole-resistant IA is challenging. Potential options, based on limited clinical data, include the use of L-AMB or combination therapy with an azole and echinocandin. However, in vitro findings have demonstrated the combination of posaconazole and an echinocandin may or may not be effective based on the mutation responsible for the resistance. Similarly, isavuconazole exhibits higher MICs in the presence of the TR34/L98H and TR46/Y121F/T289A mutations and it is, therefore, recommended that during the care of a patient with a resistant isolate, susceptibility testing to multiple antifungals be performed in an attempt to optimize pharmacokinetic-pharmacodynamic parameters.

BREAKTHROUGH INFECTIONS

Breakthrough infection describes IA developing in a patient already receiving prophylactic or therapeutic antifungal therapy. As previously discussed, the diagnosis in these cases can be challenging due to a reduction in the sensitivity of noninvasive testing in patients previously receiving antifungals. The development of resistance is of concern, as well as subtherapeutic drug levels. In allogeneic HSCT recipients, breakthrough fungal infections were more common among those individuals receiving posaconazole, with suboptimal serum levels (<400 ng/mL).[93]

Management of these breakthrough infections has not been extensively studied but consideration must be given to the use of drug level optimization, a change in antifungal class, or even combination therapy.[94]

SUMMARY

Cases of aspergillosis continue to increase as a consequence of the continually growing immunosuppressed population. Diagnostic and treatment practices are also evolving and substantial progress has been made during the last decade. Early therapy remains critical in attempts to improve outcomes. The growing number of antifungal medications offers the potential for more effective and less toxic therapeutic options. Future work focusing on diagnosis using emerging noninvasive methodologies, such as breath analysis, and treatment with newer agents will provide additional insight and assistance in this fight against this lethal pathogen.

REFERENCES

1. Walsh TJ, Anaissie EJ, Denning DW, et al. Treatment of aspergillosis: Clinical practice guidelines of the Infectious Diseases Society of America. Clin Infect Dis 2008;46(3):327–60.
2. Pagano L, Akova M, Dimopoulos G, et al. Risk assessment and prognostic factors for mould-related diseases in immunocompromised patients. J Antimicrob Chemother 2011;66(Suppl 1):i5–14.
3. Summerbell R. Ascomycetes. *Aspergillus, fusarium, sporothrix, piedraia*, and their relatives. In: Howard DH, editor. Pathogenic fungi in humans and animals. 2nd edition. New York: Marcel Dekker; 2003. p. 237–498.
4. Balajee SA, Houbraken J, Verweij PE, et al. *Aspergillus* species identification in the clinical setting. Stud Mycol 2007;59:39–46.
5. Patterson TF, Kirkpatrick WR, White M, et al. Invasive aspergillosis. Disease spectrum, treatment practices, and outcomes. I3 *Aspergillus* Study Group. Medicine (Baltimore) 2000;79(4):250–60.

6. Balajee SA, Nickle D, Varga J, et al. Molecular studies reveal frequent misidentification of *Aspergillus fumigatus* by morphotyping. Eukaryot Cell 2006;5(10): 1705–12.
7. Klich M, Pitt J. A laboratory guide to common *Aspergillus* species and their teleomorphs. North Ryde, New South Wales, (Australia): Commonwealth Scientific and Industrial Research Organization; 1988.
8. O'Gorman CM, Fuller HT, Dyer PS. Discovery of a sexual cycle in the opportunistic fungal pathogen *Aspergillus fumigatus*. Nature 2009;457(7228):471–4.
9. Pitt JI, Samson RA. Nomenclatural considerations in naming species of *Aspergillus* and its teleomorphs. Stud Mycol 2007;59:67–70.
10. Nedel WL, Pasqualotto AC. Treatment of infections by cryptic *Aspergillus* species. Mycopathologia 2014;178(5–6):441–5.
11. Howard SJ, Harrison E, Bowyer P, et al. Cryptic species and azole resistance in the *Aspergillus niger* complex. Antimicrob Agents Chemother 2011;55(10): 4802–9.
12. Neofytos D, Horn D, Anaissie E, et al. Epidemiology and outcome of invasive fungal infection in adult hematopoietic stem cell transplant recipients: Analysis of multicenter prospective antifungal therapy (path) alliance registry. Clin Infect Dis 2009;48(3):265–73.
13. Panackal AA, Li H, Kontoyiannis DP, et al. Geoclimatic influences on invasive aspergillosis after hematopoietic stem cell transplantation. Clin Infect Dis 2010; 50(12):1588–97.
14. Nucci M, Anaissie E. Fungal infections in hematopoietic stem cell transplantation and solid-organ transplantation–focus on aspergillosis. Clin Chest Med 2009; 30(2):295–306, vii.
15. Nucci M, Portugal RD, Garnica M. Index to predict invasive mold infection in high-risk neutropenic patients based on the area over the neutrophil curve. J Clin Oncol 2009;27(23):3849–54.
16. Patterson JE, Peters J, Calhoon JH, et al. Investigation and control of aspergillosis and other filamentous fungal infections in solid organ transplant recipients. Transpl Infect Dis 2000;2(1):22–8.
17. Singh N, Paterson DL. *Aspergillus* infections in transplant recipients. Clin Microbiol Rev 2005;18(1):44–69.
18. Paterson DL, Singh N. Invasive aspergillosis in transplant recipients. Medicine 1999;78(2):123–38.
19. Denning DW. Aspergillosis in "nonimmunocompromised" critically ill patients. Am J Respir Crit Care Med 2004;170(6):580–1.
20. Lat A, Bhadelia N, Miko B, et al. Invasive aspergillosis after pandemic (H1N1) 2009. Emerg Infect Dis 2010;16(6):971–3.
21. Meersseman W, Vandecasteele SJ, Wilmer A, et al. Invasive aspergillosis in critically ill patients without malignancy. Am J Respir Crit Care Med 2004;170(6):621–5.
22. Koulenti D, Garnacho-Montero J, Blot S. Approach to invasive pulmonary aspergillosis in critically ill patients. Curr Opin Infect Dis 2014;27(2):174–83.
23. Warris A, Bjorneklett A, Gaustad P. Invasive pulmonary aspergillosis associated with infliximab therapy. N Engl J Med 2001;344(14):1099–100.
24. Cohen MS, Isturiz RE, Malech HL, et al. Fungal infection in chronic granulomatous disease. The importance of the phagocyte in defense against fungi. Am J Med 1981;71(1):59–66.
25. Chai LY, de Boer MG, van der Velden WJ, et al. The Y238X stop codon polymorphism in the human beta-glucan receptor dectin-1 and susceptibility to invasive aspergillosis. J Infect Dis 2011;203(5):736–43.

26. Bochud PY, Chien JW, Marr KA, et al. Toll-like receptor 4 polymorphisms and aspergillosis in stem-cell transplantation. N Engl J Med 2008;359(17):1766–77.

27. Denning DW, Riniotis K, Dobrashian R, et al. Chronic cavitary and fibrosing pulmonary and pleural aspergillosis: Case series, proposed nomenclature change, and review. Clin Infect Dis 2003;37(Suppl 3):S265–80.

28. Greenberger PA, Bush RK, Demain JG, et al. Allergic bronchopulmonary aspergillosis. J Allergy Clin Immunol Pract 2014;2(6):703–8.

29. Binder RE, Faling LJ, Pugatch RD, et al. Chronic necrotizing pulmonary aspergillosis: a discrete clinical entity. Medicine 1982;61(2):109–24.

30. Gefter WB, Weingrad TR, Epstein DM, et al. "Semi-invasive" pulmonary aspergillosis: a new look at the spectrum of *Aspergillus* infections of the lung. Radiology 1981;140(2):313–21.

31. Hope WW, Walsh TJ, Denning DW. The invasive and saprophytic syndromes due to *Aspergillus* spp. Med Mycol 2005;43(Suppl 1):S207–38.

32. Felton TW, Baxter C, Moore CB, et al. Efficacy and safety of posaconazole for chronic pulmonary aspergillosis. Clin Infect Dis 2010;51(12):1383–91.

33. Gerson SL, Talbot GH, Hurwitz S, et al. Prolonged granulocytopenia: the major risk factor for invasive pulmonary aspergillosis in patients with acute leukemia. Ann Intern Med 1984;100(3):345–51.

34. Wald A, Leisenring W, van Burik JA, et al. Epidemiology of *Aspergillus* infections in a large cohort of patients undergoing bone marrow transplantation. J Infect Dis 1997;175(6):1459–66.

35. Thompson GR 3rd, Patterson TF. Pulmonary aspergillosis: recent advances. Semin Respir Crit Care Med 2011;32(6):673–81.

36. Denning DW. Invasive aspergillosis. Clin Infect Dis 1998;26(4):781–803 [quiz: 804–5].

37. Caillot D, Couaillier JF, Bernard A, et al. Increasing volume and changing characteristics of invasive pulmonary aspergillosis on sequential thoracic computed tomography scans in patients with neutropenia. J Clin Oncol 2001;19(1):253–9.

38. Greene R. The radiological spectrum of pulmonary aspergillosis. Med Mycol 2005;43(Suppl 1):S147–54.

39. Miceli MH, Maertens J, Buve K, et al. Immune reconstitution inflammatory syndrome in cancer patients with pulmonary aspergillosis recovering from neutropenia: Proof of principle, description, and clinical and research implications. Cancer 2007;110(1):112–20.

40. Baddley JW, Andes DR, Marr KA, et al. Factors associated with mortality in transplant patients with invasive aspergillosis. Clin Infect Dis 2010;50(12):1559–67.

41. von Eiff M, Roos N, Schulten R, et al. Pulmonary aspergillosis: Early diagnosis improves survival. Respiration 1995;62(6):341–7.

42. Denning DW, Follansbee SE, Scolaro M, et al. Pulmonary aspergillosis in the acquired immunodeficiency syndrome. N Engl J Med 1991;324(10):654–62.

43. Kramer MR, Denning DW, Marshall SE, et al. Ulcerative tracheobronchitis after lung transplantation. A new form of invasive aspergillosis. Am Rev Respir Dis 1991;144(3 Pt 1):552–6.

44. Fernandez-Ruiz M, Silva JT, San-Juan R, et al. *Aspergillus tracheobronchitis*: Report of 8 cases and review of the literature. Medicine (Baltimore) 2012;91(5): 261–73.

45. Thompson GR 3rd, Patterson TF. Fungal disease of the nose and paranasal sinuses. J Allergy Clin Immunol 2012;129(2):321–6.

46. Chang C, Gershwin ME, Thompson GR 3rd. Fungal disease of the nose and sinuses: an updated overview. Curr Allergy Asthma Rep 2013;13(2):152–61.

47. Duggal P, Wise SK. Chapter 8: invasive fungal rhinosinusitis. Am J Rhinol Allergy 2013;27(Suppl 1):S28–30.
48. Prajna NV, Krishnan T, Mascarenhas J, et al. The mycotic ulcer treatment trial: a randomized trial comparing natamycin vs voriconazole. JAMA Ophthalmol 2013; 131(4):422–9.
49. Gabrielli E, Fothergill AW, Brescini L, et al. Osteomyelitis caused by *Aspergillus* species: a review of 310 reported cases. Clin Microbiol Infect 2014;20(6):559–65.
50. Munoz P, Alcala L, Sanchez Conde M, et al. The isolation of *Aspergillus fumigatus* from respiratory tract specimens in heart transplant recipients is highly predictive of invasive aspergillosis. Transplantation 2003;75(3):326–9.
51. Horvath JA, Dummer S. The use of respiratory-tract cultures in the diagnosis of invasive pulmonary aspergillosis. Am J Med 1996;100(2):171–8.
52. Herbrecht R, Letscher-Bru V, Oprea C, et al. *Aspergillus* galactomannan detection in the diagnosis of invasive aspergillosis in cancer patients. J Clin Oncol 2002;20(7):1898–906.
53. Maertens J, Verhaegen J, Lagrou K, et al. Screening for circulating galactomannan as a noninvasive diagnostic tool for invasive aspergillosis in prolonged neutropenic patients and stem cell transplantation recipients: a prospective validation. Blood 2001;97(6):1604–10.
54. Verweij PE, Mennink-Kersten MA. Issues with galactomannan testing. Med Mycol 2006;44(Suppl):179–83.
55. Duarte RF, Sanchez-Ortega I, Cuesta I, et al. Serum galactomannan-based early detection of invasive aspergillosis in hematology patients receiving effective anti-mold prophylaxis. Clin Infect Dis 2014;59(12):1696–702.
56. Hope WW, Petraitis V, Petraitiene R, et al. The initial 96 hours of invasive pulmonary aspergillosis: histopathology, comparative kinetics of galactomannan and (1->3) beta-d-glucan and consequences of delayed antifungal therapy. Antimicrob Agents Chemother 2010;54(11):4879–86.
57. Koo S, Bryar JM, Baden LR, et al. Prognostic features of galactomannan antigenemia in galactomannan-positive invasive aspergillosis. J Clin Microbiol 2010; 48(4):1255–60.
58. Maertens J, Maertens V, Theunissen K, et al. Bronchoalveolar lavage fluid galactomannan for the diagnosis of invasive pulmonary aspergillosis in patients with hematologic diseases. Clin Infect Dis 2009;49(11):1688–93.
59. Odabasi Z, Mattiuzzi G, Estey E, et al. Beta-D-glucan as a diagnostic adjunct for invasive fungal infections: validation, cutoff development, and performance in patients with acute myelogenous leukemia and myelodysplastic syndrome. Clin Infect Dis 2004;39(2):199–205.
60. Obayashi T, Yoshida M, Mori T, et al. Plasma (1->3)-beta-D-glucan measurement in diagnosis of invasive deep mycosis and fungal febrile episodes. Lancet 1995; 345(8941):17–20.
61. Aguado JM, Vazquez L, Fernandez-Ruiz M, et al. Serum galactomannan versus a combination of galactomannan and polymerase chain reaction-based *Aspergillus* DNA detection for early therapy of invasive aspergillosis in high-risk hematological patients: a randomized controlled trial. Clin Infect Dis 2015;60(3): 405–14.
62. White PL, Wingard JR, Bretagne S, et al. *Aspergillus* polymerase chain reaction: Systematic review of evidence for clinical use in comparison with antigen testing. Clin Infect Dis 2015;61(8):1293–303.
63. White PL, Posso RB, Barnes RA. Analytical and Clinical Evaluation of the Patho-Nostics AsperGenius Assay for Detection of Invasive Aspergillosis and

Resistance to Azole Antifungal Drugs during Testing of Serum Samples. J Clin Microbiol 2015;53(7):2115–21.

64. Caramalho R, Gusmao L, Lackner M, et al. SNaPAfu: A novel single nucleotide polymorphism multiplex assay for aspergillus fumigatus direct detection, identification, and genotyping in clinical specimens. PLoS One 2013;8(10):e75968.

65. Wiederhold NP, Patterson TF. What's new in antifungals: an update on the in-vitro activity and in-vivo efficacy of new and investigational antifungal agents. Curr Opin Infect Dis 2015;28:539–45.

66. Lat A, Thompson GR 3rd. Update on the optimal use of voriconazole for invasive fungal infections. Infect Drug Resist 2011;4:43–53.

67. Herbrecht R, Denning DW, Patterson TF, et al. Voriconazole versus amphotericin B for primary therapy of invasive aspergillosis. N Engl J Med 2002;347(6):408–15.

68. Eiden C, Peyriere H, Cociglio M, et al. Adverse effects of voriconazole: Analysis of the French Pharmacovigilance Database. Ann Pharmacother 2007;41(5):755–63.

69. Park WB, Kim NH, Kim KH, et al. The effect of therapeutic drug monitoring on safety and efficacy of voriconazole in invasive fungal infections: a randomized controlled trial. Clin Infect Dis 2012;55(8):1080–7.

70. Ashbee HR, Barnes RA, Johnson EM, et al. Therapeutic drug monitoring (TDM) of antifungal agents: guidelines from the British Society for Medical Mycology. J Antimicrob Chemother 2014;69(5):1162–76.

71. Alvarez-Lerma F, Allepuz-Palau A, Garcia MP, et al. Impact of intravenous administration of voriconazole in critically ill patients with impaired renal function. J Chemother 2008;20(1):93–100.

72. Thompson GR 3rd, Lewis JS 2nd. Pharmacology and clinical use of voriconazole. Expert Opin Drug Metab Toxicol 2010;6(1):83–94.

73. Ullmann AJ, Lipton JH, Vesole DH, et al. Posaconazole or fluconazole for prophylaxis in severe graft-versus-host disease. N Engl J Med 2007;356(4):335–47.

74. Cornely OA, Maertens J, Winston DJ, et al. Posaconazole vs. fluconazole or itraconazole prophylaxis in patients with neutropenia. N Engl J Med 2007;356(4): 348–59.

75. Dolton MJ, Ray JE, Chen SC, et al. Multicenter study of posaconazole therapeutic drug monitoring: exposure-response relationship and factors affecting concentration. Antimicrob Agents Chemother 2012;56(11):5503–10.

76. De Beule K, Van Gestel J. Pharmacology of itraconazole. Drugs 2001;61(Suppl 1):27–37.

77. Andes D, Pascual A, Marchetti O. Antifungal therapeutic drug monitoring: established and emerging indications. Antimicrob Agents Chemother 2009;53(1): 24–34.

78. Thompson GR 3rd, Wiederhold NP. Isavuconazole: a comprehensive review of spectrum of activity of a new triazole. Mycopathologia 2010;170(5):291–313.

79. Maertens J, Patterson TF, Rahav G, et al. A phase 3 randomized, double-blind trial evaluating isavuconazole vs voriconazole for the primary treatment of invasive fungal disease caused by *Aspergillus* spp. or other filamentous fungi (SECURE). 24th ECCMID. Barcelona, Spain, 10–13 May, 2014.

80. Miceli MH, Kauffman CA. Isavuconazole: a new broad-spectrum triazole antifungal agent. Clin Infect Dis 2015;61(10):1558–65.

81. Bennett JE. Echinocandins for candidemia in adults without neutropenia. N Engl J Med 2006;355(11):1154–9.

82. Viscoli C, Herbrecht R, Akan H, et al. An EORTC phase II study of caspofungin as first-line therapy of invasive aspergillosis in haematological patients. J Antimicrob Chemother 2009;64(6):1274–81.

83. Kohno S, Izumikawa K, Ogawa K, et al. Intravenous micafungin versus voriconazole for chronic pulmonary aspergillosis: a multicenter trial in Japan. J Infect 2010;61(5):410–8.

84. Denning DW, Marr KA, Lau WM, et al. Micafungin (FK463), alone or in combination with other systemic antifungal agents, for the treatment of acute invasive aspergillosis. J Infect 2006;53(5):337–49.

85. Hiemenz JW, Raad II, Maertens JA, et al. Efficacy of caspofungin as salvage therapy for invasive aspergillosis compared to standard therapy in a historical cohort. Eur J Clin Microbiol Infect Dis 2010;29(11):1387–94.

86. Kontoyiannis DP, Ratanatharathorn V, Young JA, et al. Micafungin alone or in combination with other systemic antifungal therapies in hematopoietic stem cell transplant recipients with invasive aspergillosis. Transpl Infect Dis 2009;11(1):89–93.

87. Anderson TM, Clay MC, Cioffi AG, et al. Amphotericin forms an extramembranous and fungicidal sterol sponge. Nat Chem Biol 2014;10(5):400–6.

88. Patterson TF, Boucher HW, Herbrecht R, et al. Strategy of following voriconazole versus amphotericin B therapy with other licensed antifungal therapy for primary treatment of invasive aspergillosis: impact of other therapies on outcome. Clin Infect Dis 2005;41(10):1448–52.

89. Bates DW, Su L, Yu DT, et al. Mortality and costs of acute renal failure associated with amphotericin B therapy. Clin Infect Dis 2001;32(5):686–93.

90. Cornely OA, Maertens J, Bresnik M, et al. Liposomal amphotericin B as initial therapy for invasive mold infection: a randomized trial comparing a high-loading dose regimen with standard dosing (AmBiLoad trial). Clin Infect Dis 2007; 44(10):1289–97.

91. Marr KA, Schlamm HT, Herbrecht R, et al. Combination antifungal therapy for invasive aspergillosis: a randomized trial. Ann Intern Med 2015;162(2):81–9.

92. van der Linden JW, Arendrup MC, Warris A, et al. Prospective multicenter international surveillance of azole resistance in Aspergillus fumigatus. Emerg Infect Dis 2015;21(6):1041–4.

93. Winston DJ, Bartoni K, Territo MC, et al. Efficacy, safety, and breakthrough infections associated with standard long-term posaconazole antifungal prophylaxis in allogeneic stem cell transplantation recipients. Biol Blood Marrow Transplant 2011;17(4):507–15.

94. Maschmeyer G, Patterson TF. Our 2014 approach to breakthrough invasive fungal infections. Mycoses 2014;57(11):645–51.

Mucormycoses

Dimitrios Farmakiotis, MD[a],*, Dimitrios P. Kontoyiannis, MD, ScD[b]

KEYWORDS

- Amphotericin • Antifungal • Diabetes • Hematopoietic stem cell transplantation
- Immunocompromised • Ketoacidosis • Isavuconazole • Leukemia

KEY POINTS

- The clinician should have a high index of suspicion when a breakthrough mold infection develops in an immunosuppressed patient who has been on antifungals that have only anti-*Aspergillus* activity (eg, voriconazole prophylaxis), especially when the negative fungal biomarkers (*Aspergillus* galactomannan antigen and β-D-glucan) are negative.
- On chest computed tomography scan, the reversed halo sign, an area of central ground-glass necrosis surrounded by a ring of consolidation, is suggestive of pulmonary mucormycosis, especially in neutropenic patients with leukemia.
- Timely initiation of amphotericin-B lipid formulation monotherapy is the first-line treatment of mucormycosis. Posaconazole and isavuconazole are acceptable salvage and long-term treatment options, which can also be used as initial therapy in patients at high risk of amphotericin-induced nephrotoxicity.
- Surgical debridement or resection should be pursued when feasible.
- Resolution of immunologic and metabolic abnormalities is important for outcome.

INTRODUCTION

The term zygomycosis has been commonly used to describe invasive fungal infections (IFI) by the Zygomycetes, a term formerly used to describe molds with aseptate or pauciseptate, irregularly branching ribbonlike hyphae that reproduce sexually via formation of zygospores.[1-3] However, those species were reclassified into 2 orders, Mucorales and Entomophthorales.[4] Entomophthorales molds are uncommon pathogens, typically restricted to tropical areas, and usually cause chronic sinus and skin infections that rarely disseminate to internal organs.[5] One important exception is

Disclosures: D.P. Kontoyiannis has received research support and honoraria from Astellas US, Pfizer, Gilead, and Merck & Co., Inc. D. Farmakiotis has nothing to disclose.
[a] Division of Infectious Diseases, Rhode Island Hospital, Warren Alpert Medical School of Brown University, 593 Eddy Street, Providence, RI 02903, USA; [b] Department of Infectious Diseases, Infection Control and Employee Health, The University of Texas MD Anderson Cancer Center, 1515 Holcombe Boulevard, Houston, TX 77030, USA
* Corresponding author.
E-mail address: dimitrios.farmakiotis@lifespan.org

gastrointestinal basidiobolomycosis, which has been reported in Arizona and usually presents with chronic abdominal pain mimicking Crohn disease, but in rare cases (diabetics and the immunocompromised), can progress rapidly across tissue planes, with evidence of angioinvasion.[6-8]

The term mucormycoses is herein used to describe the spectrum of subacute, acute, and often rapidly progressing infections, caused by angiotropic fungi of the order Mucorales, which are associated with high mortalities, particularly among immunosuppressed patients. In the present review, recent advances in the understanding of the pathophysiology, diagnosis, and treatment of mucormycoses are summarized.

EPIDEMIOLOGY

The most common fungal organisms causing mucormycosis are summarized in **Table 1**. Seasonal variations affect the incidence of mucormycoses, with most infections occurring from late August to November.[9] Because the Mucorales are ubiquitous environmental fungi found in decaying organic substrates,[2] mucormycoses with uncommon species, even in immunocompetent adults, have been associated with major natural disasters: wound infections due to *Apophysomyces elegans* were reported after the tsunami in Sri-Lanka[10]; *Syncephalastrum racemosum* was isolated from respiratory samples following Hurricane Katrina[11]; and *Apophysomyces trapeziformis* caused soft tissue infections in patients with traumatic injuries associated with the tornado in Joplin, Missouri.[12] Furthermore, death by drowning is a well-described risk factor for donor-derived pulmonary mucormycosis (PM) in solid organ transplant (SOT) recipients.[13-15]

Table 1 Most common fungal organisms causing mucormycosis (approximate percentage frequency) and entomophthoramycosis	
Mucormycosis	**%**
Rhizopus arrhizus (R oryzae) *Rhizopus microspores* *Rhizopus stolonifer*	47
Mucor circinelloides *Mucor velutinosus*	18
Cunninghamella bertholletiae	7
Apophysomyces elegans	5
Saksenaea vasiformis	5
Lichtheimia (Absidia) corymbifera	5
Rhizomucor pusillus	4
Syncephalastrum racemosum	—
Actinomucor elegans	—
Cokeromyces recurvatus	—
Mortierella wolfii	—
Entomophthoramycosis	**%**
Conidiobolus coronatus	—
Conidiobolus incongruous	—
Basidiobolus ranarum	—

Data from Refs.[3,4,16,187]

Until the past 2 decades, most published cases of mucormycosis had been in diabetic patients.[16] However, there has been a notable increase in the rates of mucormycosis in the growing and vulnerable population of patients with impaired immune defenses, primarily those with hematological malignancies (HM) and recipients of hematopoietic stem cell transplants (HSCT) or SOTs.[16–22] The exact incidence of mucormycosis is not known, but in a 1992 to 1993 US population-based survey, was estimated at 1.7 cases per 1 million people-years (500 cases per year).[23] More recent surveys from Europe have reported annual rates between 0.43 and 1.2 cases per million.[24,25] On the contrary, in a review of autopsy data in patients with HM from 1999 to 2003 at MD Anderson Cancer Center (Houston, TX), there were approximately 30 cases per 1000 autopsies,[26] with mucormycosis being 60- to 300-fold more common than in older autopsy series in the general population.[23] Among patients with HM and HSCT recipients, mucormycosis is the second most common invasive mold infection (IMI) after invasive aspergillosis (IA).[17] Data from the Centers for Disease Control and Prevention Transplant Associated Infection Surveillance Network, acquired from prospective surveys of 25 US transplantation centers from 2001 to 2006, reported 1-year incidence rates for mucormycosis of 0.29% in allogeneic-HSCT[27] and 0.07% in SOT,[28] accounting for 8% and 2%, respectively, of all IFIs. In some hospitals, investigators have noted a shift in mucormycosis cases from HSCT recipients to the acute leukemia population.[22,29]

The increasing number of mucormycosis cases breaking through antifungal prophylaxis or treatment effective against *Aspergillus* but not the Mucorales (voriconazole, echinocandins) is concerning.[17,30–32] In the most recent autopsy study of IFI among all patients with HM from MD Anderson (1998–2008), the incidence of *Aspergillus* spp decreased significantly, whereas only Mucorales accounted for an increasing proportion of IFIs,[33] which could be due to the increasing use of voriconazole and echinocandins. The authors' prior[17] and most recent[34] experience with leukemia and HSCT patients suggests that mucormycosis is the most likely in cases of fungal sinusitis when the patient has been receiving *Aspergillus*-active antifungal prophylaxis.

Breakthrough mucormycosis in patients with cancer receiving voriconazole prophylaxis has been associated with a crude mortality of 73%.[17] Also, evidence from animal models suggests that voriconazole may increase the virulence of certain Mucorales, although the mechanism is unclear.[35] Such factors, along with a shift to more immunocompromised patient populations, and delayed diagnosis, likely account for the relatively stable high mortalities, despite major advances in antifungal chemotherapy.[36]

Outside of the HM patient population,[37] risk factors for mucormycosis are poorly controlled diabetes, especially in the setting of ketoacidosis,[38,39] high-dose glucocorticoids, penetrating trauma or burns, and chelation therapy with deferoxamine in hemodialysis or transfusion-dependent patients.[16,36] Less frequently,[16,36] mucormycosis occurs in the setting of renal failure, malnutrition in low-birth-weight infants, surgical wounds (from contaminated bandages),[37,40,41] and blast combat injuries.[42] In intravenous drug users, fatal cerebral mucormycosis has been described and should be considered in cases of rapidly progressing brain abscesses or in the absence of response to antibacterials.[16,43]

PATHOGENESIS

The primary mode of infection in sino-PMs is through inhalation of fungal spores.[36,44,45] Most Mucorales form spores that are sufficiently small (3–11 μm) to reach the distal alveolar spaces. Larger spores (>10 μm) may lodge in the nasal turbinates, causing sinusitis.[2,3] Inhalation of a high-spore inoculum, such as with construction in contaminated air ducts, can lead to subacute sino-PM even in immunocompetent hosts.[46] However, to establish infection, fungal spores must generally overcome phagocytosis by macrophages and neutrophils to germinate into hyphae—the angioinvasive form of infection (**Fig. 1**).[9,45] Therefore, mucormycosis rarely affects humans with healthy innate immune response, but it can be rapidly progressive and lethal in neutropenic patients, particularly those with HM, who also have no monocyte reserve.[44]

Glucocorticoids are known to impair macrophage migration, ingestion, and phagolysosome fusion; therefore, patients on high-dose steroids represent another high-risk group for mucormycoses.[47,48] Moreover, neutrophils collected from patients with hyperglycemia and ketoacidosis show impaired chemotaxis and diminished fungicidal mechanisms against the Mucorales spores and hyphae, partially accounting for the well-known predisposition of patients with diabetes to mucormycosis.[39,49] Obese normoglycemic immunocompetent *Drosophila melanogaster* flies succumb faster to *Rhizopus oryzae* infection and have higher tissue fungal burdens compared with normal-weight flies.[50] Notably, obese flies also had significantly higher glucose levels shortly after infection, even before the establishment of diabetes (elevated glucose levels in the absence of stress).[50] In another recent study of HM patients with PM, hyperglycemia was associated with significantly higher 4-week mortality (>200 mg/dL, 56% vs <200 mg/dL, 28%, $P<.05$), although the prevalence of known diabetes was similar in patients who survived for greater than 4 weeks (30%) and those who did not (32%).[51] These data highlight the importance of (stress-induced) hyperglycemia as a predisposing factor and one associated with unfavorable outcomes in patients with mucormycosis.

In cases of primary cutaneous mucormycosis, subcutaneous inoculation of spores through breach of the skin barrier can lead to infection, even with minor trauma, such as insect bites and tattooing.[52,53] Stress-induced hyperglycemia further contributes to the increased susceptibility of burn patients to mucormycosis.[54] Health care–associated cases of mucormycosis[41,55] have been described with the use of contaminated needles, bandages,[56,57] even tongue depressors.[3,9]

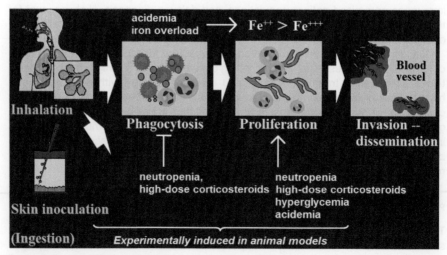

Fig. 1. Pathogenesis of mucormycosis.

Little is known about mechanisms of attachment to and invasion of mucosal surfaces by fungi causing mucormycosis. Recent studies have suggested that sporangiospores are able to adhere to subendothelial matrix proteins and invade intact endothelial barriers.[58,59] Intriguingly, live spores are not essential for causing tissue damage, and injection of heat-killed *Rhizopus* kills diabetic mice, suggesting that secreted components may be toxic to endothelial cells.[58,60] Some mycotoxins may not be directly produced by the fungus itself, but by endosymbiotic intracellular bacteria of the genus *Burkholderia*.[61] It is, therefore, possible that adaptation of toxin-producing endosymbiotic bacteria in response to antibacterial pressure may influence the virulence of molds causing mucormycosis.

The relationship between iron overload and mucormycosis is of particular interest.[44,45,62] Fungi acquire iron from the host by using siderophores (low-molecular-weight iron chelators) or high-affinity iron permeases (ferrirhizoferrin), the latter being likely more important for adaptation and survival inside the human host.[62] However, in mammalian hosts, iron is strongly bound to transferrin; therefore, a limited amount is available to micro-organisms, and iron starvation was recently found to induce *R oryzae* apoptosis.[63] Diabetic ketoacidosis is associated with increased free iron, because of the low pH, which is another mechanism explaining its strong association with mucormycosis.[64,65] Also, the ability of Mucorales to extract iron from desferrioxamine,[48,66–69] especially in the setting of uremia,[70] explains the susceptibility of hemodialysis patients receiving desferrioxamine to mucormycosis in the past, which nowadays has almost disappeared, with use of new chelating agents and erythropoietin instead of blood transfusions.[70]

CLINICAL MANIFESTATIONS

The mucormycoses are usually grouped according to clinical presentation and anatomic predilection into 1 of 6 syndromes, although some overlap exists (**Table 2**)[9,24,36]: 1. sinusitis (rhino-orbital or rhinocerebral) (**Fig. 2**); 2. pulmonary (**Fig. 3**); 3. cutaneous; 4. gastrointestinal; 5. disseminated; 6. other (uncommon) presentations, such as peritonitis (especially in the setting of peritoneal dialysis),[71–73] tracheitis,[74] mediastinitis,[75–77] renal abscess,[78] osteomyelitis,[79] myocarditis,[80] endocarditis,[81] otitis externa,[82] keratitis,[82] and isolated brain abscess in intravenous drug users.[43]

Sinusitis occurs more frequently in patients with poorly controlled diabetes, whereas PM is more common in patients with HM.[9,21] Necrotic eschars in the nasal

Table 2
Clinical manifestations of mucormycosis in different hosts

Host	Sinus	Pulmonary	Cutaneous	Gastrointestinal	Disseminated	Rare Manifestations
Diabetes	+	(+)*	(+)	—	—	*Endobronchial
HM, HSCT	+	+	(+)	(+)	+	(+)
SOT, steroids	+	+	(+)	(+)	(+)	(+)
Intravenous drug use	—	—	(+)	—	(+)	Endocarditis Brain abscess
Malnutrition	—	—	—	+	(+)	(+)
Trauma	—	—	+	—	(+)	(+)

+, common; (+), less frequent; *, endobronchial.

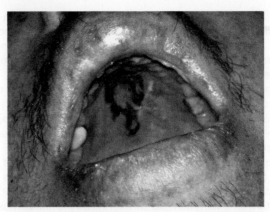

Fig. 2. Black necrotic eschar in the palate of a patient with rhinosinus mucormycosis.

cavity, the palate, or even the face can be early diagnostic signs (see **Fig. 2**)[83–85]; nevertheless, they are present in only 50% of patients, within 3 days of the onset of infection.[86] Contiguous extension to the orbit may lead to preseptal or orbital cellulitis, subperiosteal and orbital abscess, with resultant eyelid edema, chemosis, ptosis, proptosis, ophthalmoplegia, and loss of vision.[87,88] Trigeminal and facial cranial nerve palsies are not uncommon.[89] Intracranial complications include epidural and subdural abscess, cavernous and, less frequently, sagittal sinus thrombosis,[90] but frank meningitis is rarely observed.[9]

The clinical presentation of PM is similar to pulmonary IA, that is, pneumonia refractory to antibacterials.[9,21,91] Fungal invasion of blood vessels leads to hemoptysis, which can be massive and fatal.[92–94] Atypical presentations of PM include chronic infection with subacute constitutional symptoms in apparently immunocompetent hosts, multiple mycotic pulmonary artery aneurysms and pseudoaneurysms, bronchial obstruction, or asymptomatic solitary nodules.[9] Patients with diabetes have a predilection for the development of endobronchial lesions, which can occasionally progress to obstruction of major airways or erosion into pulmonary blood vessels.[2,9,24] Like *Aspergillus* spp, the Mucorales in rare instances can form mycetomas in pre-existing lung cavities or cause slowly necrotizing pneumonia and hypersensitivity syndromes. *Rhizopus* spp have also been implicated in an allergic alveolitis described in farm and sawmill workers (wood-trimmer's disease).[95,96]

Cutaneous zygomycosis, typically associated with trauma, starts with erythema and induration[97,98] and, if untreated, progresses to necrosis, extension to the subcutaneous tissue, and necrotizing fasciitis.[10,12,99–107] Necrotic skin lesions in immunocompromised patients have a very broad differential diagnosis; therefore, skin biopsy is required.[108] Unlike other fungal pathogens (*Candida* and *Fusarium* spp),[108] the skin appears to be a much less common site of involvement in disseminated mucormycosis.

Gastrointestinal mucormycosis affects mostly patients with malnutrition, or it can be secondary to disseminated infection.[9] Depending on host and anatomic location, it can present as peptic ulceration, neutropenic typhlitis, appendiceal or ileal mass, or, in premature neonates, necrotizing enterocolitis.[109,110] Ingestion of herbal medications contaminated with *Mucor indicus* has been described to cause liver abscess.[111] Neutropenic patients with leukemia and HSCT recipients are the main groups at risk for disseminated mucormycosis, usually with PM as the primary source.[21]

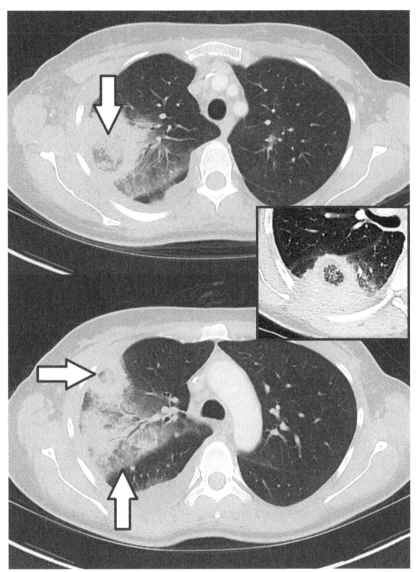

Fig. 3. Single (*inset*) and multiple (*arrows*) reversed halo signs in patients with PM. (*Courtesy of* Sophia Koo, MD, SM, Brigham and Women's Hospital and Dana-Farber Cancer Institute, Harvard Medical School, Boston, MA.)

DIAGNOSIS

Diagnosis of mucormycosis is challenging, because clinical symptoms and signs are nonspecific, but delayed initiation of appropriate treatment can be detrimental: In a case series of leukemia and HSCT patients with fungal pneumonia, 84% of patients who were eventually diagnosed with PM were receiving ineffective antifungal therapy at the time of diagnosis.[112] Furthermore, in a classification and regression tree analysis of HM patients with PM who received appropriate antifungal therapy, a delay in the administration of amphotericin-B (AMB) for 6 days or more was associated with doubling of all-cause mortalities.[113]

In susceptible hosts, evidence of pulmonary infarction in high-resolution pulmonary computed tomographic (CT) angiography is highly diagnostic of IMIs.[114–116] Such clinical and radiographic syndromes of IFI while on voriconazole prophylaxis should be approached as mucormycosis unless proven otherwise.[30–32,36,117] A chest CT can provide further useful information early in the course of the disease, mainly the reversed halo sign, an area of central ground-glass necrosis, surrounded by a ring of consolidation (see **Fig. 3**), reflecting central lung infarction with dense peripheral hemorrhage.[118–122] This finding was first described in cryptogenic organizing pneumonia and can be present in various pulmonary syndromes.[121,123,124] Nonetheless, in a recent series of neutropenic patients with leukemia and PM, 15 of 16 patients (94%) had the reversed halo sign early in sequential chest CTs, and the investigators concluded that it is a pathognomonic early sign of PM in this patient population.[120] Other radiographic findings that might favor PM over IA are multiple ($\geq$10) nodules and pleural effusions[91]; however, they seem to appear later in the course of PM.[120]

The presence of sinusitis, especially pansinusitis, along with pulmonary infiltrates is consistent with PM rather than IA.[91] Among patients with mold sinusitis, those with diabetes or receiving high-dose corticosteroids were more likely to have mucormycosis.[34] Negative fungal markers (β-D-glucan or galactomannan) with clinical or radiographic presentation consistent with IFI are strongly suggestive of mucormycosis, given that both are virtually absent from the fungal wall of the Mucorales.[125]

Definitive diagnosis of mucormycosis requires histopathological evidence of fungal invasion of tissue.[3,126] Hyphae of the Mucorales are broad (3–25 μm), thin-walled, mostly aseptate, with nondichotomous, irregular branching, occasionally at right angles (**Fig. 4**).[1,9] However, histopathological sections occasionally show twisted and compressed hyphae, which may be mistaken for septae, similar to *Aspergillus* (see **Fig. 4**). Perineural invasion, which is found in 90% of tissues that contain nerves, can be a useful diagnostic clue.[9,89] Compared with other filamentous fungi, the Mucorales do not stain as deeply with specialized fungal stains, such as Gomori methenamine silver (GMS) or periodic acid-Schiff stain, but they can often be detected in tissue sections stained with hematoxylin and eosin (H&E). Costaining with H&E intensifies GMS staining of hyphae, potentially providing a unique clue for identification of Mucorales. Calcofluor white, Blankofluor, or Uvitex may enhance detection of hyphae and improve the discrimination between septate and aseptate molds during microscopic examination.[45,113]

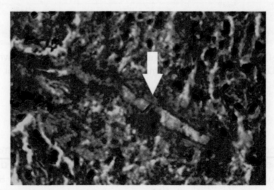

Fig. 4. Characteristic appearance of an aseptate, broad-angled *Cunninghamella* hyphal form in H&E (original magnification ×400) tissue stain. Note central fragmentation resembling a septum (*arrow*).

It should be noted that needle biopsy is not always diagnostic, even when a pathogen is identified, as exemplified in the "green herring" syndrome, a term recently used to describe bacterial superinfection masking PM in patients with HM.[127] Also, because of the ubiquitous nature of the fungus in the environment, positive cultures may occasionally reflect culture contamination rather than true infection, especially in nonimmunocompromised hosts.[9]

Identification to the genus and species level requires cultivation in fungal culture media, such as Sabouraud dextrose agar incubated at 25°C to 30° C, to examine reproductive fruiting structures. The level of development of the rhizoids, the shape of the sporangium, and the location of the sporangiospores are the morphologic features used to identify different genera of Mucorales. Molecular identification techniques (polymerase chain reaction [PCR]), and MALDI-TOF (matrix-assisted laser desorption ionization time-of-flight) mass spectrometry[128] could be of utility as adjunctive diagnostics, or for confirmation of pathogen genus when histopathology is positive but cultures are negative.[9,129]

Another potential diagnostic tool is the identification of Mucorales-specific T cells in the blood.[130] Mucorales-specific CD4+ or CD8+ cells were detected in 3 HM patients with mucormycosis, both at diagnosis and throughout the entire course of PM, but neither before nor after resolution of the infection. In the same study, none of 25 patients with HM and other clinical syndromes had Mucorales-specific T cells.[130] Similar to PCR, these results require further validation in larger-scale studies, before those methods are established as adjunctive diagnostic tests for mucormycosis.[131]

ANTIFUNGAL TREATMENT

AMB is the most active antifungal agent against mucormycosis.[3,36,132,133] AMB lipid formulations (liposomal AMB [LAMB, Ambisome] and AMB lipid complex [ABLC, Abelcet]) are better tolerated than AMB-deoxycholate, but their use is still hampered by nephrotoxicity and infusion reactions.[133,134] The latter do not seem to represent a class effect, and patients with severe infusion reactions to one AMB lipid formulation can often tolerate the other.[135,136] The standard dose of LAMB and ABLC is 5 mg/kg, but higher doses of LAMB (7.5–10 mg/kg) have been proposed for the treatment of mucormycosis.[36] Nevertheless, in a recent series, high-dose LAMB (10 mg/kg) was not more effective compared with prior studies (36% success rate at 6 weeks, 45% at 12), but was associated with a high rate (40%) of kidney injury, defined as doubling of serum creatinine while on LAMB treatment.[137]

Posaconazole has potent activity against the Mucorales.[138] In an open-label salvage trial, the success rate of posaconazole oral solution (800 mg in 4 divided doses) was 70% in 24 patients. The drug was well-tolerated with only minimal gastrointestinal side effects.[139] Similarly, a retrospective review of posaconazole-based salvage therapy in 91 patients who had refractory mucormycosis showed a success rate of 61% (65% in patients with PM). An additional 21% of subjects had stable disease after 12 weeks of treatment.[140] The recent introduction of an extended release tablet (300 mg daily after a loading dose of 300 mg twice a day for 2 doses) overcomes the tenuous absorption of the liquid suspension, independent of gastric acidity.[141] The tablet cannot be crushed for administration through a gastric or enteric tube, but an intravenous formulation is available.[142] Although steady-state serum levels are usually greater than 1000 ng/mL,[141] until more clinical data are available, the authors favor therapeutic drug monitoring, given the concern for hepatotoxicity with high concentrations, subtherapeutic drug levels in obese individuals, and drug-drug interactions.[143] It should be noted that, in a small series of leukemia patients, switching from posaconazole suspension to tablets significantly increased serum drug levels without apparent hepatotoxicity.[144]

Isavuconazole is another triazole that was recently approved by the US Food and Drug Administration for the management of IMI, including mucormycosis.[145–147] It is available in oral and intravenous formulations and is administered with a loading dose of 200 mg 3 times a day for 2 days and 200 mg daily thereafter. Isavuconazole is a substrate, but, unlike the other azoles, is not an inhibitor of cytochrome P450 enzymes, and, therefore, has only few drug-drug interactions. Its oral bioavailability is excellent (98%), independent of gastric acidity and intake with food, and it does not cause QT prolongation.[145–147]

Isavuconazole was administered to an HSCT recipient with clinical and radiographic improvement after 29 weeks of treatment.[148] Also, a patient with ulcerative colitis on high-dose steroids and sino-orbital mucormycosis responded to salvage treatment with isavuconazole, despite clinical failure of AMB + posaconazole for 3 months prior, and had a durable (>2 years) clinical response, despite high (>8 µg/mL) in vitro minimum inhibitory concentrations.[149]

The VITAL study was a multicenter, phase III noncomparator trial of isavuconazole for the treatment of IFIs.[150] Among 37 patients with mucormycosis, 21 received isavuconazole as primary treatment and 16 received isavuconazole as salvage treatment. Treatment success was 31% (11 of 35 evaluable patients), which is comparable to a series of AMB-based treatments. Stable disease, regarded as failure, was achieved in 10 additional patients (27%). Complete response was achieved in 5 patients (14%), after 86 to 735 days of treatment. The remarkably long treatment durations in all of the above studies speak for the safety and tolerability of the 2 triazoles for the treatment of mucormycosis.[145,146]

Successful treatment of mucormycosis with combinations of AMB, terbinafine, and rifampin has been described in case reports.[151–154] In one retrospective analysis, the combination of AMB + echinocandin was associated with improved therapeutic success in diabetic patients with rhino-orbital or rhinocerebral mucormycosis, in that 6 of 7 patients started on the combination of LAMB/ABLC + caspofungin were successfully treated, compared with only 7 of 22 on ABLC (P = .02).[155] This observation is in agreement with in vitro studies and animal experiments that showed evidence of synergism between polyenes and echinocandins, presumably due to degradation of the small amount of glucan, with unmasking of immune epitopes and facilitation of phagocytosis.[156–160] However, a recent study of 106 HM patients with mucormycosis failed to show any benefit from combination treatment, compared with AMB monotherapy, in unadjusted analysis, and after robust propensity score–based adjustment for confounding factors.[161]

Based on these data, the authors deem that early (within 4–6 days) initiation of AMB lipid formulation monotherapy should be considered adequate first-line treatment of mucormycosis. Posaconazole and isavuconazole are acceptable salvage and long-term treatment options, which can also be used as initial therapy in patients at high risk from polyene-induced nephrotoxicity. In vitro minimal inhibitory concentrations to isavuconazole tend to be high[145,162,163] and should be taken into consideration in the appropriate clinical context.

ADJUNCTIVE MANAGEMENT

In rhinosinusitis, surgical debridement of infected tissue is crucial and should be urgently performed to limit the aggressive spread of infection. Repeated removal of necrotic tissue or radical surgical resection, even orbit exenteration, with subsequent reconstructive surgeries, may be required.[164] However, rhinosinus mucormycosis has been treated successfully in select patients without radical resection.[165] In PM, surgical treatment in conjunction with systemic antifungal therapy has been shown to significantly improve survival compared with antifungal therapy alone.[92,164] Cavitation of lesions near hilar vessels can lead to fatal hemoptysis, providing an additional reason for resection.[9,92] Overall, although study outcomes may reflect a selection bias in offering surgery to less severely ill patients with localized disease, the authors deem that timely removal of devitalized tissue provides significant benefit.

The increased oxygen pressure achieved with hyperbaric oxygen (HBO) treatment appears to improve the ability of neutrophils to kill organisms. Furthermore, by reversing acidosis, treatment with HBO promotes the AMB action. In addition, high oxygen pressure inhibits fungal growth and improves the rate of wound healing by elevating tissue oxygen levels and releasing growth factors. Thus, treatment with HBO may be a beneficial adjunct to surgical and antifungal therapy for mucormycosis, particularly in patients with diabetes who have sinusitis, or in cutaneous mucormycosis.[85,166–170]

Unlike deferoxamine, the newer chelator agent deferasirox, which does not act as xenosiderophore to the Mucorales, showed protective effects in animal models of mucormycosis[66,171] and case reports.[172] However, in a small study of patients with probable or proven mucormycosis, those treated with deferasirox + LAMB had significantly higher 90-day mortality compared with patients treated with LAMB alone.[173] Therefore, adjunctive iron chelation therapy cannot be recommended in patients with mucormycosis.

Immune-augmentation strategies, such as administration of granulocyte (macrophage) colony-stimulating factor or interferon-γ, alone or in combination with granulocyte transfusions, have shown promise in vitro and in case reports.[174,175] However, granulocyte transfusions also carry some risk for inflammatory lung injury.[176] Statins were found to have in vitro[177] and in vivo (Dimitrios P. Kontoyiannis, MD, ScD, unpublished data, 2015) activity against *Rhizopus* spp and have been described as promising drugs for mucormycosis treatment.[39] Given the limited evidence, the relative benefit of adjunctive strategies must be balanced against the cost and potential for harm, on an individual patient basis.

SUMMARY AND FUTURE DIRECTIONS

Advances in diagnosis and the recent availability of nontoxic active antifungals have improved the prospects for control and even cure of mucormycosis. However, many fundamental issues are still unresolved[178]: What is the optimal initial antifungal therapy, balancing efficacy with toxicity and drug-drug interactions: AMB, posaconazole, or isavuconazole? Which patients will benefit from broad-spectrum antifungal prophylaxis, in the era of antifungal stewardship and selective pressure from prolonged use of azoles, leading to worrisome rates of antifungal resistance among *Candida* spp[143,179–184]? What are the most appropriate timing and extent of surgical intervention? Is there a role for adoptive immunotherapy for IMI,[185] including mucormycosis? Do the Mucorales have a volatome signature, like *Aspergillus* spp,[186] which could be detected in patient breath, and lead to early and accurate bedside diagnosis? These important questions remain to be answered through translational research, standardized, prospective data collection, and multi-institutional collaborations.

ACKNOWLEDGMENTS

D.P. Kontoyiannis acknowledges the Frances King Black Endowment for Cancer Research.

REFERENCES

1. Larone DH. Medically important fungi—a guide to identification. 3rd edition. Washington, DC: ASM Press; 1995.
2. Ribes JA, Vanover-Sams CL, Baker DJ. Zygomycetes in human disease. Clin Microbiol Rev 2000;13(2):236–301.
3. Kontoyiannis DP, Lewis RE. Agents of mucormycosis and entomophthoramycosis. In: Mandell GE, Bennett JE, Dolin R, editors. Mandell, Douglas and Bennett's principles and practice of infectious diseases, vol. 1, 7th edition. Philadephia: Chuchill-- Livingstone; 2010. p. 3257–69.
4. Kwon-Chung KJ. Taxonomy of fungi causing mucormycosis and entomophthoramycosis (zygomycosis) and nomenclature of the disease: molecular mycologic perspectives. Clin Infect Dis 2012;54(Suppl 1):S8–15.
5. Spellberg B, Edwards J Jr, Ibrahim A. Novel perspectives on mucormycosis: pathophysiology, presentation, and management. Clin Microbiol Rev 2005; 18(3):556–69.
6. Bigliazzi C, Poletti V, Dell'Amore D, et al. Disseminated basidiobolomycosis in an immunocompetent woman. J Clin Microbiol 2004;42(3):1367–9.
7. Vikram HR, Smilack JD, Leighton JA, et al. Emergence of gastrointestinal basidiobolomycosis in the United States, with a review of worldwide cases. Clin Infect Dis 2012;54(12):1685–91.
8. Lyon GM, Smilack JD, Komatsu KK, et al. Gastrointestinal basidiobolomycosis in Arizona: clinical and epidemiological characteristics and review of the literature. Clin Infect Dis 2001;32(10):1448–55.
9. Kontoyiannis DP, Lewis RE. Invasive zygomycosis: update on pathogenesis, clinical manifestations, and management. Infect Dis Clin North Am 2006; 20(3):581–607.
10. Andresen D, Donaldson A, Choo L, et al. Multifocal cutaneous mucormycosis complicating polymicrobial wound infections in a tsunami survivor from Sri Lanka. Lancet 2005;365(9462):876–8.
11. Rao CY, Kurukularatne C, Garcia-Diaz JB, et al. Implications of detecting the mold syncephalastrum in clinical specimens of New Orleans residents after hurricanes Katrina and Rita. J Occup Environ Med 2007;49(4):411–6.
12. Neblett Fanfair R, Benedict K, Bos J, et al. Necrotizing cutaneous mucormycosis after a tornado in Joplin, Missouri, in 2011. N Engl J Med 2012;367(23):2214–25.
13. Gomez CA, Singh N. Donor-derived filamentous fungal infections in solid organ transplant recipients. Curr Opin Infect Dis 2013;26(4):309–16.
14. Singh N, Huprikar S, Burdette SD, et al. Donor-derived fungal infections in organ transplant recipients: guidelines of the American Society of Transplantation, Infectious Diseases Community of Practice. Am J Transplant 2012;12(9): 2414–28.
15. Alexander BD, Schell WA, Siston AM, et al. Fatal Apophysomyces elegans infection transmitted by deceased donor renal allografts. Am J Transplant 2010;10(9):2161–7.
16. Roden MM, Zaoutis TE, Buchanan WL, et al. Epidemiology and outcome of zygomycosis: a review of 929 reported cases. Clin Infect Dis 2005;41(5): 634–53.
17. Kontoyiannis DP, Lionakis MS, Lewis RE, et al. Zygomycosis in a tertiary-care cancer center in the era of Aspergillus-active antifungal therapy: a case-control observational study of 27 recent cases. J Infect Dis 2005;191(8): 1350–60.

18. Marr KA, Carter RA, Crippa F, et al. Epidemiology and outcome of mould infections in hematopoietic stem cell transplant recipients. Clin Infect Dis 2002;34(7): 909–17.

19. Pagano L, Girmenia C, Mele L, et al. Infections caused by filamentous fungi in patients with hematologic malignancies. A report of 391 cases by GIMEMA Infection Program. Haematologica 2001;86(8):862–70.

20. Pagano L, Ricci P, Tonso A, et al. Mucormycosis in patients with haematological malignancies: a retrospective clinical study of 37 cases. GIMEMA Infection Program (Gruppo Italiano Malattie Ematologiche Maligne dell'Adulto). Br J Haematol 1997;99(2):331–6.

21. Kontoyiannis DP, Wessel VC, Bodey GP, et al. Zygomycosis in the 1990s in a tertiary-care cancer center. Clin Infect Dis 2000;30(6):851–6.

22. Hammond SP, Baden LR, Marty FM. Mortality in hematologic malignancy and hematopoietic stem cell transplant patients with mucormycosis, 2001 to 2009. Antimicrob Agents Chemother 2011;55(11):5018–21.

23. Rees JR, Pinner RW, Hajjeh RA, et al. The epidemiological features of invasive mycotic infections in the San Francisco Bay Area, 1992-1993: results of population-based laboratory active surveillance. Clin Infect Dis 1998;27(5): 1138–47.

24. Petrikkos G, Skiada A, Lortholary O, et al. Epidemiology and clinical manifestations of mucormycosis. Clin Infect Dis 2012;54(Suppl 1):S23–34.

25. Petrikkos G, Skiada A, Drogari-Apiranthitou M. Epidemiology of mucormycosis in Europe. Clin Microbiol Infect 2014;20(Suppl 6):67–73.

26. Chamilos G, Luna M, Lewis RE, et al. Invasive fungal infections in patients with hematologic malignancies in a tertiary care cancer center: an autopsy study over a 15-year period (1989-2003). Haematologica 2006;91(7):986–9.

27. Kontoyiannis DP, Marr KA, Park BJ, et al. Prospective surveillance for invasive fungal infections in hematopoietic stem cell transplant recipients, 2001-2006: overview of the Transplant-Associated Infection Surveillance Network (TRANSNET) Database. Clin Infect Dis 2010;50(8):1091–100.

28. Pappas PG, Alexander BD, Andes DR, et al. Invasive fungal infections among organ transplant recipients: results of the Transplant-Associated Infection Surveillance Network (TRANSNET). Clin Infect Dis 2010;50(8):1101–11.

29. Woolley AE, Farmakiotis D, Liakos A, et al. ID week 2015 abstract 1211: temporal trends in stem cell transplant and hematologic malignancy patients with mucormycosis, 2001-2014. San Diego (CA): Infectious Diseases Society of America; 2015.

30. Marty FM, Cosimi LA, Baden LR. Breakthrough zygomycosis after voriconazole treatment in recipients of hematopoietic stem-cell transplants. N Engl J Med 2004;350(9):950–2.

31. Imhof A, Balajee SA, Fredricks DN, et al. Breakthrough fungal infections in stem cell transplant recipients receiving voriconazole. Clin Infect Dis 2004;39(5): 743–6.

32. Siwek GT, Dodgson KJ, de Magalhaes-Silverman M, et al. Invasive zygomycosis in hematopoietic stem cell transplant recipients receiving voriconazole prophylaxis. Clin Infect Dis 2004;39(4):584–7.

33. Lewis RE, Cahyame-Zuniga L, Leventakos K, et al. Epidemiology and sites of involvement of invasive fungal infections in patients with haematological malignancies: a 20-year autopsy study. Mycoses 2013;56(6):638–45.

34. Davoudi S, Kumar VA, Jiang Y, et al. Invasive mould sinusitis in patients with haematological malignancies: a 10 year single-centre study. J Antimicrob Chemother 2015;70(10):2899–905.

35. Lamaris GA, Ben-Ami R, Lewis RE, et al. Increased virulence of zygomycetes organisms following exposure to voriconazole: a study involving fly and murine models of zygomycosis. J Infect Dis 2009;199(9):1399–406.
36. Kontoyiannis DP, Lewis RE. How I treat mucormycosis. Blood 2011;118(5): 1216–24.
37. Sims CR, Ostrosky-Zeichner L. Contemporary treatment and outcomes of zygomycosis in a non-oncologic tertiary care center. Arch Med Res 2007;38(1):90–3.
38. Peleg AY, Weerarathna T, McCarthy JS, et al. Common infections in diabetes: pathogenesis, management and relationship to glycaemic control. Diabetes Metab Res Rev 2007;23(1):3–13.
39. Rammaert B, Lanternier F, Poiree S, et al. Diabetes and mucormycosis: a complex interplay. Diabetes Metab 2012;38(3):193–204.
40. Skiada A, Petrikkos G. Cutaneous mucormycosis. Skinmed 2013;11(3):155–9 [quiz: 159–60].
41. Davoudi S, Graviss LS, Kontoyiannis DP. Healthcare-associated outbreaks due to Mucorales and other uncommon fungi. Eur J Clin Invest 2015;45(7):767–73.
42. Warkentien T, Rodriguez C, Lloyd B, et al. Invasive mold infections following combat-related injuries. Clin Infect Dis 2012;55(11):1441–9.
43. Clark D, Al Mohajer M, Broderick J. Pearls & Oy-sters: isolated cerebral zygomycosis in an intravenous drug user. Neurology 2011;76(1):e1–2.
44. Ibrahim AS, Spellberg B, Walsh TJ, et al. Pathogenesis of mucormycosis. Clin Infect Dis 2012;54(Suppl 1):S16–22.
45. Ibrahim AS, Kontoyiannis DP. Update on mucormycosis pathogenesis. Curr Opin Infect Dis 2013;26(6):508–15.
46. England AC 3rd, Weinstein M, Ellner JJ, et al. Two cases of rhinocerebral zygomycosis (mucormycosis) with common epidemiologic and environmental features. Am Rev Respir Dis 1981;124(4):497–8.
47. Lionakis MS, Kontoyiannis DP. Glucocorticoids and invasive fungal infections. Lancet 2003;362(9398):1828–38.
48. Chamilos G, Lewis RE, Hu J, et al. Drosophila melanogaster as a model host to dissect the immunopathogenesis of zygomycosis. Proc Natl Acad Sci U S A 2008;105(27):9367–72.
49. Waldorf AR, Ruderman N, Diamond RD. Specific susceptibility to mucormycosis in murine diabetes and bronchoalveolar macrophage defense against Rhizopus. J Clin Invest 1984;74(1):150–60.
50. Shirazi F, Farmakiotis D, Yan Y, et al. Diet modification and metformin have a beneficial effect in a fly model of obesity and mucormycosis. PLoS One 2014; 9(9):e108635.
51. Lewis RE, Georgiadou SP, Sampsonas F, et al. Risk factors for early mortality in haematological malignancy patients with pulmonary mucormycosis. Mycoses 2014;57(1):49–55.
52. Prevoo RL, Starink TM, de Haan P. Primary cutaneous mucormycosis in a healthy young girl. Report of a case caused by Mucor hiemalis Wehmer. J Am Acad Dermatol 1991;24(5 Pt 2):882–5.
53. Parker C, Kaminski G, Hill D. Zygomycosis in a tattoo, caused by Saksenaea vasiformis. Australas J Dermatol 1986;27(3):107–11.
54. Chinn RY, Diamond RD. Generation of chemotactic factors by Rhizopus oryzae in the presence and absence of serum: relationship to hyphal damage mediated by human neutrophils and effects of hyperglycemia and ketoacidosis. Infect Immun 1982;38(3):1123–9.

55. Rammaert B, Lanternier F, Zahar JR, et al. Healthcare-associated mucormycosis. Clin Infect Dis 2012;54(Suppl 1):S44–54.
56. Paparello SF, Parry RL, MacGillivray DC, et al. Hospital-acquired wound mucormycosis. Clin Infect Dis 1992;14(1):350–2.
57. Chakrabarti A, Kumar P, Padhye AA, et al. Primary cutaneous zygomycosis due to Saksenaea vasiformis and Apophysomyces elegans. Clin Infect Dis 1997; 24(4):580–3.
58. Ibrahim AS, Spellberg B, Avanessian V, et al. Rhizopus oryzae adheres to, is phagocytosed by, and damages endothelial cells in vitro. Infect Immun 2005; 73(2):778–83.
59. Bouchara JP, Oumeziane NA, Lissitzky JC, et al. Attachment of spores of the human pathogenic fungus Rhizopus oryzae to extracellular matrix components. Eur J Cell Biol 1996;70(1):76–83.
60. Chayakulkeeree M, Ghannoum MA, Perfect JR. Zygomycosis: the re-emerging fungal infection. Eur J Clin Microbiol Infect Dis 2006;25(4):215–29.
61. Partida-Martinez LP, Hertweck C. Pathogenic fungus harbours endosymbiotic bacteria for toxin production. Nature 2005;437(7060):884–8.
62. Howard DH. Acquisition, transport, and storage of iron by pathogenic fungi. Clin Microbiol Rev 1999;12(3):394–404.
63. Shirazi F, Kontoyiannis DP, Ibrahim AS. Iron starvation induces apoptosis in rhizopus oryzae in vitro. Virulence 2015;6(2):121–6.
64. Artis WM, Patrusky E, Rastinejad F, et al. Fungistatic mechanism of human transferrin for Rhizopus oryzae and Trichophyton mentagrophytes: alternative to simple iron deprivation. Infect Immun 1983;41(3):1269–78.
65. Artis WM, Fountain JA, Delcher HK, et al. A mechanism of susceptibility to mucormycosis in diabetic ketoacidosis: transferrin and iron availability. Diabetes 1982;31(12):1109–14.
66. Boelaert JR, Van Cutsem J, de Locht M, et al. Deferoxamine augments growth and pathogenicity of Rhizopus, while hydroxypyridinone chelators have no effect. Kidney Int 1994;45(3):667–71.
67. Boelaert JR, de Locht M, Schneider YJ. The effect of deferoxamine on different zygomycetes. J Infect Dis 1994;169(1):231–2.
68. de Locht M, Boelaert JR, Schneider YJ. Iron uptake from ferrioxamine and from ferrirhizoferrin by germinating spores of Rhizopus microsporus. Biochem Pharmacol 1994;47(10):1843–50.
69. Boelaert JR, de Locht M, Van Cutsem J, et al. Mucormycosis during deferoxamine therapy is a siderophore-mediated infection. In vitro and in vivo animal studies. J Clin Invest 1993;91(5):1979–86.
70. Verpooten GA, D'Haese PC, Boelaert JR, et al. Pharmacokinetics of aluminoxamine and ferrioxamine and dose finding of desferrioxamine in haemodialysis patients. Nephrol Dial Transplant 1992;7(9):931–8.
71. Branton MH, Johnson SC, Brooke JD, et al. Peritonitis due to Rhizopus in a patient undergoing continuous ambulatory peritoneal dialysis. Rev Infect Dis 1991; 13(1):19–21.
72. Nakamura M, Weil WB Jr, Kaufman DB. Fatal fungal peritonitis in an adolescent on continuous ambulatory peritoneal dialysis: association with deferoxamine. Pediatr Nephrol 1989;3(1):80–2.
73. Polo JR, Luno J, Menarguez C, et al. Peritoneal mucormycosis in a patient receiving continuous ambulatory peritoneal dialysis. Am J Kidney Dis 1989; 13(3):237–9.

74. Schwartz JR, Nagle MG, Elkins RC, et al. Mucormycosis of the trachea: an unusual cause of acute upper airway obstruction. Chest 1982;81(5):653–4.
75. Connor BA, Anderson RJ, Smith JW. Mucor mediastinitis. Chest 1979;75(4):525–6.
76. Marwaha RK, Banerjee AK, Thapa BR, et al. Mediastinal zygomycosis. Postgrad Med J 1985;61(718):733–5.
77. Puthanakit T, Pongprot Y, Borisuthipandit T, et al. A mediastinal mass resembling lymphoma: an unusual manifestation of probable case of invasive zygomycosis in an immunocompetent child. J Med Assoc Thai 2005; 88(10):1430–3.
78. Lussier N, Laverdiere M, Weiss K, et al. Primary renal mucormycosis. Urology 1998;52(5):900–3.
79. Echols RM, Selinger DS, Hallowell C, et al. Rhizopus osteomyelitis. A case report and review. Am J Med 1979;66(1):141–5.
80. Roy TM, Anderson KC, Farrow JR. Cardiac mucormycosis complicating diabetes mellitus. J Diabet Complications 1990;4(3):132–5.
81. Mishra B, Mandal A, Kumar N. Mycotic prosthetic-valve endocarditis. J Hosp Infect 1992;20(2):122–5.
82. Tierney MR, Baker AS. Infections of the head and neck in diabetes mellitus. Infect Dis Clin North Am 1995;9(1):195–216.
83. DeWeese DD, Schleuning AJ 2nd, Robinson LB. Mucormycosis of the nose and paranasal sinuses. Laryngoscope 1965;75(9):1398–407.
84. Ferguson BJ. Mucormycosis of the nose and paranasal sinuses. Otolaryngol Clin North Am 2000;33(2):349–65.
85. Ferguson BJ, Mitchell TG, Moon R, et al. Adjunctive hyperbaric oxygen for treatment of rhinocerebral mucormycosis. Rev Infect Dis 1988;10(3):551–9.
86. Yohai RA, Bullock JD, Aziz AA, et al. Survival factors in rhino-orbital-cerebral mucormycosis. Surv Ophthalmol 1994;39(1):3–22.
87. Onyango JF, Kayima JK, Owen WO. Rhinocerebral mucormycosis: case report. East Afr Med J 2002;79(7):390–3.
88. Ochiai H, Iseda T, Miyahara S, et al. Rhinocerebral mucormycosis–case report. Neurol Med Chir (Tokyo) 1993;33(6):373–6.
89. Frater JL, Hall GS, Procop GW. Histologic features of zygomycosis: emphasis on perineural invasion and fungal morphology. Arch Pathol 2001;125(3): 375–8.
90. Tsai TC, Hou CC, Chou MS, et al. Rhinosino-orbital mucormycosis causing cavernous sinus thrombosis and internal carotid artery occlusion: radiological findings in a patient with treatment failure. Kaohsiung J Med Sci 1999;15(9): 556–61.
91. Chamilos G, Marom EM, Lewis RE, et al. Predictors of pulmonary zygomycosis versus invasive pulmonary aspergillosis in patients with cancer. Clin Infect Dis 2005;41(1):60–6.
92. Lee FY, Mossad SB, Adal KA. Pulmonary mucormycosis: the last 30 years. Arch Intern Med 1999;159(12):1301–9.
93. Gupta KL, Khullar DK, Behera D, et al. Pulmonary mucormycosis presenting as fatal massive haemoptysis in a renal transplant recipient. Nephrol Dial Transplant 1998;13(12):3258–60.
94. Funada H, Matsuda T. Pulmonary mucormycosis in a hematology ward. Intern Med 1996;35(7):540–4.
95. O'Connell MA, Pluss JL, Schkade P, et al. Rhizopus-induced hypersensitivity pneumonitis in a tractor driver. J Allergy Clin Immunol 1995;95(3):779–80.

96. Hedenstierna G, Alexandersson R, Belin L, et al. Lung function and Rhizopus antibodies in wood trimmers. A cross-sectional and longitudinal study. Int Arch Occup Environ Health 1986;58(3):167–77.

97. Nouri-Majalan N, Moghimi M. Skin mucormycosis presenting as an erythema-nodosum-like rash in a renal transplant recipient: a case report. J Med Case Rep 2008;2:112.

98. Vernon SE, Dave SP. Cutaneous zygomycosis associated with urate panniculitis. Am J Dermatopathol 2006;28(4):327–30.

99. Chander J, Kaur J, Attri A, et al. Primary cutaneous zygomycosis from a tertiary care centre in north-west India. Indian J Med Res 2010;131:765–70.

100. Devi SC, Kanungo R, Barreto E, et al. Favorable outcome of amphotericin B treatment of zygomycotic necrotizing fascitis caused by Apophysomyces elegans. Int J Dermatol 2008;47(4):407–9.

101. De Decker K, Van Poucke S, Wojciechowski M, et al. Successful use of posaconazole in a pediatric case of fungal necrotizing fasciitis. Pediatr Crit Care Med 2006;7(5):482–5.

102. Jain D, Kumar Y, Vasishta RK, et al. Zygomycotic necrotizing fasciitis in immunocompetent patients: a series of 18 cases. Mod Pathol 2006;19(9):1221–6.

103. Kordy FN, Al-Mohsen IZ, Hashem F, et al. Successful treatment of a child with posttraumatic necrotizing fasciitis caused by Apophysomyces elegans: case report and review of literature. Pediatr Infect Dis J 2004;23(9):877–9.

104. Thami GP, Kaur S, Bawa AS, et al. Post-surgical zygomycotic necrotizing subcutaneous infection caused by Absidia corymbifera. Clin Exp Dermatol 2003; 28(3):251–3.

105. Mathews MS, Raman A, Nair A. Nosocomial zygomycotic post-surgical necrotizing fasciitis in a healthy adult caused by Apophysomyces elegans in south India. J Med Vet Mycol 1997;35(1):61–3.

106. Lakshmi V, Rani TS, Sharma S, et al. Zygomycotic necrotizing fasciitis caused by Apophysomyces elegans. J Clin Microbiol 1993;31(5):1368–9.

107. Patino JF, Castro D, Valencia A, et al. Necrotizing soft tissue lesions after a volcanic cataclysm. World J Surg 1991;15(2):240–7.

108. Farmakiotis D, Ciurea AM, Cahuayme-Zuniga L, et al. The diagnostic yield of skin biopsy in patients with leukemia and suspected infection. J Infect 2013; 67(4):265–72.

109. Song KY, Kang WK, Park CW, et al. Mucormycosis resulting in gastric perforation in a patient with acute myelogenous leukemia: report of a case. Surg Today 2006;36(9):831–4.

110. Park YS, Lee JD, Kim TH, et al. Gastric mucormycosis. Gastrointest Endosc 2002;56(6):904–5.

111. Oliver MR, Van Voorhis WC, Boeckh M, et al. Hepatic mucormycosis in a bone marrow transplant recipient who ingested naturopathic medicine. Clin Infect Dis 1996;22(3):521–4.

112. Lass-Florl C, Resch G, Nachbaur D, et al. The value of computed tomography-guided percutaneous lung biopsy for diagnosis of invasive fungal infection in immunocompromised patients. Clin Infect Dis 2007;45(7):e101–4.

113. Chamilos G, Lewis RE, Kontoyiannis DP. Delaying amphotericin B-based frontline therapy significantly increases mortality among patients with hematologic malignancy who have zygomycosis. Clin Infect Dis 2008;47(4):503–9.

114. Stanzani M, Sassi C, Lewis RE, et al. High resolution computed tomography angiography improves the radiographic diagnosis of invasive mold disease in patients with hematological malignancies. Clin Infect Dis 2015;60(11):1603–10.

115. Stanzani M, Lewis RE, Fiacchini M, et al. A risk prediction score for invasive mold disease in patients with hematological malignancies. PLoS One 2013; 8(9):e75531.
116. Stanzani M, Battista G, Sassi C, et al. Computed tomographic pulmonary angiography for diagnosis of invasive mold diseases in patients with hematological malignancies. Clin Infect Dis 2012;54(5):610–6.
117. Kontoyiannis DP, Lewis RE. Treatment principles for the management of mold infections. Cold Spring Harb Perspect Med 2015;5(4).
118. Moosavi Movahed M, Hosamirudsari H, Mansouri F, et al. Spontaneous pneumothorax followed by reversed halo sign in immunocompromised patient with pulmonary mucormycosis. Med Mycol Case Rep 2015;9:22–5.
119. Sharma P, Beltran AD. Reversed halo sign—look for the mold within. J Gen Intern Med 2015;30(1):138.
120. Legouge C, Caillot D, Chretien ML, et al. The reversed halo sign: pathognomonic pattern of pulmonary mucormycosis in leukemic patients with neutropenia? Clin Infect Dis 2014;58(5):672–8.
121. Georgiadou SP, Sipsas NV, Marom EM, et al. The diagnostic value of halo and reversed halo signs for invasive mold infections in compromised hosts. Clin Infect Dis 2011;52(9):1144–55.
122. Wahba H, Truong MT, Lei X, et al. Reversed halo sign in invasive pulmonary fungal infections. Clin Infect Dis 2008;46(11):1733–7.
123. Souza AS Jr, Souza AS, Soares-Souza L, et al. Reversed halo sign in acute schistosomiasis. J Bras Pneumol 2015;41(3):286–8.
124. Zhan X, Zhang L, Wang Z, et al. Reversed halo sign: presents in different pulmonary diseases. PLoS One 2015;10(6):e0128153.
125. Marty FM, Koo S. Role of (1–>3)-beta-d-glucan in the diagnosis of invasive aspergillosis. Med Mycol 2009;47(Suppl 1):S233–s240.
126. Walsh TJ, Gamaletsou MN, McGinnis MR, et al. Early clinical and laboratory diagnosis of invasive pulmonary, extrapulmonary, and disseminated mucormycosis (zygomycosis). Clin Infect Dis 2012;54(Suppl 1):S55–s60.
127. Peixoto D, Hammond SP, Issa NC, et al. Green herring syndrome: bacterial infection in patients with mucormycosis cavitary lung disease. Open Forum Infect Dis 2014;1(1):ofu014.
128. Cassagne C, Ranque S, Normand AC, et al. Mould routine identification in the clinical laboratory by matrix-assisted laser desorption ionization time-of-flight mass spectrometry. PLoS One 2011;6(12):e28425.
129. Hammond SP, Bialek R, Milner DA, et al. Molecular methods to improve diagnosis and identification of mucormycosis. J Clin Microbiol 2011;49(6):2151–3.
130. Potenza L, Vallerini D, Barozzi P, et al. Mucorales-specific T cells emerge in the course of invasive mucormycosis and may be used as a surrogate diagnostic marker in high-risk patients. Blood 2011;118(20):5416–9.
131. Skiada A, Lanternier F, Groll AH, et al. Diagnosis and treatment of mucormycosis in patients with hematological malignancies: guidelines from the 3rd European Conference on Infections in Leukemia (ECIL 3). Haematologica 2013;98(4):492–504.
132. Lewis RE, Lortholary O, Spellberg B, et al. How does antifungal pharmacology differ for mucormycosis versus aspergillosis? Clin Infect Dis 2012;54(Suppl 1):S67–72.
133. Hamill RJ. Amphotericin B formulations: a comparative review of efficacy and toxicity. Drugs 2013;73(9):919–34.

134. Craddock C, Anson J, Chu P, et al. Best practice guidelines for the management of adverse events associated with amphotericin B lipid complex. Expert Opin Drug Saf 2010;9(1):139–47.

135. Walsh TJ, Anaissie EJ, Denning DW, et al. Treatment of aspergillosis: clinical practice guidelines of the Infectious Diseases Society of America. Clin Infect Dis 2008;46(3):327–60.

136. Farmakiotis D, Tverdek FP, Kontoyiannis DP. The safety of amphotericin B lipid complex in patients with prior severe intolerance to liposomal amphotericin B. Clin Infect Dis 2013;56(5):701–3.

137. Lanternier F, Poiree S, Elie C, et al. Prospective pilot study of high-dose (10 mg/kg/day) liposomal amphotericin B (L-AMB) for the initial treatment of mucormycosis. J Antimicrob Chemother 2015;70:3116–23.

138. Torres HA, Hachem RY, Chemaly RF, et al. Posaconazole: a broad-spectrum triazole antifungal. Lancet Infect Dis 2005;5(12):775–85.

139. Greenberg RN, Mullane K, van Burik JA, et al. Posaconazole as salvage therapy for zygomycosis. Antimicrob Agents Chemother 2006;50(1):126–33.

140. van Burik JA, Hare RS, Solomon HF, et al. Posaconazole is effective as salvage therapy in zygomycosis: a retrospective summary of 91 cases. Clin Infect Dis 2006;42(7):e61–5.

141. Krishna G, Ma L, Martinho M, et al. A new solid oral tablet formulation of posaconazole: a randomized clinical trial to investigate rising single- and multiple-dose pharmacokinetics and safety in healthy volunteers. J Antimicrob Chemother 2012;67(11):2725–30.

142. Maertens J, Cornely OA, Ullmann AJ, et al. Phase 1b study of the pharmacokinetics and safety of posaconazole intravenous solution in patients at risk for invasive fungal disease. Antimicrob Agents Chemother 2014;58(7):3610–7.

143. Farmakiotis D, Kontoyiannis DP. Emerging issues with diagnosis and management of fungal infections in solid organ transplant recipients. Am J Transplant 2015;15(5):1141–7.

144. Jung DS, Tverdek FP, Kontoyiannis DP. Switching from posaconazole suspension to tablets increases serum drug levels in leukemia patients without clinically relevant hepatotoxicity. Antimicrob Agents Chemother 2014;58(11):6993–5.

145. Chitasombat MN, Kontoyiannis DP. The 'cephalosporin era' of triazole therapy: isavuconazole, a welcomed newcomer for the treatment of invasive fungal infections. Expert Opin Pharmacother 2015;16(10):1543–58.

146. Ananda-Rajah MR, Kontoyiannis D. Isavuconazole: a new extended spectrum triazole for invasive mold diseases. Future Microbiol 2015;10(5):693–708.

147. Miceli MH, Kauffman CA. Isavuconazole: a new broad-spectrum triazole antifungal agent. Clin Infect Dis 2015;61:1558–65.

148. Peixoto D, Gagne LS, Hammond SP, et al. Isavuconazole treatment of a patient with disseminated mucormycosis. J Clin Microbiol 2014;52(3):1016–9.

149. Ervens J, Ghannoum M, Graf B, et al. Successful isavuconazole salvage therapy in a patient with invasive mucormycosis. Infection 2014;42(2):429–32.

150. Marty FM, Perfect JR, Cornely OA, et al. ID Week 2014 abstract 824: an open-label phase 3 study of isavuconazole (VITAL): focus on mucormycosis. Open Forum Infect Dis 2014;1:3(Suppl 1):S235–6.

151. Francis P, Walsh TJ. Approaches to management of fungal infections in cancer patients. Oncology 1992;6(5):133–44 [discussion: 144, 147–8].

152. Francis P, Walsh TJ. Current approaches to the management of fungal infections in cancer patients: part 1. Oncology 1992;6(4):81–92 [discussion: 97–100].

153. Walsh TJ, Skiada A, Cornely OA, et al. Development of new strategies for early diagnosis of mucormycosis from bench to bedside. Mycoses 2014;57(Suppl 3): 2–7.
154. Ng TT, Campbell CK, Rothera M, et al. Successful treatment of sinusitis caused by Cunninghamella bertholletiae. Clin Infect Dis 1994;19(2):313–6.
155. Reed C, Bryant R, Ibrahim AS, et al. Combination polyene-caspofungin treatment of rhino-orbital-cerebral mucormycosis. Clin Infect Dis 2008;47(3): 364–71.
156. Rickerts V, Loeffler J, Bohme A, et al. Diagnosis of disseminated zygomycosis using a polymerase chain reaction assay. Eur J Clin Microbiol Infect Dis 2001; 20(10):744–5.
157. Ibrahim AS, Bowman JC, Avanessian V, et al. Caspofungin inhibits Rhizopus oryzae 1,3-beta-D-glucan synthase, lowers burden in brain measured by quantitative PCR, and improves survival at a low but not a high dose during murine disseminated zygomycosis. Antimicrob Agents Chemother 2005;49(2): 721–7.
158. Ibrahim AS, Gebremariam T, Fu Y, et al. Combination echinocandin-polyene treatment of murine mucormycosis. Antimicrob Agents Chemother 2008;52(4): 1556–8.
159. Lamaris GA, Lewis RE, Chamilos G, et al. Caspofungin-mediated beta-glucan unmasking and enhancement of human polymorphonuclear neutrophil activity against aspergillus and non-aspergillus hyphae. J Infect Dis 2008;198(2): 186–92.
160. Spellberg B, Ibrahim A, Roilides E, et al. Combination therapy for mucormycosis: why, what, and how? Clin Infect Dis 2012;54(Suppl 1):S73–8.
161. Kyvernitakis A, Torres HA, Jiang Y, et al. ICAAC 2015 oral presentation: initial use of combination treatment does not impact early survival of 106 patients with hematologic malignancies and mucormycosis: a propensity score analysis. San Diego (CA): Infectious Diseases Society of America; 2015.
162. Chowdhary A, Kathuria S, Singh PK, et al. Molecular characterization and in vitro antifungal susceptibility of 80 clinical isolates of mucormycetes in Delhi, India. Mycoses 2014;57(Suppl 3):97–107.
163. Seyedmousavi S, Verweij PE, Mouton JW. Isavuconazole, a broad-spectrum triazole for the treatment of systemic fungal diseases. Expert Rev Anti Infect Ther 2015;13(1):9–27.
164. Tedder M, Spratt JA, Anstadt MP, et al. Pulmonary mucormycosis: results of medical and surgical therapy. Ann Thorac Surg 1994;57(4):1044–50.
165. Hamilton JF, Bartkowski HB, Rock JP. Management of CNS mucormycosis in the pediatric patient. Pediatr Neurosurg 2003;38(4):212–5.
166. Shafer MR. Use of hyperbaric oxygen as adjunct therapy to surgical debridement of complicated wounds. Semin Perioper Nurs 1993;2(4):256–62.
167. Price JC, Stevens DL. Hyperbaric oxygen in the treatment of rhinocerebral mucormycosis. Laryngoscope 1980;90(5 Pt 1):737–47.
168. Kajs-Wyllie M. Hyperbaric oxygen therapy for rhinocerebral fungal infection. J Neurosci Nurs 1995;27(3):174–81.
169. Couch L, Theilen F, Mader JT. Rhinocerebral mucormycosis with cerebral extension successfully treated with adjunctive hyperbaric oxygen therapy. Arch Otolaryngol Head Neck Surg 1988;114(7):791–4.
170. Barratt DM, Van Meter K, Asmar P, et al. Hyperbaric oxygen as an adjunct in zygomycosis: randomized controlled trial in a murine model. Antimicrob Agents Chemother 2001;45(12):3601–2.

171. Ibrahim AS, Gebermariam T, Fu Y, et al. The iron chelator deferasirox protects mice from mucormycosis through iron starvation. J Clin Invest 2007;117(9): 2649–57.
172. Reed C, Ibrahim A, Edwards JE Jr, et al. Deferasirox, an iron-chelating agent, as salvage therapy for rhinocerebral mucormycosis. Antimicrob Agents Chemother 2006;50(11):3968–9.
173. Spellberg B, Ibrahim AS, Chin-Hong PV, et al. The deferasirox-ambisome therapy for mucormycosis (DEFEAT MUCOR) study: a randomized, double-blinded, placebo-controlled trial. J Antimicrob Chemother 2012;67(3):715–22.
174. Abzug MJ, Walsh TJ. Interferon-gamma and colony-stimulating factors as adjuvant therapy for refractory fungal infections in children. Pediatr Infect Dis J 2004; 23(8):769–73.
175. Gil-Lamaignere C, Simitsopoulou M, Roilides E, et al. Interferon-gamma and granulocyte-macrophage colony-stimulating factor augment the activity of polymorphonuclear leukocytes against medically important zygomycetes. J Infect Dis 2005;191(7):1180–7.
176. Hubel K, Dale DC, Engert A, et al. Current status of granulocyte (neutrophil) transfusion therapy for infectious diseases. J Infect Dis 2001;183(2):321–8.
177. Chamilos G, Lewis RE, Kontoyiannis DP. Lovastatin has significant activity against zygomycetes and interacts synergistically with voriconazole. Antimicrob Agents Chemother 2006;50(1):96–103.
178. Kontoyiannis DP, Lewis RE, Lortholary O, et al. Future directions in mucormycosis research. Clin Infect Dis 2012;54(Suppl 1):S79–85.
179. Farmakiotis D, Kyvernitakis A, Tarrand JJ, et al. Early initiation of appropriate treatment is associated with increased survival in cancer patients with Candida glabrata fungaemia: a potential benefit from infectious disease consultation. Clin Microbiol Infect 2015;21(1):79–86.
180. Farmakiotis D, Tarrand JJ, Kontoyiannis DP. Drug-resistant Candida glabrata infection in cancer patients. Emerg Infect Dis 2014;20(11):1833–40.
181. Wang E, Farmakiotis D, Yang D, et al. The ever-evolving landscape of candidaemia in patients with acute leukaemia: non-susceptibility to caspofungin and multidrug resistance are associated with increased mortality. J Antimicrob Chemother 2015;70(8):2362–8.
182. Cowen LE, Sanglard D, Howard SJ, et al. Mechanisms of antifungal drug resistance. Cold Spring Harb Perspect Med 2015;5(7):a019752.
183. Perlin DS. Mechanisms of echinocandin antifungal drug resistance. Ann N Y Acad Sci 2015;1354:1–11.
184. Perlin DS, Shor E, Zhao Y. Update on antifungal drug resistance. Curr Clin Microbiol Rep 2015;2(2):84–95.
185. Kumaresan PR, Manuri PR, Albert ND, et al. Bioengineering T cells to target carbohydrate to treat opportunistic fungal infection. Proc Natl Acad Sci U S A 2014; 111(29):10660–5.
186. Koo S, Thomas HR, Daniels SD, et al. A breath fungal secondary metabolite signature to diagnose invasive aspergillosis. Clin Infect Dis 2014;59(12): 1733–40.
187. Gomes MZ, Lewis RE, Kontoyiannis DP. Mucormycosis caused by unusual mucormycetes, non-Rhizopus, -Mucor, and -Lichtheimia species. Clin Microbiol Rev 2011;24(2):411–45.

Dematiaceous Molds

Eunice H. Wong, MD, Sanjay G. Revankar, MD*

KEYWORDS

- Dematiaceous • Phaeohyphomycosis • Amphotericin B • Itraconazole
- Voriconazole • Isavuconazole • Posaconazole

KEY POINTS

- Phaeohyphomycosis refers to infections due to dematiaceous, or darkly pigmented fungi that are distinguished from other fungal species by the presence of melanin.
- They are ubiquitous and commonly found in soil. Transmission is generally by inhalation or by direct contact in the presence of trauma to skin or mucous membrane.
- Although they are rare causes of infection, they can cause superficial and disseminated infection in both immunocompromised and immunocompetent individuals and are often difficult to treat, requiring both surgical intervention and prolonged medical therapy.
- Standard therapies are lacking; management is based on in vitro data, animal studies, and clinical experience and expert opinions derived primarily from descriptive case studies.

INTRODUCTION

Dematiaceous, or darkly pigmented fungi, are the cause of phaeohyphomycosis, the general term used to describe a variety of infections ranging from superficial infections, allergic disease, pneumonia, brain abscess, and disseminated infection. These fungi are uncommon causes of human disease but can be responsible for life-threatening infections in both immunocompromised and immunocompetent individuals. They are commonly found in the soil and are generally distributed worldwide, which suggests that most if not all individuals are exposed to them, presumably from inhalation. However, phaeohyphomycosis should be distinguished from other specific pathologic conditions associated with dematiaceous fungi, which include chromoblastomycosis and mycetoma. Chromoblastomycosis is caused by a small group of fungi that produce characteristic sclerotic bodies in tissue and is usually seen in tropical regions.[1] Mycetoma is a deep tissue infection, typically of the lower

Disclosure statement: research grant from Merck, Gilead, Astellas (S.G. Revankar); none (E. Wong).
Division of Infectious Diseases, Harper University Hospital, Wayne State University, 3990 John R., 5 Hudson, Detroit, MI 48201, USA
* Corresponding author.
E-mail address: srevankar@med.wayne.edu

Infect Dis Clin N Am 30 (2016) 165–178
http://dx.doi.org/10.1016/j.idc.2015.10.007   **id.theclinics.com**

extremities, characterized by the presence of mycotic granules.[1] These clinical syndromes are discussed in detail in other reviews.[1–3]

Dematiaceous molds have become increasingly recognized as important pathogens. The spectrum of diseases they are associated with has also broadened. Although they are commonly seen in immunocompromised patients, for some infectious syndromes in immunocompetent individuals, such as allergic fungal sinusitis and brain abscess, they are among the most common etiologic fungi.

MYCOLOGY

More than 150 species and 70 genera of dematiaceous fungi have been implicated in human disease.[3] As the number of immunocompromised patients increases because of conditions, such as diabetes, organ transplantation, and novel medical therapy (eg, monoclonal antibodies), additional species are being reported as causes of human disease, expanding an already long list of potential pathogens.[4–6] Common genera associated with specific clinical syndromes are listed in **Table 1**. The distinguishing characteristic common to all these various species is the presence of melanin in their cell walls, which imparts the dark color to their conidia or spores and hyphae. The colonies are typically brown to black in color as well. In tissue, they will stain strongly with the Fontana-Masson stain, which is specific for melanin.[2] This stain can be helpful in distinguishing these fungi from other species, particularly *Aspergillus*. In addition, hyphae typically appear more fragmented in tissue than seen with *Aspergillus*, with irregular septate hyphae and yeastlike forms.[2]

Guidelines are available regarding the handling of potentially infectious fungi in the laboratory setting. It is suggested that cultures of certain well-known fungi, such as *Coccidioides immitis* and *Histoplasma capsulatum*, are to be worked with in a biosafety level 3 facility, which requires a separate negative pressure room. Recently agents of phaeohyphomycosis, in particular *Cladophialophora bantiana*, have been included in the list of fungi that should be kept under biosafety level 2 containment.[7] This requirement seems reasonable given their propensity, albeit rarely, for causing life-threatening infection in normal individuals.

Table 1
MIC distribution of isavuconazole tested against dematiaceous fungi based on CLSI broth microdilution M38-A2 method

Organism (Number of Isolates)	Range	MIC$_{50}$ (μg/mL)	MIC$_{90}$ (μg/mL)	Mean
Cladophialophora carrionii (81)	0.016–1.0	0.125	0.25	0.136
Cladophialophora bantiana (37)	0.008–1.0	0.25	0.5	0.259
Fonsecaea monophora (25)	0.063–1.0	0.125	0.25	0.184
Fonsecaea pedrosoi (21)	0.063–0.25	0.25	0.25	0.226
Madurella mycetomatis	≤0.016–0.125	0.031	0.063	0.037
Scedosporium prolificans (6)	>32.0	—	—	—
Exophiala sp environmental (106)	0.25–16.0	2.0	4.0	1.78
Exophiala dermatitidis (66)	0.031–1.0	0.5	1.0	0.418
Exophiala jeanselmei	0.25–>2.0	2.0	—	—
Exophiala spinifera	2.0	—	—	—

Abbreviation: CLSI, clinical & laboratory standards institute; MIC, minimal inhibitory concentration.
Data from Ref.[75–84]

DIAGNOSIS

The diagnosis of phaeohyphomycosis currently relies on pathologic examination of clinical specimens and expert gross and microscopic examination of cultures, occasionally requiring referral to a mycology reference laboratory. As many of these are rarely seen in practice, a high degree of clinical suspicion is required when interpreting culture results. Unlike other common mycoses that cause human disease, there are no simple serologic or antigen tests available to detect these fungi in blood or tissue. Polymerase chain reaction (PCR) is being studied as an aid to the diagnosis of fungal infections but as yet does not reliably distinguish between dematiaceous fungi and other more common mycoses and is not widely available. Different components of fungal rRNA, namely, internal transcribed spacer (ITS), small subunit, and large subunit, have been compared with regions of the representative protein-binding gene (RPB1) in species discrimination based on barcode gap (ie, where interspecies variation exceeds intraspecies variation). Although ITS only follows second to RPB1 in the greatest indication of barcode gap, ITS has a high PCR and sequencing success rate across a broad range of fungi; thus, it has been used widely in species identification in clinical studies.[8]

PATHOGENESIS

The pathogenic mechanisms by which these fungi cause disease, particularly in immunocompetent individuals, remain largely unknown. One of the likely candidate virulence factors is the presence of melanin in the cell wall, which is common to all dematiaceous fungi. There are several mechanisms proposed by which melanin may act as a virulence factor.[9–11] It is thought to confer a protective advantage by scavenging free radicals and hypochlorite that are produced by phagocytic cells in their oxidative burst and that would normally kill most organisms.[9] In addition, melanin may bind to hydrolytic enzymes, thereby preventing their action on the plasma membrane.[9] These multiple functions may help explain the pathogenic potential of some dematiaceous fungi, even in immunocompetent hosts. Considerable work has been done in several fungi that contain melanin. Specifically, in the yeasts *Cryptococcus neoformans* and *Wangiella dermatitidis*, disruption of melanin production leads to markedly reduced virulence in animal models.[12,13] Melanin has also been shown to reduce the susceptibility of *Cryptococcus neoformans* and *Histoplasma capsulatum* to amphotericin B and caspofungin, possibly by binding these drugs.[14,15] This effect is not apparent with azole drugs.[14]

Recent studies have linked certain genetic immunodeficiencies with disseminated *Exophiala* infection and other severe fungal diseases caused by *Candida* species, dermatophytes, and *Phialophora verrucosa*. Mutations in the caspase activation and recruitment domains (CARD), specifically CARD9, leading to functional CARD9 deficiency have been hypothesized to cause an impairment of fungal killing by monocytes, macrophages, and/or microglial cells at the blood-brain barrier due to impaired production of certain inflammatory markers.[16] This mutation is the first specific genetic mutation associated with infection due to dematiaceous fungi.

In addition, almost all allergic disease and eosinophilia is caused by 2 genera, *Bipolaris* and *Curvularia*. These organisms are very common in the environment, though the virulence factors in these fungi that are responsible for eliciting allergic reactions are unclear at present.

IN VITRO SUSCEPTIBILITY

Although in vitro antifungal testing has become more routine in the past several years with the development of standardized methods for testing yeasts and molds,[17,18] the available in vitro data for dematiaceous fungi are relatively sparse and often rely on small numbers of isolates per species. Recent years have seen an increased interest in dematiaceous fungi and reports of in vitro testing.

Azoles were the first oral, broad-spectrum antifungal agents available and are widely used. Itraconazole, voriconazole, and posaconazole have the most consistent activity against dematiaceous fungi. Apart from *Scedosporium prolificans* and *Scopulariopsis brumptii*, all demonstrate good activity against most of the dematiaceous fungi tested.[19–23] Minimal inhibitory concentrations (MICs) are generally 0.125 µg/mL or less for this group of fungi. However, MICs are usually slightly higher for voriconazole, though the clinical significance of this is unclear. Fluconazole has negligible activity against dematiaceous molds, and use of ketoconazole is negligible.

Isavuconazole is a novel broad-spectrum azole recently approved by the Food and Drug Administration for treatment of aspergillosis and mucormycosis, with a tolerability profile comparable to fluconazole and less drug interactions than voriconazole and itraconazole.[24] Although there are no published clinical data for the treatment of phaeohyphomycosis, in vitro susceptibility data are available for dematiaceous fungi as listed in **Table 1**.

Amphotericin B is usually rapidly fungicidal against susceptible species in vitro, and generally has good activity against most clinically important dematiaceous fungi.[21] However, some species have been consistently resistant (minimum inhibitory concentration [MIC] ≥ 2 µg/mL) in vitro, including *Scedosporium prolificans* and *Scopulariopsis brumptii*.[19]

Limited data are available for other agents. Terbinafine is the only oral allylamine available for systemic use. However, its extensive binding to serum proteins and distribution into skin and adipose tissue have diminished enthusiasm for its use in treating serious systemic fungal infections.[25,26] In vitro studies against dematiaceous fungi are emerging, and fairly broad-spectrum activity is seen. The echinocandins are the latest group of antifungal agents to be developed and have a unique mechanism of action, inhibiting β-1,3 glucan synthesis and thereby disrupting the fungal cell wall.[27] Caspofungin, micafungin, and anidulafungin are available for clinical use, though in vitro studies with dematiaceous fungi are limited. In general, MICs for dematiaceous fungi are higher than for *Aspergillus* sp.[28] Flucytosine (5-FC) is unique in its mechanism of action, inhibiting DNA and RNA synthesis. It has a limited role in the therapy for these fungi, though some species are susceptible.[29]

Use of antifungal combinations is a potentially useful strategy for refractory infections, though it has not been studied extensively in phaeohyphomycosis. The combination of itraconazole and terbinafine has been studied against *Scedosporium prolificans*, which is otherwise generally resistant to all agents. In vitro, synergistic activity was found against most isolates of this species, and no antagonism was noted.[30] Voriconazole and terbinafine also display similar synergy in vitro.[31] The mechanism is presumably potent inhibition of ergosterol synthesis at 2 different steps of the pathway by these agents. However, this should be interpreted with caution, as terbinafine is not generally used for systemic infections. Other reports suggest synergy for *Scedosporium prolificans* with voriconazole and caspofungin and improved outcomes for brain abscess with 3 or more combinations of antifungals.[3,32]

CLINICAL SYNDROMES AND THERAPY

There are no standard therapies for infections caused by dematiaceous fungi, with regard to choice of agent or duration of therapy. Recommendations from clinical guidelines are based partly on in vitro data and animal studies and mostly on results from uncontrolled experiments, opinions of respected authorities, clinical experience, descriptive case studies, or reports from expert committees.[33] Nevertheless, far more experience has accumulated with itraconazole than for any other single drug, though newer agents may have specific advantages. Length of therapy is generally based on clinical response and ranges from several weeks to several months or longer. A summary of suggested therapies is presented in **Table 2**, whereas a summary of clinical and microbiologic data on some of the more clinically important dematiaceous fungi is presented on **Table 3**.

Superficial Infections

Superficial infections are the most common form of infection due to dematiaceous fungi. These cases are generally associated with minor trauma or other environmental exposure. Although many pathogens have been reported, relatively few are responsible for most infections. Although they rarely lead to life-threatening disease, significant morbidity can occur depending on the site of infection and response to therapy.

Onychomycosis

Dematiaceous fungi are rare causes of onychomycosis. Clinical features may include a history of trauma, involvement of only one or 2 toenails, and lack of response to standard systemic therapy.[34] *Onychocola* and *Alternaria* have been reported, with the former being highly resistant to therapy.[34,35] Itraconazole and terbinafine are the most commonly used systemic agents and may be combined with topical therapy for refractory cases.[35] Sparse data are available for the newer azole agents.

Table 2
Clinical syndromes associated with phaeohyphomycosis

Clinical Syndrome	Commonly Associated Fungal Genera[a]	Suggested Therapy
Onychomycosis	*Onychocola* *Alternaria*	Itra or Terb +/− topical agents
Subcutaneous nodules	*Exophiala* *Alternaria* *Phialophora*	Surgery +/− Vori
Keratitis	*Curvularia* *Bipolaris* *Exserohilum* *Lasiodiplodia*	Topical natamycin +/− Vori
Allergic disease	*Bipolaris* *Curvularia*	Steroids +/− itra
Pneumonia	*Ochroconis* *Exophiala* *Chaetomium*	Vori (AmB if severe)
Brain abscess	*Cladophialophora (C bantiana)* *Ramichloridium (R mackenziei)* *Ochroconis*	High-dose azole + lipid AmB +/− 5-FC
Disseminated disease	*Scedosporium (S prolificans)* *Bipolaris* *Wangiella*	Lipid AmB + azole +/− echinocandin

Abbreviations: AmB, amphotericin B; azole, itraconazole, voriconazole, posaconazole; Itra, itraconazole; Terb, terbinafine; Vori, voriconazole.
[a] Taxonomy notes: *Bipolaris* = *Dreschlera* or *Helminthosporium* (older terms), *Ochroconis* = *Dactylaria* (older term), *Cladophialophora* = *Xylohypha* or *Cladosporium* (older terms).

Table 3
Clinical and microbiologic data on some clinically important dematiaceous fungi

Organism	Clinical Syndrome	Microscopic Features	In Vitro Antifungal Susceptibility	Management
Alternaria	Subcutaneous, disseminated	Brown hyphae with elongated, septate conidia	Amphotericin B, itraconazole, voriconazole, posaconazole	Wide excision, antifungal therapy
Bipolaris	Pansinusitis, necrotizing pneumonia, allergic bronchopulmonary mycosis, peritonitis, encephalitis	Brown hyphae with oval, septate conidia	Amphotericin B, itraconazole, voriconazole, posaconazole	Surgical debridement and antifungal therapy with amphotericin B or azole
Cladophialophora	Cerebral	Brown hyphae with long, delicate, branching chains of small conidia	Itraconazole, posaconazole, voriconazole, flucytosine, echinocandins, lipid amphotericin B	Surgery with combination antifungal therapy (see text)
Exophiala	Cerebral, subcutaneous, disseminated	Dark brown yeast cells	Posaconazole, itraconazole, voriconazole, amphotericin B	Surgery with antifungal therapy

Subcutaneous lesions

There are numerous case reports of subcutaneous infection due to a wide variety of species.[36-38] *Exophiala, Alternaria, Phialophora,* and *Bipolaris* are among the more common etiologic agents.[39] Minor trauma is the usual inciting factor, though it may be unrecognized by patients. Lesions typically occur on exposed areas of the body and often appear as isolated cystic or papular lesions. Immunocompromised patients are at increased risk of subsequent dissemination, though rare cases have been described in apparently immunocompetent patients as well. Occasionally, infection may involve joints or bone requiring more extensive surgery or prolonged antifungal therapy.

As for many of the infectious syndromes associated with dematiaceous fungi, therapy is not standardized. Surgical excision alone has been successful in several cases.[40] Oral systemic therapy with an azole antifungal agent in conjunction with surgery is frequently used and has been used successfully. Two cases of refractory bone and joint infection due to *Scedosporium prolificans* were treated effectively with voriconazole and the combination of voriconazole and caspofungin.[32,41]

Keratitis

Fungal keratitis is an important ophthalmologic problem, particularly in tropical areas of the world. In one large series, 40% of all infectious keratitis was caused by fungi, almost exclusively molds.[42] The most common fungi are *Fusarium* and *Aspergillus,* followed by dematiaceous fungi (up to 8%–17% of cases).[43] Approximately half the cases are associated with trauma; prior eye surgery, diabetes, and contact lens use have also been noted as important risk factors.[42,43] Diagnosis rests on potassium hydroxide smear and culture.

Some of the largest case series with dematiaceous fungi have come from India.[44,45] In a large experience of keratitis due to dematiaceous fungi, 88 cases were examined.[44] The most common dematiaceous genus causing keratitis was *Curvularia,* followed by *Bipolaris, Exserohilum,* and *Lasiodiplodia.* Almost half the cases were associated with trauma. Most patients received topical agents only (5% natamycin +/− azole), though more severe cases also received oral ketoconazole. The overall response was 72% in those available for follow-up. Surgery was needed in 13 patients, with an additional 6 requiring enucleation because of poor response.

In a study from the United States of 43 cases of *Curvularia* keratitis, almost all were associated with trauma.[46] Plants were the most common source, though several cases of metal injury were seen as well. Topical natamycin was used almost exclusively, with only a few severe cases requiring adjunctive therapy, usually with an azole. Of the oral agents, itraconazole had the best in vitro activity. Surgery, including penetrating keratoplasty, was required in 19% of patients. At the end of therapy, only 78% had a visual acuity of 20/40 or better.

Topical polyenes, such as amphotericin B and natamycin, are commonly used; but oral and topical itraconazole has also been found to be useful.[42,47] Voriconazole is a potentially useful agent, but published clinical experience is primarily limited to cases due to *Scedosporium apiospermum* (teleomorph: *Pseudallescheria boydii*).[48] However, many patients are left with residual visual deficits at the end of therapy, suggesting that further advances in therapy are needed for this debilitating disease.

Allergic Disease

Fungal sinusitis

Patients with this condition usually present with chronic sinus symptoms that are not responsive to antibiotics. Previously, *Aspergillus* was thought to be the most common fungus responsible for allergic sinusitis; but it is now appreciated that disease due to dematiaceous fungi actually compose most of the cases.[49,50] The most common species isolated are *Bipolaris* and *Curvularia*. Criteria have been suggested for this disease and include (1) nasal polyps; (2) presence of allergic mucin, containing Charcot-Leyden crystals and eosinophils; (3) hyphal elements in the mucosa without evidence of tissue invasion; (4) positive skin test to fungal allergens; and (5) on computed tomography scans, characteristic areas of central hyperattenuation within the sinus cavity.[51] Diagnosis generally depends on demonstration of allergic mucin, with or without actual culture of the organism. Therapy consists of surgery to remove the mucin, which is often tenacious, and systemic steroids. Antifungal therapy, usually in the form of itraconazole, may play a role in reducing the requirement for steroids; but this is not routinely recommended.[52] Other azoles have only rarely been used for this disease.

Allergic bronchopulmonary mycosis

This disease is similar in presentation to allergic bronchopulmonary aspergillosis (ABPA), which is typically seen in patients with asthma or cystic fibrosis.[53] There is a suggestion that allergic fungal sinusitis and allergic bronchopulmonary mycosis may actually be a continuum of disease and should be referred to as sinobronchial allergic mycosis.[54] Criteria for the diagnosis of ABPA in patients with asthma include (1) asthma, (2) positive skin test for fungal allergens, (3) elevated immunoglobulin E (IgE) levels, (4) *Aspergillus*-specific IgE, and (5) proximal bronchiectasis.[53] Similar criteria for ABPM are not established but may include elevated IgE levels, positive skin tests, and response to systemic steroids.

In reviewing cases of ABPM due to dematiaceous fungi, essentially all cases are due to *Bipolaris* or *Curvularia*.[55] These two genera are commonly found in the environment, and their spores are large (20–30 μm × 8–12 μm) compared with *Aspergillus* (2–3 μm). Asthma was common in these cases; but bronchiectasis was often not present, perhaps reflecting somewhat different pathogenic mechanisms. All cases had either eosinophilia or elevated IgE levels. Therapy was primarily systemic steroids, usually prednisone at 0.5 mg/kg/d for 2 weeks, followed by a slow taper over 2 to 3 months or longer, if necessary. Itraconazole has been used as a steroid-sparing agent; but its efficacy is not clear, and routine use of itraconazole is not generally recommended.[53,56]

Pneumonia

Nonallergic pulmonary disease is usually seen in immunocompromised patients and may be due to a wide variety of species, in contrast to allergic disease.[57–60] Clinical manifestations include pneumonia, asymptomatic solitary pulmonary nodules, and endobronchial lesions, which may cause hemoptysis. Therapy consists of systemic antifungal agents, usually amphotericin B or itraconazole initially, followed by itraconazole for a more prolonged period. Mortality rates are high in immunocompromised patients. Experience with the newer azoles is anecdotal.

Brain Abscess

This condition is a rare but frequently fatal manifestation of phaeohyphomycosis, often in immunocompetent individuals.[61] In a review of 101 cases of central nervous system (CNS) infection due to dematiaceous fungi, 87 were found to be brain abscess.[62] More than half of the cases were in patients with no risk factor or immunodeficiency. The most common species was *Cladophialophora bantiana*, accounting for half the cases. Other species included *Ramichloridium mackenziei*, *Ochroconis gallopavum*, and

W dermatitidis. Symptoms included headache, neurologic deficits, and seizures. The pathogenesis may be hematogenous spread from an initial, presumably subclinical pulmonary focus. It remains unclear why these fungi preferentially cause CNS disease in immunocompetent individuals.

Therapy varied depending on the case report. A retrospective analysis of reported cases suggested that the combination of amphotericin B, flucytosine, and itraconazole may be associated with improved survival, though it was not frequently used. Complete excision of brain abscesses seemed to have better outcomes than aspiration or partial excision. Outcomes were poor, with an overall mortality greater than 70%.

The newer azoles (voriconazole and the investigational posaconazole) were not used in the aforementioned case series. However, more recent reports have used both agents. Voriconazole was unsuccessful in treating 3 cases of *Cladophialophora bantiana* brain abscess, though 2 of these patients were immunocompromised.[63-65] However, clinical improvement was seen in one of the severely immunosuppressed patients while receiving voriconazole, despite later succumbing to the infection.[65] Despite these reports, voriconazole may have a role in the therapy for dematiaceous fungal brain abscess, as it has been successfully used in cases of *Aspergillus* and *Scedosporium apiospermum* brain abscess.[66,67] Posaconazole has been reported effective in a case of *R mackenziei* brain abscess, which represents the first reported survival of infection due to this species.[68] In addition, use of lipid formulations of amphotericin B may allow for better efficacy by administration of much higher doses than possible with standard amphotericin B, though this has not been systematically studied for these infections.[69] Finally, triple antifungal combinations may be useful based on animal studies.[3]

Disseminated Infection

This is the most uncommon manifestation of infection seen with dematiaceous fungi. In a recent review, most patients were immunocompromised, though occasional patients without known immunodeficiency or risk factors developed disseminated disease as well.[70] Based on a study of patients with probable and proven phaeohyphomycosis using data from the Transplant Associated Infection Surveillance Network, *Alternaria* was the most frequent genus followed by *Exophiala*.[71] In contrast to most invasive mold infections, blood cultures were positive in more than half the cases. The most common isolate was *Scedosporium prolificans*, accounting for more than a third of cases. This species should be distinguished from *Scedosporium apiospermum* (teleomorph *Pseudallescheria boydii*), which some experts do not consider truly dematiaceous and which has different antifungal susceptibilities.

The mortality rate was greater than 70%, despite aggressive antifungal therapy. There were no antifungal regimens associated with improved survival in disseminated infection. Infection with *Scedosporium prolificans* was associated with nearly 100% mortality in the absence of recovery from neutropenia, as it is generally resistant to all available antifungal agents. However, recent case reports have suggested that the combination of itraconazole or voriconazole with terbinafine may be synergistic against this species and improve outcomes.[30,72]

Other combinations or therapies have not been shown to be effective, though clinical experience is limited and will likely be confined to anecdotal reports, given the rarity of this infection. More recently, a case of disseminated *Exophiala spinifera* infection was treated successfully with posaconazole after failing itraconazole and amphotericin B.[73]

Miscellaneous

Fungal infections of the genitourinary tract have been reported in immunocompromised patients, usually caused by *Candida*, rarely by other fungi, such as *Aspergillus* or *Cryptococcus*. A case of unilateral pyelonephritis with pyonephrosis caused by *Alternaria alternata* has been reported in a 21-year-old man with undiagnosed insulin-dependent diabetes mellitus, who presented with 1-year history of dysuria and inguinal pain. Therapy involved radical nephrectomy with concomitant amphotericin B administration.[74]

SUMMARY

Phaeohyphomycosis is an uncommon infection but has become increasingly recognized in a wide variety of clinical syndromes. Many species are associated with human infection, though relatively few are responsible for most of the cases. As these are typically soil organisms and common laboratory contaminants, they are often disregarded from clinical specimens as nonpathogenic. However, the clinical setting in which they are isolated should always be carefully considered before making decisions regarding therapy. *Bipolaris* and *Curvularia* are often associated with allergic disease. Diagnosis depends on a high degree of clinical suspicion and appropriate pathologic and mycologic examination of clinical specimens. Therapy is evolving for many of the clinical syndromes described, and randomized clinical trials are unlikely given the sporadic nature of cases. Case reporting of both successful and unsuccessful clinical experiences will be important in attempting to better define optimal therapy for the more refractory infections, though recent guidelines have been published. Itraconazole, voriconazole, posaconazole, and, most recently, isavuconazole demonstrate the most consistent in vitro activity against this group of fungi. Voriconazole should be considered the drug of choice for most situations, given the greater clinical experience associated with its use for these infections in recent years. Much additional work is needed in order to better understand the pathogenic mechanisms underlying phaeohyphomycosis and to optimize therapy for these often-refractory infections.

REFERENCES

1. McGinnis MR. Chromoblastomycosis and phaeohyphomycosis: new concepts, diagnosis, and mycology. J Am Acad Dermatol 1983;8:1–16.
2. Rinaldi MG. Phaeohyphomycosis. Dermatol Clin 1996;14:147–53.
3. Revankar SG, Sutton DA. Melanized fungi in human disease. Clin Microbiol Rev 2010;23(4):884–928.
4. Wang L, Wang C, Shen Y, et al. Phaeohyphomycosis caused by Exophiala sinifera: an increasing disease in young females in mainland China? Two case reports and review of five cases reported from mainland China. Mycoses 2015;58(3):193–6.
5. Bonifaz A, Davoudi MM, de Hoog GS, et al. Severe disseminated phaeohyphomycosis in an immunocompetent patient caused by Veronaea botryosa. Mycopathologia 2013;175(5–6):497–503.
6. Mazzurco JD, Ramirez J, Fivenson DP. Phaeohyphomycosis caused by Phaeoacremonium species in a patient taking infliximab. J Am Acad Dermatol 2012; 66(2):333–5.
7. Padhye AA, Bennett JE, McGinnis MR, et al. Biosafety considerations in handling medically important fungi. Med Mycol 1998;36(Suppl 1):258–65.
8. Schoch C, Seifert K, Huhndorf S, et al. Nuclear ribosomal internal transcribed spacer (ITS) region as a universal DNA barcode marker for Fungi. Proc Natl Acad Sci U S A 2012;109(16):6241–6.

9. Jacobson ES. Pathogenic roles for fungal melanins. Clin Microbiol Rev 2000;13: 708–17.

10. Butler MJ, Day AW. Fungal melanins: a review. Can J Microbiol 1998;44:1115–36.

11. Hamilton AJ, Gomez BL. Melanins in fungal pathogens. J Med Microbiol 2002;51: 189–91.

12. Dixon DM, Polak A, Szaniszlo PJ. Pathogenicity and virulence of wild-type and melanin-deficient Wangiella dermatitidis. J Med Vet Mycol 1987;25:97–106.

13. Kwon-Chung KJ, Polacheck I, Popkin TJ. Melanin-lacking mutants of Cryptococcus neoformans and their virulence for mice. J Bacteriol 1982;150:1414–21.

14. van Duin D, Casadevall A, Nosanchuk JD. Melanization of Cryptococcus neoformans and Histoplasma capsulatum reduces their susceptibilities to amphotericin B and caspofungin. Antimicrob Agents Chemother 2002;46:3394–400.

15. Ikeda R, Sugita T, Jacobson ES, et al. Effects of melanin upon susceptibility of Cryptococcus to antifungals. Microbiol Immunol 2003;47:271–7.

16. Lanternier F, Barbati E, Meinzer U, et al. Inherited CARD9 deficiency in 2 unrelated patients with invasive Exophiala infection. J Infect Dis 2015;211:1241–50.

17. National Committe for Clinical Laboratory Standards. Reference method for broth dilution antifungal susceptibility testing of yeasts. Approved standard M27-A2. 2nd edition. Villanova (PA): National Committe for Clinical Laboratory Standards; 2002.

18. National Committe for Clinical Laboratory Standards. Reference method for broth dilution antifungal susceptibility testing of conidium-forming filamentous fungi. Approved M38-A. Wayne (PA): National Committe for Clinical Laboratory Standards; 2002.

19. McGinnis MR, Pasarell L. In vitro testing of susceptibilities of filamentous ascomycetes to voriconazole, itraconazole, and amphotericin B, with consideration of phylogenetic implications. J Clin Microbiol 1998;36:2353–5.

20. Meletiadis J, Meis JF, Mouton JW, et al. In vitro activities of new and conventional antifungal agents against clinical Scedosporium isolates. Antimicrob Agents Chemother 2002;46:62–8.

21. Espinel-Ingroff A, Boyle K, Sheehan DJ. In vitro antifungal activities of voriconazole and reference agents as determined by NCCLS methods: review of the literature. Mycopathologia 2001;150:101–15.

22. McGinnis MR, Pasarell L. In vitro evaluation of terbinafine and itraconazole against dematiaceous fungi. Med Mycol 1998;36:243–6.

23. Espinel-Ingroff A. In vitro fungicidal activities of voriconazole, itraconazole, and amphotericin B against opportunistic moniliaceous and dematiaceous fungi. J Clin Microbiol 2001;39:954–8.

24. Falci DR, Pasqualotto AC. Profile of isavuconazole and its potential in the treatment of severe invasive fungal infections. Infect Drug Resist 2013;6:163–74.

25. Hosseini-Yeganeh M, McLachlan AJ. Physiologically based pharmacokinetic model for terbinafine in rats and humans. Antimicrob Agents Chemother 2002;46:2219–28.

26. Ryder NS, Frank I. Interaction of terbinafine with human serum and serum proteins. J Med Vet Mycol 1992;30:451–60.

27. Deresinski SC, Stevens DA. Caspofungin. Clin Infect Dis 2003;36:1445–57.

28. Espinel-Ingroff A. In vitro antifungal activities of anidulafungin and micafungin, licensed agents and the investigational triazole posaconazole as determined by NCCLS methods for 12,052 fungal isolates: review of the literature. Rev Iberoam Micol 2003;20:121–36.

29. Vermes A, Guchelaar HJ, Dankert J. Flucytosine: a review of its pharmacology, clinical indications, pharmacokinetics, toxicity and drug interactions. J Antimicrob Chemother 2000;46:171–9.

30. Meletiadis J, Mouton JW, Rodriguez-Tudela JL, et al. In vitro interaction of terbinafine with itraconazole against clinical isolates of Scedosporium prolificans. Antimicrob Agents Chemother 2000;44:470–2.
31. Meletiadis J, Mouton JW, Meis JF, et al. In vitro drug interaction modeling of combinations of azoles with terbinafine against clinical Scedosporium prolificans isolates. Antimicrob Agents Chemother 2003;47:106–17.
32. Steinbach WJ, Schell WA, Miller JL, et al. Scedosporium prolificans osteomyelitis in an immunocompetent child treated with voriconazole and caspofungin, as well as locally applied polyhexamethylene biguanide. J Clin Microbiol 2003;41: 3981–5.
33. Chowdhary A, Meis JF, Guarro J, et al. European Society of Clinical Microbiology and Infectious Diseases (ESCMID) and European Confederation of Medical Mycology (ECMM) joint clinical guidelines for the diagnosis and management of systemic phaeohyphomycosis: diseases caused by black fungi. Clin Microbiol Infect 2014;20(Suppl 3):47–75.
34. Gupta AK, Ryder JE, Baran R, et al. Non-dermatophyte onychomycosis. Dermatol Clin 2003;21:257–68.
35. Tosti A, Piraccini BM, Lorenzi S, et al. Treatment of nondermatophyte mold and Candida onychomycosis. Dermatol Clin 2003;21:491–7.
36. Kimura M, Goto A, Furuta T, et al. Multifocal subcutaneous phaeohyphomycosis caused by Phialophora verrucosa. Arch Pathol Lab Med 2003;127:91–3.
37. Agarwal A, Singh SM. A case of cutaneous phaeohyphomycosis caused by Exserohilum rostratum, its in vitro sensitivity and review of literature. Mycopathologia 1995;131:9–12.
38. Chuan MT, Wu MC. Subcutaneous phaeohyphomycosis caused by Exophiala jeanselmei: successful treatment with itraconazole. Int J Dermatol 1995;34:563–6.
39. Koga T, Matsuda T, Matsumoto T, et al. Therapeutic approaches to subcutaneous mycoses. Am J Clin Dermatol 2003;4:537–43.
40. Summerbell RC, Krajden S, Levine R, et al. Subcutaneous phaeohyphomycosis caused by Lasiodiplodia theobromae and successfully treated surgically. Med Mycol 2004;42:543–7.
41. Studahl M, Backteman T, Stalhammar F, et al. Bone and joint infection after traumatic implantation of Scedosporium prolificans treated with voriconazole and surgery. Acta Paediatr 2003;92:980–2.
42. Gopinathan U, Garg P, Fernandes M, et al. The epidemiological features and laboratory results of fungal keratitis: a 10-year review at a referral eye care center in South India. Cornea 2002;21:555–9.
43. Srinivasan M. Fungal keratitis. Curr Opin Ophthalmol 2004;15:321–7.
44. Garg P, Gopinathan U, Choudhary K, et al. Keratomycosis: clinical and microbiologic experience with dematiaceous fungi. Ophthalmology 2000;107:574–80.
45. Chowdhary A, Singh K. Spectrum of fungal keratitis in North India. Cornea 2005; 24:8–15.
46. Wilhelmus KR, Jones DB. Curvularia keratitis. Trans Am Ophthalmol Soc 2001;99: 111–30.
47. Thomas PA. Fungal infections of the cornea. Eye 2003;17:852–62.
48. Hernandez PC, Llinares TF, Burgos SJ, et al. Voriconazole in fungal keratitis caused by Scedosporium apiospermum. Ann Pharmacother 2004;38:414–7.
49. Ferguson BJ. Definitions of fungal rhinosinusitis. Otolaryngol Clin North Am 2000; 33:227–35.
50. Schubert MS. Allergic fungal sinusitis: pathogenesis and management strategies. Drugs 2004;64:363–74.

51. Houser SM, Corey JP. Allergic fungal rhinosinusitis: pathophysiology, epidemiology, and diagnosis. Otolaryngol Clin North Am 2000;33:399–409.
52. Kuhn FA, Javer AR. Allergic fungal rhinosinusitis: perioperative management, prevention of recurrence, and role of steroids and antifungal agents. Otolaryngol Clin North Am 2000;33:419–33.
53. Greenberger PA. Allergic bronchopulmonary aspergillosis. J Allergy Clin Immunol 2002;110:685–92.
54. Venarske DL, deShazo RD. Sinobronchial allergic mycosis: the SAM syndrome. Chest 2002;121:1670–6.
55. Lake FR, Froudist JH, McAleer R, et al. Allergic bronchopulmonary fungal disease caused by Bipolaris and Curvularia. Aust N Z J Med 1991;21:871–4.
56. Wark PAB, Gibson PG. Allergic bronchopulmonary aspergillosis: new concepts of pathogenesis and treatment. Respirology 2001;6:1–7.
57. Burns KE, Ohori NP, Iacono AT. Dactylaria gallopava infection presenting as a pulmonary nodule in a single-lung transplant recipient. J Heart Lung Transplant 2000;19:900–2.
58. Odell JA, Alvarez S, Cvitkovich DG, et al. Multiple lung abscesses due to Ochroconis gallopavum, a dematiaceous fungus, in a nonimmunocompromised wood pulp worker. Chest 2000;118:1503–5.
59. Tamm M, Malouf M, Glanville A. Pulmonary Scedosporium infection following lung transplantation. Transpl Infect Dis 2001;3:189–94.
60. Mazur JE, Judson MA. A case report of a Dactylaria fungal infection in a lung transplant patient. Chest 2001;119:651–3.
61. Carter E, Boudreaux C. Fatal cerebral phaeohyphomycosis due to Curvularia lunata in an immunocompetent patient. J Clin Microbiol 2004;42:5419–23.
62. Revankar SG, Sutton DA, Rinaldi MG. Primary central nervous system phaeohyphomycosis: a review of 101 cases. Clin Infect Dis 2004;38:206–16.
63. Levin TP, Baty DE, Fekete T, et al. Cladophialophora bantiana brain abscess in a solid-organ transplant recipient: case report and review of the literature. J Clin Microbiol 2004;42:4374–8.
64. Fica A, Diaz MC, Luppi M, et al. Unsuccessful treatment with voriconazole of a brain abscess due to Cladophialophora bantiana. Scand J Infect Dis 2003;35:892–3.
65. Trinh JV, Steinbach WJ, Schell WA, et al. Cerebral phaeohyphomycosis in an immunodeficient child treated medically with combination antifungal therapy. Med Mycol 2003;41:339–45.
66. de Lastours V, Lefort A, Zappa M, et al. Two cases of cerebral aspergillosis successfully treated with voriconazole. Eur J Clin Microbiol Infect Dis 2003;22:297–9.
67. Nesky MA, McDougal EC, Peacock JE Jr. Pseudallescheria boydii brain abscess successfully treated with voriconazole and surgical drainage: case report and literature review of central nervous system pseudallescheriasis. Clin Infect Dis 2000;31:673–7.
68. Al Abdely HM, Alkhunaizi AM, Al Tawfiq JA, et al. Successful therapy of cerebral phaeohyphomycosis due to Ramichloridium mackenziei with the new triazole posaconazole. Med Mycol 2005;43:91–5.
69. Walsh TJ, Goodman JL, Pappas P, et al. Safety, tolerance, and pharmacokinetics of high-dose liposomal amphotericin B (AmBisome) in patients infected with Aspergillus species and other filamentous fungi: maximum tolerated dose study. Antimicrob Agents Chemother 2001;45(12):3487–96.
70. Revankar SG, Patterson JE, Sutton DA, et al. Disseminated phaeohyphomycosis: review of an emerging mycosis. Clin Infect Dis 2002;34:467–76.

71. McCarty TP, Baddley JW, Walsh TJ, et al. Phaeohyphomycosis in transplant recipients: results from the Transplant Associated Infection Surveillance Network (TRANSNET). Med Mycol 2015;53(5):440–6.
72. Howden BP, Slavin MA, Schwarer AP, et al. Successful control of disseminated Scedosporium prolificans infection with a combination of voriconazole and terbinafine. Eur J Clin Microbiol Infect Dis 2003;22:111–3.
73. Negroni R, Helou SH, Petri N, et al. Case study: posaconazole treatment of disseminated phaeohyphomycosis due to Exophiala spinifera. Clin Infect Dis 2004;38:e15–20.
74. Raza H, Khan RU, Anwar K, et al. Visceral phaeohyphomycosis caused by Alternaria alternata offering a diagnostic as well as a therapeutic challenge. Saudi J Kidney Dis Transpl 2015;26(2):339–43.
75. Deng S, de Hoog GS, Badali H, et al. In vitro antifungal susceptibility of Cladophialophora carrionii, an agent of human chromoblastomycosis. Antimicrob Agents Chemother 2013;57(4):1974–7.
76. Badali H, de Hoog GS, Curf-Breuker I, et al. Use of amplified fragment length polymorphism to identify 42 Cladophialophora strains related to cerebral phaeohyphomycosis with in vitro antifungal susceptibility. J Clin Microbiol 2010;48(7):2350–6.
77. Najafzadeh JM, Keisari MS, Vicente VA, et al. In vitro activities of eight antifungal drugs against 106 waterborne and cutaneous Exophiala species. Antimicrob Agents Chemother 2013;57(12):6395–8.
78. Badali H, de Hoog GS, Sudhadham M, et al. Microdilution in vitro antifungal susceptibility of Exophiala dermatitidis, a systemic opportunist. Med Mycol 2011;49:819–24.
79. Badali H, Najafzadeh MJ, Van Esbroecke M, et al. The clinical spectrum of Exophiala jeanselmei, with a case report and in vitro antifungal susceptibility of the species. Med Mycol 2010;48:318–27.
80. Najafzadeh MJ, Badali H, Illnait-Zaragozi MT, et al. In vitro activities of eight antifungal drugs against 55 clinical isolates of Fonsecaea spp. Antimicrob Agents Chemother 2010;54(4):1636–8.
81. Guinea J, Pelaez T, Recio S, et al. In vitro antifungal activities of isavuconazole (BAL4815), voriconazole, and fluconazole against 1007 isolates of Zygomycete, Candida, Aspergillus, Fusarium, and Scedosporium species. Antimicrob Agents Chemother 2008;52(4):1396–400.
82. Pfaller MA, Messer SA, Rhomberg PR, et al. In vitro activities of isavuconazole and comparator antifungal agents tested against a global collection of opportunistic yeasts and molds. J Clin Microbiol 2013;51(8):2608–16.
83. Feng P, Najafzadeh MJ, Sun J, et al. In vitro activities of nine antifungal drugs against 81 Phialophora and Cyphellophora isolates. Antimicrob Agents Chemother 2012;56(110):6044–7.
84. Kloezen W, Meis JF, Curfs-Breuker I, et al. In vitro antifungal activity of isavuconazole against Madurella mycetomatis. Antimicrob Agents Chemother 2012;56(11):6054–6.

Cryptococcosis

Eileen K. Maziarz, MD*, John R. Perfect, MD

KEYWORDS

- Cryptococcosis • Opportunistic mycoses • HIV/AIDS
- Solid organ transplantation (SOT) • Central nervous system (CNS) infection
- Immune reconstitution inflammatory syndrome (IRIS)

KEY POINTS

- Cryptococcosis is a major invasive fungal infection that is capable of widespread disease outbreaks in both immunocompromised and apparently immunocompetent hosts.
- Molecular advances continue to enhance our understanding of *Cryptococcus* and provide insight into its evolution into a pathogen of global importance.
- Diagnosis has improved with the introduction of point-of-care diagnostic assays.
- Screening and preemptive antifungal therapy offer great promise in making a significant impact in this highly deadly opportunistic mycosis.

INTRODUCTION

Cryptococcosis is an infectious disease with worldwide distribution and wide array of clinical presentations caused by pathogenic encapsulated yeasts in the genus *Cryptococcus*. Currently, there are 2 species of *Cryptococcus* that commonly cause disease in humans: *Cryptococcus neoformans* and *Cryptococcus gattii*. *C neoformans* was first identified as a human pathogen in the late 19th century, but was not recognized as a common cause of human disease until the late 1970s.[1,2] Over the last several decades, as vulnerable populations have expanded, cryptococcal meningitis became an infection of global importance, with up to 1 million new infections annually and significant attributable morbidity and mortality, especially among patients with human immunodeficiency virus (HIV) infection and AIDS.[3] Although *C neoformans and C gattii* share many features of a highly evolved, environmentally savvy yeast, there are important species- and strain-specific differences with respect to geographic distribution, environmental niches, host predilection, and clinical manifestations that

Disclosure Statement: Dr J.R. Perfect is a Principal Investigator for the following companies: Amplyx, Astellas, Cidara, Merck, Pfizer, Schering-Plough, Tokoyama, and Viamet.
Division of Infectious Diseases and International Health, Department of Medicine, Duke University Medical Center, DUMC Box 102359, 315 Trent Drive, Durham, NC 27710, USA
* Corresponding author.
E-mail address: eileen.maziarz@dm.duke.edu

Infect Dis Clin N Am 30 (2016) 179–206
http://dx.doi.org/10.1016/j.idc.2015.10.006
0891-5520/16/$ – see front matter © 2016 Elsevier Inc. All rights reserved.
id.theclinics.com

should be emphasized. As molecular techniques of identification have evolved, we have gained further insight into the pathobiology of these encapsulated yeasts, and their capacity to adapt to environmental pressures, exploit new geographic environments, and cause disease in both immunocompromised and apparently immunocompetent hosts.[4] Despite increased availability of and success with antiretroviral therapy (ART), the worldwide burden of and mortality associated cryptococcal disease remains unacceptably high, and novel strategies of screening and preemptive therapy offer great promise at making a sustained and much needed impact on this sugar-coated opportunistic mycosis.

THE PATHOGENS: *CRYPTOCOCCUS NEOFORMANS* AND *CRYPTOCOCCUS GATTII*

Cryptococcus is a genus of basidiomycetous fungi with more than 30 species ubiquitously distributed in the environment. There are only 2 species commonly known to cause human disease, *C neoformans* and *C gattii*. The epidemiology of *C neoformans* is well-characterized and this organism causes disease in both immunocompromised and apparently immunocompetent hosts. *C gattii*, conversely, has historically been regarded as a pathogen of apparently immunocompetent patients. However, preexisting conditions and immunocompromised states, including subclinical immune defects, are also reported as risk factors for infection with this species.[5–8] These species differences in clinical presentation may be primarily determined by variable host predilections, but may also be better characterized as we further our understanding of molecular subtypes.[9–12]

Historically, the genus was further classified into 3 varieties, 5 serotypes (based on structural differences in the polysaccharide capsule), and 8 molecular subtypes (**Table 1**). Molecular methods of identification have enhanced our appreciation for the significant genetic diversity among the *C gattii–C neoformans* complex and have called into question the current 2 species classification system. Recent proposed taxonomy changes based on the understanding of molecular studies have divided the pathogenic cryptococcal species from their classic divisions into better-defined molecular and genetic divisions. At present, the following divisions have been proposed: *C neoformans* var. *grubii* (serotype A) with 3 genotypes (VNI, VNII, VNB); *C neoformans* var. *neoformans* (serotype D or VNIV); and 5 other cryptic species, *C gattii*, *C bacillisporus*, *C deuterogattii*, *C tetragattii*, and *C decagattii* (serotypes B/C or VGI-IV).[13] Phylogenetic analyses, combined with recognized heterogeneity with respect to virulence, host preference, and antifungal susceptibility do provide evidence to support

Table 1		
Current classification of pathogenic *Cryptococcus* species		
Serotype	**Species and Varieties**	**Molecular Types**
A	*C neoformans* var. *grubii*[a]	VN I, VN II
B	*C gattii*	VG I, VG II, VG III, VG IV
C	*C gattii*	VG I, VG II, VG III, VG IV
D	*C neoformans* var. *neoformans*	VN IV
AD	*C neoformans*	VN III

[a] Responsible for the vast majority of disease owing to C neoformans worldwide.
Adapted from Hagen F, Khayhan K, Theelen B, et al. Recognition of seven species in the *Cryptococcus gatti/Cryptococcus neoformans* species complex. Fungal Genet Biol 2015;78:17.

further taxonomic classification into a 7-species/4 hybrid species scheme (**Table 2**). The molecular taxonomy of cryptococcal species is a vibrant area of evolution that has allowed for a greater understanding of specific strain characteristics, including fitness and predilection for certain environmental niches[13]; clinical correlations have yet to match this molecular precision, however, and for this review we will tend to lump the yeasts into their historical species designations, *C neoformans* and *C gattii*.

Approximately 95% of cryptococcal infections are caused by *C neoformans* (serotype A) strains with the remaining 4% to 5% of infections caused by *C neoformans* (serotype D) or *C gattii* (serotypes B/C strains). Whereas *C neoformans* var. *grubii* (serotype A) is found worldwide, *C neoformans* var *neoformans* (serotype D) is primarily observed in European countries and *C gattii* has historically been geographically restricted to tropical and subtropical regions, such as southern California, Hawaii, Brazil, Australia, Southeast Asia, and central Africa. More recently, *C gattii* has been identified in temperate climates such as Vancouver Island and the Pacific Northwest region of the United States and parts of Europe, suggesting an ecological shift possibly related to global temperature and moisture changes.[4,10–12] Although *C gattii* causes up to 15% of all cases of cryptococcosis in Australia and New Zealand, *C neoformans* remains the predominant species even in these endemic areas.[14] In certain areas of Africa around Botswana, where *C neoformans* and *C gattii* live together in the environment, active sexual recombination has been reported.[15] Although outbreaks of cryptococcosis are ongoing among immunocompromised populations worldwide, to date only *C gattii* strains have been reported to produce a geographically defined outbreak of disease.[4]

C neoformans is found throughout the world in association with excreta from certain birds such as pigeons,[16] environmental scavengers such as ameba and sowbugs,[17,18] and in a variety of tree species in their hollows. *C gattii* is commonly associated with

Table 2
Proposed taxonomy changes for the *Cryptococcus neoformans/C gattii* complex

Current Species Name	Genotype by RFLP	Proposed Species Name
C neoformans var. *grubii*	VNI VNII VNIII	*C neoformans*
C neoformans var. *neoformans*	VNIV	*C deneoformans*
C neoformans intervariety hybrid	VNIII	*C neoformans* × *C deneoformans* hybrid
C gattii	VGI VGIII VGII VGIV VGIV/VGIIIc	*C gattii* *C bacillisporus* *C deuterogattii* *C tetragattii* *C decagattii*
C neoformans var. *neoformans* × *C gattii* AFLP4/VGI hybrid	—	*C deneoformans* × *C gattii* hybrid
C neoformans var. *grubii* × *C gattii* AFLP4/VGI hybrid	—	*C neoformans* × *C gattii* hybrid
C neoformans var. *grubii* × *C gattii* AFLP6/VGII hybrid	—	*C deneoformans* × *C deuterogattii* hybrid

Adapted from Hagen F, Khayhan K, Theelen B, et al. Recognition of seven species in the *Cryptococcus gatti/Cryptococcus neoformans* species complex. Fungal Genet Biol 2015;78:17.

several species of eucalyptus trees in tropical and subtropical climates.[19] However, recently as it has emerged as an important pathogen capable of widespread outbreaks within new geographic niches including British Columbia and the Pacific Northwest United States,[4,10-12] it has been associated with temperate trees, such as firs and oaks.[9,20-22]

The life cycle of *Cryptococcus* involves both asexual and sexual forms.[23] The asexual form is the haploid encapsulated yeast that reproduces by mitosis with narrow-based budding and is found in clinical and environmental specimens. The sexual state is observed at present under certain laboratory conditions, resulting in meiosis between 2 mating types (MATa and MATα) to form clamp connections, basidia and basidiospores. The α mating type strains represent the vast majority of clinical and environmental isolates, probably related to their ability to produce haploid fruiting. Even same sex mating between 2 strains of the same type (MATα–MATα) does occur and is thought to produce the infectious spores that cause human infection.[24,25] This nonclassical mating between 2 α–α strains allows for further genetic diversity and is implicated in the production of hypervirulent, clonal strains responsible for the *C gattii* outbreak on Vancouver Island, suggesting that such mechanisms may confer the yeast the ability to exploit new geographic niches.[26,27] Furthermore, there are locations in Botswana where there are equal proportions of MATα and MATa isolates in both environmental and clinical populations, providing evidence that sexual recombination remains active even with the spread worldwide of relatively clonal strains.[15,28]

EPIDEMIOLOGY AND RISK FACTORS

Cryptococcosis was considered an uncommon infection before the AIDS pandemic; however, it was an awakening mycosis giant in the 1970s because it was associated with malignancy, organ transplantation, and certain immunosuppressive treatments. The incidence of disease increased significantly in the mid 1980s, with HIV/AIDS accounting for more than 80% of cryptococcosis cases worldwide.[29-31] Cryptococcal meningitis preferentially occurs in persons with impaired cell-mediated immunity and is a major AIDS-related opportunistic infection as the CD4$^+$ cell count falls below 100 cells/μL. With widespread implementation of successful antiretroviral therapy (ART), the incidence of HIV-associated cryptococcosis has decreased significantly in most developed nations, although the incidence in other at-risk populations has not changed (**Table 3**).[32] Furthermore, the prevalence of and morbidity and mortality associated with cryptococcal meningitis remain unacceptably high in settings where access to ART and other necessary health care resources are limited, specifically sub-Saharan Africa and parts of Asia. In fact, mortality peaked at approximately 600,000 deaths per year in the first decade of the 21st century; even today, it is likely that cryptococcal meningitis–related deaths approach several hundred thousand per year.[3] Although both *C neoformans* and *C gattii* can also cause disease in apparently immunocompetent hosts, the percentage of infections owing to *C gattii* in such patients is significantly higher than for *C neoformans*.

Pathogenesis and Host Immunity

Cryptococcal infection occurs primarily by inhalation of the infectious propagules (either poorly encapsulated yeast cells or basidiospores) from environmental reservoirs with deposition into pulmonary alveoli. Traumatic inoculation into tissues has been described[33] and may occur infrequently. The yeast may potentially enter via the gastrointestinal tract, although this entry is less consistent. Primary pulmonary infection is generally thought to be asymptomatic or minimally symptomatic despite

Table 3	
Risk factors for *Cryptococcus* infection	
HIV infection	Rheumatologic diseases[a]
	Systemic lupus erythematosus
	Rheumatoid arthritis
Corticosteroid and/or immunosuppressive therapies	Idiopathic CD4[+] lymphopenia
Solid organ transplantation[a]	Chronic liver disease (decompensated)[b]
Malignant and lymphoproliferative disorders[a,b]	Renal failure and/or peritoneal dialysis
Sarcoidosis	Hyper-IgM syndrome or hyper-IgE syndrome
Treatment with monoclonal antibodies (etanercept, infliximab, alemtuzumab)	*Diabetes mellitus[c]*
Anti-GM CSF antibodies	—

Abbreviations: GM CSF, granulocyte macrophage colony stimulating factor; HIV, human immuno-deficiency virus; Ig, immunoglobulin.
  [a] Immunosuppression for these conditions may influence risk.
  [b] Poor prognosis especially among patients with hematologic malignancy.[32]
  [c] Historically considered a risk factor but may reflect the frequency of condition rather than specific risk to an individual. Not found to be a risk factor in.[190,191]
  Adapted from Casadevall A, Perfect JR. Cryptococcus neoformans. Washington, DC: ASM Press; 1998.

high rates of serologic reactivity in children in certain urban settings.[34] Clearance of the infection by the host may occur. However, in many individuals, after yeasts are deposited in alveoli, they encounter alveolar macrophages, which play a central role in the immune response.[35] Host response to cryptococcal infection primarily involves a helper T cell response with cytokines including tumor necrosis factor (TNF), interferon-γ, and interleukin-2, resulting in granulomatous inflammation.[36] In many circumstances, this yeast will establish a latent infection within phagolysosome, with dormant (yet viable) yeasts within the thoracic lymph nodes or a pulmonary granuloma that can persist in an asymptomatic individual for years. When local immunity is suppressed, the yeast can grow and disseminate outside these pulmonary lymph node complexes similar to the pathophysiology that is observed in cases of reactivation tuberculosis or histoplasmosis.[31,37] In some hosts, *C gattii* disease seems to be more likely than *C neoformans* disease to present as a progressive granulomatous pulmonary infection, but less likely to disseminate to the central nervous system (CNS). This general observation has been made in human outbreaks and characterized in mouse models, but there remains substantial overlap between species.[12,31,38] In a patient with severely compromised cellular immunity, the yeasts reactivate and can proliferate at the site of initial infection and can disseminate within phagocytes or as yeast cells and gain access to other body sites.[39] Both direct invasion of the blood–brain barrier via transcytosis of free yeast forms through a series of mechanisms between yeast and host factors[40] and/or transport via macrophages into the CNS (the "Trojan horse" mechanism) seem to occur.[41–43] Whether certain immune states permit additional body sites of latency (eg, the CNS or prostate) have not yet been elucidated fully.

Advances in the molecular biology of *Cryptococcus* have confirmed multiple yeast virulence factors.[44] The 3 classical and prominent virulence factors of *C neoformans* include capsule formation, melanin pigment production, and thermotolerance.[23,36] The prominent antiphagocytic polysaccharide capsule, which is composed of glucuronoxylomannan, is unique to *Cryptococcus* species and is considered an essential virulence factor that has multiple effects on host immunity and can increase in size with exposure to body tissues and fluids.[45,46] In addition, *C neoformans* possesses an enzyme that catalyzes the conversion of diphenolic compounds to form melanin, which, when expressed, may have a biological role to protect the yeasts from host oxidative stresses and which may partially explain the organism's neurotropism into sites with high concentrations of the diphenolic catecholamines. Finally, the ability to grow at 37°C is a basic part of the virulence composite for most pathogenic fungi in humans including *Cryptococcus*, and molecular studies have linked high temperature growth with multiple signaling pathways and enzymes that this yeast has acquired or adapted to over time to retain or enhance its mammalian pathogenicity. Other virulence factors include phospholipase and urease production and multiple enzymes associated with protection against oxidative stresses, conferring survival within the phagolysosome.[44] It is estimated that more than 100 genes are important for optimal fitness of the yeast in mammalian hosts. The yeast has even adapted sophisticated mechanisms to escape the intracellular environment by modifying the permeability of the phagosome membrane and via nonlytic exocytosis (vomocytosis), allowing cell-to-cell or host compartment transfer of yeast ant its virulence factors without damage to the host macrophages.[47,48]

The many factors in the immunologic responses to *Cryptococcus* cannot be covered completely in this review, but several observations can be made. First, exposure is frequent and the healthy immunocompetent individual is generally resistant to cryptococcal disease. In fact, even in this group, some apparently normal hosts with cryptococcosis have been found to possess anti-granulocyte macrophage colony stimulating factor antibodies as a potential immune defect.[7,8] Second, the effective immune response is through a helper T cell–supported reaction and anything that weakens it may let cryptococci survive and thrive. This includes destruction of CD4+ cells by HIV, reduction of TNF activity by anti-TNF inhibitors, or the multifaceted immune suppressant effect of corticosteroids. From activated macrophages and not alternative macrophages to the development of protective antibodies over nonprotective antibodies, immunity changes over the course of cryptococcal infections. In fact, even some of our protective host mechanisms might be used against us as surfactant D may be coopted by *Cryptococcus* to gain entry into the lung.[49] Clearly, cryptococcosis emphasizes the Goldilocks paradigm of immunity. It produces disease when immunity is too little or too much, but when the human host immunity is just right, disease does not appear.

CLINICAL MANIFESTATIONS

C neoformans and *C gattii* have a major predilection for establishing clinical disease in the lungs and CNS. Other less frequent body sites of infection include skin, prostate, eyes, and bone/joints. However, it should be emphasized that this yeast can widely disseminate and infect most organs in severely immunosuppressed patients and thus has the ability to appear at any human body site.

Pulmonary Infection

The respiratory tract serves as the most important portal of entry for *Cryptococcus*. Clinical manifestations of pulmonary cryptococcosis range from asymptomatic colonization of the airways or a simple pulmonary nodule on a chest radiograph to life-threatening pneumonia with the presence of an acute respiratory distress syndrome.[50,51] In a normal host, asymptomatic, isolated pulmonary infection can occur in about one-third of patients and can be identified simply by an abnormal chest radiograph. In fact, the most common radiologic findings of cryptococcosis include well-defined single or multiple noncalcified nodules and pulmonary infiltrates (**Fig. 1**), although pleural effusions, hilar lymphadenopathy, and lung cavitation may also be observed. Patients with pulmonary cryptococcosis can present acutely with symptoms of pneumonia.[50] For example, in the recent outbreak of *C gattii* infections in Vancouver Island area, several cases of severe, symptomatic pulmonary cryptococcosis in apparently immunocompetent individuals occurred.[12] In an immunocompromised patient, however, cryptococcal pneumonia is usually symptomatic and in some cases can progress rapidly to acute respiratory distress syndrome, even in the absence of CNS involvement. Pulmonary involvement ranges from 10% to 55% of patients with AIDS-associated cryptococcal meningoencephalitis, although CNS symptoms usually predominate the clinical picture.[51]

Serum cryptococcal polysaccharide antigen testing is usually negative in cases of true isolated pulmonary cryptococcosis, but at times can be positive in the absence of CNS involvement or other apparent sites of infection. In immunocompromised individuals with *Cryptococcus* isolated from the lung or other sterile body site, however, a lumbar puncture to rule out CNS disease should be considered regardless of a patient's symptoms or serum antigen titer results. The only setting wherein a screening lumbar puncture may not necessarily be required is a patient with *Cryptococcus* isolated from the lung in the apparently immunocompetent patient without referable CNS symptoms and disease that clinically seems to be limited to the lungs.

Central Nervous System Infection

Clinical manifestations of CNS cryptococcosis include a myriad of signs and symptoms, such as headache, fever, cranial neuropathies, altered mentation, lethargy, memory loss, and signs of meningeal irritation.[2,30,31] Symptoms usually develop over a period of several weeks. However, on some occasions, patients present more acutely or lack typical features, such as headache. In severely immunocompromised, HIV-infected patients with CNS cryptococcosis, the burden of fungal organisms is usually high and can reach levels of more than 1 million yeasts per milliliter of cerebrospinal fluid (CSF). These patients may consequently have a shorter onset of signs and symptoms, greater CSF polysaccharide antigen titers, and higher intracranial pressures than other more immunocompetent individuals.

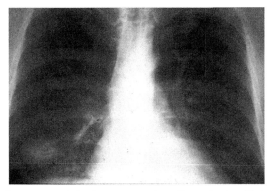

Fig. 1. Solitary pulmonary nodule. In an asymptomatic patient with isolated pulmonary cryptococcosis. (*Courtesy of* J. R. Perfect, MD, Durham, NC.)

Although disease severity is determined primarily by host immune factors, different species and/or strains of *Cryptococcus* may produce unique clinical manifestations, which can have implications for management. For instance, in certain areas of the world, *C gattii* has been observed to cause cerebral cryptococcomas and/or obstructive hydrocephalus with or without large pulmonary mass lesions more frequently than *C neoformans*.[12,52,53] These patients with parenchymal brain involvement may have a high intracranial pressure and present with cranial neuropathies. In such patients, who have been observed to respond poorly to antifungal therapy, early neurosurgical intervention to control pressure or ensure a correct diagnosis and longer antifungal treatment courses may be required for a successful outcome.[9,54]

Skin Infection

Cutaneous infections are the third most common clinical manifestations of cryptococcosis and patients can present with a variety of skin lesions. Lesions are often indistinguishable from those owing to other infections; as such, a skin biopsy with culture and histopathology are absolutely essential for definitive diagnosis. Primary cutaneous cryptococcosis is very rare and is usually associated with skin injury and direct inoculation of the yeasts[33]; thus, the appearance of cutaneous lesions usually heralds the presence of disseminated infection. Solid organ transplant recipients on tacrolimus seem to be more likely to develop skin, soft tissue, and osteoarticular infections owing to *Cryptococcus*.[55] Tacrolimus acts on the temperature signaling molecule calcineurin in *Cryptococcus* and has anticryptococcal activity at high temperatures, but it loses this direct antifungal activity as environmental temperatures decrease; this may in part explain the increased frequency of cutaneous lesions in patients receiving calcineurin inhibitors.[56]

Prostate Infection

The prostate is not a rare site for cryptococcal infection, but prostatic cryptococcosis is usually asymptomatic. For instance, latent *C neoformans* infection has been recognized to disseminate in the bloodstream during urologic surgery on the prostate for other indications.[57] The prostate gland may thus serve as an important reservoir for disease relapse in patients with a high fungal tissue burden.[58] Cultures of urine or seminal fluid may still be positive for *Cryptococcus* after initial antifungal treatment of cryptococcal meningitis in poorly controlled AIDS patients,[59] strongly supporting the need for prolonged antifungal treatment to eradicate infection in sanctuary sites in these severely immunocompromised patients.

Eye Infection

In early reports of cryptococcal meningitis before the AIDS epidemic, ocular signs and symptoms were noted in a substantial proportion of cases,[60] such as ocular palsies and papilledema. Several other ocular manifestations of cryptococcosis have been identified, including extensive retinal disease with or without vitritis, which can lead to irreversible blindness.[61] Visual loss may be owing to optic nerve infiltration by yeasts or vascular compromise from intracranial hypertension. The former process results in rapid visual loss with limited effective treatments, whereas the latter phenomenon results in more gradual visual loss and can be interrupted with aggressive management of increased intracranial pressure.

Infection at Other Body Sites

C neoformans can cause disease in essentially any organ of the human body. In fact, the first identification of this fungus from a clinical specimen was from a patient with tibial osteomyelitis in the 19th century.[1] Bone involvement of cryptococcosis typically presents as circumscribed osteolytic lesions in any bone of the body, but most commonly the vertebrae, and cryptococcal osteomyelitis has been associated with underlying sarcoidosis.[62] Bone marrow infiltration can be observed in severely immunocompromised hosts. Fungal peritonitis[63] and cryptococcuria are also reported in several case series. An appreciation for this yeast's protean clinical manifestations is essential, both at the time of initial diagnosis, as well as when immune defects are restored during treatment and immune restoration phenomena can present.

Immune Reconstitution Inflammatory Syndrome

Restoration of pathogen-specific immunity can result in a phenomenon known as the immune reconstitution inflammatory syndrome (IRIS), an entity that can occur before ("unmasking IRIS") or during ("paradoxic IRIS") antifungal therapy. Cryptococcal IRIS is best characterized in HIV-infected patients with CNS infection and is associated with significant morbidity and mortality.[64–76] In addition, IRIS is estimated to occur in 5% to 11% of solid organ transplant recipients with cryptococcal infection and is associated with increased risk of allograft failure[77–83] and may also be observed in non-HIV, nontransplant patients.[84] Proposed criteria for IRIS in HIV-associated disease include onset of symptoms within 12 months of ART initiation (with concomitant CD4[+] recovery).[85] These criteria are imprecise and do not address all populations at risk (**Box 1**). As such, it is incumbent upon the treating provider to have a high level of suspicion for this entity, as opposed to alternative diagnoses, which include progressive infection (from inadequate antifungal therapy, direct antifungal drug resistance, or persistent immune deficits), coinfection with other opportunistic infections, malignancy, or drug toxicity.

   Cryptococcal IRIS is thought to represent a dysregulated reversal of a Th2 (anti-inflammatory) to a strong helper T cell (pro-inflammatory) immune response in the

---

Box 1
Suggested diagnostic criteria for the immune reconstitution inflammatory syndrome

New appearance or worsening of any of the following:

Clinical or radiographic manifestations consistent with an inflammatory process:
   Central nervous system: Contrast-enhancing lesions on neuroimaging (computed tomography or MRI); cerebrospinal fluid pleocytosis (ie, >5 white blood cell count per μL); increased intracranial pressure (ie, opening pressure of $\geq$20 mm H_2O), with or without hydrocephalus.
   Pulmonary: Nodules, cavities, masses or pleural effusions.
   Other: Lymphadenopathy, skin, soft tissue, osteoarticular lesions.

Histopathology showing granulomatous lesions.

Symptoms occurring during receipt of appropriate antifungal therapy[a] that cannot be explained by a newly acquired infection or another process (neoplasm, etc).

Negative results of cultures, or stable or reduced biomarkers for the initial fungal pathogen during the diagnostic workup for the inflammatory process.

All 3 criteria must be present for a positive diagnosis.
   [a] Exclude intrinsic and de novo drug resistance, and suboptimum drug concentrations.
   Adapted from Sun H, Alexander B, Huprikar S, et al. Predictors of immune reconstitution syndrome in organ transplant recipients with cryptococcosis: implications for the management of immunosuppression. Clin Infect Dis 2015;60(1):36–44; and Singh N and Perfect JR. Immune reconstitution syndrome associated with opportunistic mycoses. Lancet Infect Dis 2007; 7:398.

setting of immune recovery.[86] Multiple factors are thought to be associated with future IRIS episodes, including high yeast burden at baseline, ineffective host immune response to initial infection, and rapid restoration of immunity.[67,73] Host immune responses in various compartments may not be uniform and are likely influenced by baseline parameters at the site.[87] Differences in baseline CSF cytokine and chemokine expression are thought to facilitate the development of cryptococcal IRIS, potentially via myeloid cell trafficking to the CNS and, consequently, production of excessive inflammation.[88,89] In fact, evidence of increased macrophage activation and linked CSF pleocytosis have been observed in patients receiving early ART and may mediate increased mortality, even before recognition of the clinical syndrome of IRIS.[87]

Clinical features of cryptococcal IRIS are similar to active cryptococcal infection itself, most commonly presenting as CNS disease, although lymphadenitis, pneumonitis, multifocal disease, soft tissue involvement, and mediastinitis have all been reported.[85,90] Meningeal disease is the most serious presentation.[85] A hallmark finding is suppurative or necrotic granulomatous inflammation with yeast forms seen on histopathology of infected tissues despite negative cultures.[77,80,90,91] Despite changes in inflammatory markers, there are no reliably specific diagnostic tests for IRIS, and establishing the diagnosis presents a considerable clinical challenge, especially with atypical presentations or manifestations at distant sites.[69,92] CSF opening pressure and white blood cell count[67,68,73] at the time of an IRIS event are significantly higher than baseline values for individual patients, which combined with negative cultures, may help to distinguish IRIS from relapsed infection.[70]

Management of cryptococcal IRIS is largely based on expert opinion.[93] First, ensuring the efficacy of antifungal therapy is essential[94,95]; in the absence of disease relapse or direct antifungal drug resistance, modification of antimicrobial therapy is generally not indicated.[93] A significant proportion of minor cases simply improve without specific treatment.[65,66,76] Corticosteroids have been shown to decrease the need for hospitalization and improve short-term quality of life and functional status in paradoxic tuberculosis-associated IRIS.[96] Although steroids may be essential in treating a serious life-threatening CNS IRIS episode owing to *Cryptococcus*, they should not be used for prevention of IRIS or to control CNS pressure, and may be harmful in some cases.[97] Immunomodulatory agents including those with anti–TNF-α activity have been used in cases of steroid-refractory IRIS.[65,98–101] Other strategies, including therapeutic lumbar drainage for intracranial hypertension[93,102] and, at times, surgical drainage of suppurative lymph nodes,[86,91] are important adjunctive measures that may be considered in severe disease. Continuation of ART in the setting of IRIS is generally recommended and has been performed safely.[66,71,92,103,104]

LABORATORY DIAGNOSIS

Definitive diagnosis of cryptococcosis is made by isolation of *Cryptococcus* from a clinical specimen or direct detection of the fungus by means of India ink staining of body fluids. There are several other methods used for the diagnosis of cryptococcosis, including histopathology of infected tissues and serologic methods. Molecular methods, although available and extensively used for research purposes, are not used currently in routine clinical practice.

Direct Examination/India Ink

The most rapid method for diagnosis of cryptococcal meningitis is direct microscopic examination for encapsulated yeasts by India ink preparation of CSF. *Cryptococcus* can be visualized as a globular, encapsulated yeast cell with or without budding, ranging in size from 5 to 20 μm in diameter (**Fig. 2**). The sensitivity of India ink staining of CSF depends on fungal burden and is reported to be 30% to 50% in non–AIDS-related cryptococcal meningitis and up to 80% in AIDS-related disease. False positives can result from intact lymphocytes, other tissue cells and nonviable yeast forms, which further limits the diagnostic utility of direct microscopy of CSF for cryptococcal meningitis.[105]

Culture and Identification

Cryptococcus can be cultured readily from biologic samples such as CSF, sputum, and skin biopsy on routine fungal and bacterial culture media. In adults with HIV-associated cryptococcal meningitis, CSF and blood cultures are positive in up to 90% and 70% of patients, respectively (reviewed in[106]). Colonies are usually observed on solid agar plates after 48 to 72 hours incubation at 30°C to 35°C in aerobic conditions and will appear as opaque, white-to-cream colonies that may turn orange-tan or brown after prolonged incubation. The mucoid appearance of the colony is related to the capsule size around the yeasts. Despite relatively rapid growth for most strains, cultures should be held for up to 4 weeks, particularly for patients receiving antifungal treatment.

Cytology and Histopathology

Cryptococcus can be identified by histologic staining of tissues from the lung, skin, bone marrow, brain, and other organs.[107] Histopathologic staining and cytology of centrifuged CSF sediment and other bodily fluids are more sensitive than the India ink staining method.[108–111] The organism is observed as a yeast that reproduces by narrow-based budding. The yeast is best identified by special stains that label the polysaccharide capsule including mucicarmine, periodic acid-Schiff, and Alcian blue stains.[2] The Fontana–Masson stain identifies melanin in the yeast cell wall. Other fungal stains such as Calcofluor, which binds fungal chitin, or Gomori methenamine silver, which stains the fungal cell wall, are also used to identify the organism from clinical specimens.[2,109]

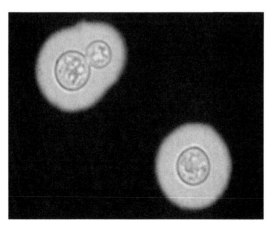

Fig. 2. India ink staining. Encapsulated yeast seen on India ink preparation of cerebrospinal fluid in a patient with cryptococcal meningitis. (*Courtesy of* J. R. Perfect, MD, Durham, NC.)

Serology

The diagnosis of cryptococcosis improved significantly with the development of serologic tests for the cryptococcal polysaccharide capsular antigen (CrAg), which is shed during infection. Latex agglutination and enzyme immunoassay techniques have been available widely (using both serum and CSF), the former of which had been the most commonly used methodology until recently, with overall sensitivities and specificities of 93% to 100% and 93% to 98%, respectively.[112,113] False-positive results of latex agglutination testing usually have initial reciprocal titers of 8 or less,[112] whereas false negatives can be seen owing to a prozone effect in the setting of extremely high antigen titers, which can be overcome with dilution.[114] Low fungal burden, as in chronic low-grade meningitis or in the very early stages of infection, and improper specimen storage can also cause false-negative results in latex agglutination tests.[115] Recently, a lateral flow assay was approved for use in serum and CSF, with sensitivity and specificity of greater than 98% in both specimen types (including whole blood from finger stick samples) and sensitivity of 85% in urine.[116–123] The semiquantitative test offers many advantages over the other serologic methods, including rapid turnaround (approximately 15 minutes), minimal requirements for laboratory infrastructure, stability at room temperature, low cost, and wider capture of *C gattii* polysaccharides.[116] Combined with these advantages, the assay's excellent performance across a broad range of clinical settings, including settings with low burden of HIV infection and high rates of *C gattii* infection,[100–104] make it an attractive option for point-of-care testing in both resource-available and resource-limited settings.[116,117,124]

Baseline cryptococcal polysaccharide antigen titers in serum and CSF correlate with fungal burden and carry prognostic significance in patients with cryptococcal meningitis.[122,125,126] However, there is limited value in serial monitoring of antigen titers acutely in assessing treatment response, because the kinetics of antigen clearance is a slower and less predictable marker of treatment response than quantitative culture.[122,127] Quantitative CSF yeast culture and its serial use for measurement of effective fungicidal activity has become a primary research tool for effectiveness of therapeutic regimens.[128] The quantitative yeast count has been correlated with outcome[129] and effective fungicidal activity has correlated with success of antifungal regimens, including survival.[95,128,130] Despite a decade of use and validation of its effectiveness in clinical studies, the use of quantitative CSF yeast culture for the determination of effective fungicidal activity has not yet become a part of routine clinical practice.

TREATMENT
Basic Principles

Amphotericin B deoxycholate (AmBd) is the cornerstone of treatment for severe cryptococcal infection, including meningoencephalitis. Treatment is summarized in **Table 4**. A standard induction dose of 0.7 to 1 mg/kg/d is recommended. Liposomal amphotericin B (3–6 mg/kg/d) has become a preferred alternative with similar outcomes and less nephrotoxicity, and is recommended specifically for primary induction in patients at risk for renal dysfunction.[93,131,132] Flucytosine (5-FC) is used in combination therapy with AmBd as first-line therapy in cryptococcal meningitis or severe pulmonary cryptococcosis at a dosage of 100 mg/kg/d in divided doses.[133,134] This combination represents the most potent fungicidal regimen, with faster CSF sterilization and fewer relapses, and is associated with lower attributable mortality.[133–139] Because the interruption of induction therapy is associated with poorer outcome, in resource-available areas the liposomal product has become the preferred polyene.

Table 4
Treatment recommendations for HIV-associated cryptococcal meningoencephalitis

	Duration
Induction therapy	
Primary regimen	
AmBd (0.7–1 mg/kg/d) plus flucytosine (5-FC) (100 mg/kg/d)[a]	2 wk
Alternative regimens[b]	
If 5-FC intolerant or unavailable: AmBd (0.7–1 mg/kg/d) or L-AMB[c] (3–4 mg/kg/d) or ABLC (5 mg/kg/d)	4–6 wk
AmBd (0.7–1 mg/kg/d) plus fluconazole (800 mg/d)	2 wk
Fluconazole ($\geq$800 mg/d, preferably 1200 mg/d) plus 5-FC (100 mg/kg/d)	6 wk
Fluconazole (800–2000 mg/d, preferably 1200 mg/d)	10–12 wk
Itraconazole (200 mg BID)	10–12 wk
Consolidation therapy	
Fluconazole (400 mg/d)	8 wk[d]
Maintenance or suppressive therapy	
Fluconazole (200 mg/d)	$\geq$1 y[e]
Alternative regimens[a]	
Itraconazole (200 mg BID)	$\geq$1 y[e]
AmBd (1 mg/kg IV per week)	$\geq$1 y

Abbreviations: 5-FC, flucytosine; ABLC, amphotericin B lipid complex; AmBd, amphotericin B deoxycholate; BID, twice daily; L-AMB, liposomal amphotericin B.
[a] L-AMB, 3–4 mg/kg/d or AmB lipid complex (ABLC; 5 mg/kg/d) for patients predisposed to renal dysfunction.
[b] Can be considered as alternative regimen when primary regimen not available but not encouraged as equivalent substitutes.
[c] L-AMB can be safely administered in doses as high as 6 mg/k/d.
[d] Initiate highly active antiretroviral therapy approximately 4 weeks after beginning antifungal regimen.
[e] After 1 year of therapy, if successful response to antiretroviral drugs (CD4 count $\geq$100 and viral load low or undetectable for >3 months), can consider discontinuation of antifungal therapy. Consider reinstitution if CD4 count is <100.
Adapted from Perfect JR, Dismukes WE, Dromer F, et al. Clinical practice guide lines for the management of cryptococcal disease: 2010 update by the Infectious Disease Society of America. Clin Infect Dis 2010;50:291–322.

Unfortunately, there are still no comparative studies with 5-FC combined with lipid formulations of amphotericin B as opposed to AmBd. Early mycological failure (defined as persistently positive CSF cultures at day 14) correlates with late treatment failure and poor outcome,[140] and lack of 5-FC is independently associated with both early[141] and late[137] mycological failure. This improved fungicidal activity of combination therapy translates into a direct survival benefit compared with AmBd monotherapy.[135] 5-FC should be dose adjusted for renal dysfunction, with therapeutic drug monitoring to decrease its primary side effect of bone marrow suppression.[142] There are emerging data that lower doses of 5-FC in combination with amphotericin may demonstrate similar fungicidal activity.[138]

Although combination induction therapy remains the recommended first-line therapy for severe cryptococcosis, 5-FC availability is limited in settings where the disease burden and mortality rates are the highest. Alternative combination therapies have been investigated, the most efficacious of which is AmBd plus fluconazole

(800 mg/d), which results in improved rates of fungal clearance, neurologic recovery, and survival compared with AmBd alone or in combination with lower doses of fluconazole.[143,144] This combination offers a more feasible and potentially viable option for effective initial therapy in settings where access to 5-FC is limited. Optimizing treatment outcomes without exhausting limited resources is critical in many settings. Standardized fluid and electrolyte supplementation protocols for patients treated with amphotericin B in these resource-limited settings have been associated with improved early survival.[145] Additionally, shorter courses of amphotericin B in combination with other agents may be considered in these settings, although clinical endpoints for such regimens have not been rigorously evaluated.[146,147] An ongoing trial evaluating the combination of intermittent dosing of high-dose of liposomal amphotericin B with high-dose fluconazole in resource-limited settings is underway to address this unanswered question (AmBition-CM, www.controlled-trials.com/ISRCTN10248064). Additional alternative induction regimens are available in the guidelines but their use is not encouraged based on limited data of the success with these regimens.[148] Fluconazole monotherapy for meningitis is not recommended for induction given its fungistatic nature, poor success, and higher relapse rates as well as increased rates of resistance in relapse.[93,94] However, in areas without access to AmBd, high doses ($\geq$1200 mg/d) of fluconazole should be commenced.

A 3-stage regimen of induction, consolidation, and maintenance is standard treatment for cryptococcal meningitis in all patients, irrespective of host risk factors.[93,133] In HIV-infected patients, initial induction treatment usually begins with combination therapy as described, followed by consolidation treatment with fluconazole (400–800 mg/d) for 8 weeks in patients who have demonstrated favorable response. Longer courses of both induction (eg, 6 weeks) and consolidation (or "eradication") therapy have been suggested in C gattii meningoencephalitis, irrespective of host immune status, owing to the observed severity of neurologic disease in this group of patients,[11,52,53] but this is not certain and in general C gattii should be treated similarly to C neoformans. After consolidation, long-term suppression is commenced with oral fluconazole (200–400 mg/d). This approach has decreased rates of relapse from approximately 40% to less than 5% in severely immunosuppressed patients.[149] Secondary prophylaxis is discontinued after 1 to 2 years of antifungal therapy in patients who respond to ART with an increase in CD4$^+$ cell counts to greater than 100 cells/µL and a decrease in HIV viral load to undetectable levels for at least 3 months.[93,150,151] The other triazoles (itraconazole, voriconazole, and posaconazole) are active against cryptococcal isolates in vitro and, in combination with AmBd, may have similar fungicidal activity to 5-FC,[144] but owing to differences in bioavailability, CSF penetration, drug interactions, cost, and lack of robust studies in cryptococcosis, these agents are not recommended as first-line agents for consolidation or maintenance therapy. However, they may have a role in refractory cases.[152–155]

Timing of Antiretroviral Therapy

In HIV-associated cryptococcal infection, ART has a major impact on long-term prognosis. However, several studies have suggested an increased risk of IRIS among HIV-infected patients initiated on ART early after the diagnosis of an opportunistic infection.[64,65,156] More contemporary studies have demonstrated conflicting results regarding outcomes of cryptococcal infection based on timing of ART initiation,[103,157,158] and studies in tuberculosis have demonstrated a survival benefit with earlier ART (despite increased rates of IRIS).[159,160] Recently, the Cryptococcal Optimal ART Timing Trial (COAT) provided some definitive guidance to delay initiation of ART in patients with cryptococcal meningitis for a minimum of 4 weeks after starting antifungal therapy. This randomized trial demonstrated improved survival in patients with cryptococcal meningitis in whom ART initiation was deferred for up to 5 weeks after diagnosis as compared with immediate ART (within 1–2 weeks).[161] Although increased rates of IRIS observed with early ART did not attain statistical significance, markers of macrophage activation were increased in this early group, suggesting that subclinical or compartmentalized IRIS may occur and influence mortality.[87,161]

Organ Transplant Recipients

Organ transplant recipients with CNS cryptococcal infection are managed similarly to HIV-infected patients, although lipid formulations of amphotericin B are preferred to limit nephrotoxicity.[93] A longer course of induction therapy is indicated if CSF cultures remain positive at 2 weeks, because this scenario is associated with an increased 6-month mortality.[162] Relapse rates among organ transplant recipients are lower than in HIV-associated disease, such that a shorter course of maintenance therapy can be pursued following standard consolidation, but generally these patients are treated for 1 year.[93,162] Drug interactions between fluconazole and immunosuppressive agents should be anticipated owing to CYP3A4 inhibition, and a preemptive reduction in calcineurin inhibitors should be considered. Management of immunosuppression in the setting of cryptococcal infection requires recognition of the increased risk of IRIS.[77,80,163] Thus, stepwise reduction in immunosuppression is recommended, although the approach should be individualized for each patient.

Non–HIV-Infected, Nontransplant Patients

Very few prospective data are available on the management of cryptococcal infection in the apparently immunocompetent host lacking classical risk factors for cryptococcosis.[134] This heterogeneous group of patients is diagnosed later, irrespective of disease severity.[32,84] Recommendations for longer induction therapy ($\geq$4 weeks) are based on the recognition of poorer outcomes and higher mortality rates in this group of patients both in early[134,164] as well as contemporary[32] studies. However, in patients with good prognostic factors and excellent antifungal induction response, 2-week induction therapy can be successful. Therapy should be extended further if 5-FC is not included (or there is limited exposure to this drug) in the induction regimen.[93] Recommendations for consolidation and maintenance parallel those for HIV-infected patients and reflect high relapse rates (30%) within the first year before the introduction of consolidation and maintenance antifungal strategies.[93,134] Criteria for stopping treatment in these patients include resolution of symptoms and at least 1 year of suppressive antifungal therapy.

Management of Intracranial Pressure

Along with the optimization of antifungal therapy, management of increased intracranial pressure is critically important in cryptococcal meningoencephalitis. Intracranial hypertension frequently corresponds with CSF fungal burden, potentially mediated by CSF outflow obstruction by clumped yeast forms even during early therapy, and is associated with increased morbidity and mortality.[97,165] Intracranial imaging should be performed before lumbar puncture if impaired mentation or focal neurologic deficits are present. A baseline CSF opening pressure should be obtained in all patients. Aggressive attempts to control increased intracranial pressure should occur when patients are symptomatic, although emerging data suggest there may be benefit to therapeutic lumbar punctures, irrespective of baseline opening pressure in resource-limited settings.[166] Treatment options for managing acutely elevated intracranial pressure include repeated lumbar punctures (daily until pressure and symptoms are stable for >2 days), lumbar drain insertion, ventriculostomy, or ventriculoperitoneal shunt, if obstructive hydrocephalus develops.[97] Consideration of early neurosurgical consultation has been recommended in cases of meningoencephalitis owing to *C gattii* where CNS inflammation is often severe.[52,53] Medical treatments such as corticosteroids (unless IRIS suspected or in cases of severe *C gattii* infection), mannitol, and acetazolamide are generally not recommended.[52,53,129,167] If shunt placement is necessary, CSF sterilization is not required before insertion, which can be performed once appropriate antifungal therapy has been commenced.[168]

Persistent and Relapsed Infection

Persistent and relapsed infection must be distinguished from IRIS. Persistent disease has been defined as persistently positive CSF cultures after 1 month of antifungal therapy, whereas relapse requires new clinical signs and symptoms and positive cultures after initial improvement and fungal sterilization.[93] Surrogate markers, including biochemical parameters, India ink staining, and cryptococcal antigen titers, are insufficient to define relapse or alter antifungal therapy. General recommendations for management in these persistent or relapsed cases include resumption of induction therapy, often for a longer duration and at increased dosages, if tolerable, and pursuance of comparative antifungal susceptibility testing.[93] Although primary direct antifungal resistance to azoles and polyenes is rare, decreased susceptibility to fluconazole has been observed in some cases of culture-positive relapse.[94] There has not yet been a convincing minimum inhibitory concentration breakpoint for cryptococcal species in antifungal susceptibility testing; thus, the importance of comparative minimum inhibitory concentration testing with the original isolate in cases where resistance is suspected cannot be overemphasized.[169,170]

Nonmeningeal Disease

Although isolation of *Cryptococcus* from respiratory tract specimens can occur in the absence of clinical disease (colonization), it is incumbent upon the treating clinician to assess for subclinical disease or potential for complications when *Cryptococcus* is isolated from any clinical specimen. In the absence of immune compromise, airway colonization carries a low risk for invasive disease and treatment can be deferred; although in most cases, given the safety profile of fluconazole, many clinicians favor treatment in all patients in whom *Cryptococcus* is isolated. In immunosuppressed patients with isolated pulmonary cryptococcosis, however, treatment is recommended to prevent dissemination.[93] This group of patients should be evaluated for systemic disease (including blood and CSF cultures as well as CrAg testing from serum and CSF) to optimize treatment. In any patient in whom cryptococcemia is identified, symptoms are severe, or CSF examination reveals asymptomatic CNS involvement, treatment for cryptococcal meningitis is recommended.[93] The potential for severe pulmonary infection owing to *C gattii* should be appreciated when *Cryptococcus* is isolated from respiratory cultures in settings where this species is endemic[11,12,52,53,171]; however, to date, there are no convincing data that species identification is required to optimally select antifungal therapy, and disease severity remains the critical factor in determining initial treatment. Cerebral cryptococcomas often can be managed with prolonged antifungal therapy without the need for surgical removal unless mass effect or other evidence of obstruction is identified. A longer induction phase with AmBd plus 5-FC, followed by 6 to 18 months of consolidation therapy with fluconazole (400–800 mg/d) is recommended. Localized infection of extrapulmonary nonmeningeal sites can occur occasionally with direct inoculation, but more commonly represents disseminated infection. Suspicion for the latter must be maintained when *Cryptococcus* is identified from a sterile body site, because management strategies differ if disseminated disease is present. Consultation with ophthalmology is indicated in cases of cryptococcal eye disease.[93]

Screening and Prevention

There is no question that early identification of HIV infection and initiation of ART in patients before progression to severe immunodeficiency is the most effective intervention at reducing the global burden of cryptococcosis and other opportunistic infections. However, despite increased access to ART worldwide, late presentations of HIV infection still occur and the burden of severe cryptococcal infection and related mortality remains disproportionately represented in these populations.

Fluconazole prophylaxis has been shown to be effective for preventing cryptococcosis in patients with advanced AIDS in endemic areas[172,173]; however, universal prophylaxis is relatively cost ineffective,[124] has not been shown to offer a survival benefit,[174] and may add to the appearance of azole-resistant strains. As such, this approach is not recommended currently.

Given that mortality from cryptococcal meningitis remains unacceptably high, alternative management strategies have been evaluated and implemented in resource-limited settings, specifically a "screen and treat" approach using serum cryptococcal antigen (CrAg) testing followed by preemptive fluconazole therapy in CrAg-positive patients. CrAg is an early marker of cryptococcal disease, detectable in serum a median of 22 days before the onset of symptoms, and is both highly predictive of incident cryptococcal meningitis and an independent risk factor for death during the first year of ART.[175–177] This approach is associated with a decreased incidence of cryptococcal meningitis and improved survival among patients with advanced HIV disease and has been successfully implemented in several resource-limited settings, with a baseline prevalence of asymptomatic cryptococcal antigenemia of 5% to 13%.[177,178] Moreover, analyses have consistently demonstrated both the cost effectiveness and survival advantage of a "screen and treat" approach, as compared with standard of care or universal fluconazole prophylaxis, at CrAg prevalences as low as 0.6%.[178–180] As access to lateral flow assay testing in these settings is increased, the cost effectiveness is likely to be greater than initially reported. The World Health Organization now recommends implementation of CrAg screening and preemptive fluconazole therapy in ART-naïve adults with a CD4 count of less than 100 cells/mm^3 before initiating ART in endemic settings.[181] Several nations in sub-Saharan Africa have since operationalized programs as a part of the existing HIV infrastructure. Several unanswered questions remain, however, including the feasibility of implementation, the dose and duration of preemptive fluconazole, the criteria for lumbar puncture in asymptomatic patients, and the potential impact on azole resistance. Some data suggest a 'screen and treat' would be cost effective, even in resource-rich settings, although this is currently not part of standard practice, despite recent reports of CrAg prevalence of more than 3% in the United States.[176,182] Routine screening for cryptococcal infection and/or prophylaxis are not recommended in solid organ transplant recipients, even when immunosuppression is augmented in patients with previously (appropriately) treated infection.[183]

In the arena of direct immune modulation for cryptococcosis management, aside from the use of ART, progress has been slow. First, although both cryptococcal glucuronoxylomannan–tetanus toxoid conjugate vaccine and specific monoclonal antibodies to cryptococci have been developed, clinical trials have not been initiated to determine their usefulness in human subjects.[184,185] The use of immune stimulation with recombinant gamma-interferon has both immunologic support and 2 positive clinical trials,[186–189] but has only been used in refractory cases and likely reflects concerns about precisely judging immune stimulation when IRIS can be a deadly problem.

REFERENCES

1. Knoke M, Schwesinger G. One hundred years ago: the history of cryptococcosis in Greifswald. Medical mycology in the nineteenth century. Mycoses 1994;37:229–33.
2. Casadevall A, Perfect JR. Cryptococcus neoformans. Washington, DC: ASM Press; 1998.
3. Park BJ, Wannemuehler KA, Marston BJ, et al. Estimation of the current global burden of cryptococcal meningitis among persons living with HIV/AIDS. AIDS 2009;23:525–30.
4. Kidd SE, Hagen F, Tscharke RL, et al. A rare genotype of *Cryptococcus gattii* caused the cryptococcosis outbreak on Vancouver Island (British Columbia, Canada). Proc Natl Acad Sci U S A 2004;101:17258–63.
5. MacDougall L, Fyfe M, Romney M, et al. Risk factors for *Cryptococcus gattii* infection, British Columbia, Canada. Emerg Infect Dis 2011;17(2):193–9.
6. Marr K, Datta K, Pirofski L, et al. *Cryptococcus gattii* Infection in healthy Hosts: A Sentinel for Subclinical Immunodeficiency? Clin Infect Dis 2012;54(1):153–4.
7. Rosen L, Freeman A, Yang L, et al. Anti-GM-CSF autoantibodies in patients with cryptococcal meningitis. J Immunol 2013;190:3959–66.
8. Saijo T, Chen J, Chen S, et al. Anti-granulocyte macrophage colony-stimulating factor autoantibodies are a risk factor for central nervous system infection by *Cryptococcus gattii* in otherwise immunocompetent patients. MBio 2014;5(2): e00912–4.
9. Mitchell D, Sorrell T, Allworth A, et al. Cryptococcal disease of the CNS in immunocompetent hosts: influence of cryptococcal variety on clinical manifestations and outcome. Clin Infect Dis 1995;20:611–6.
10. Harris J, Lockhart S, Debess E, et al. *Cryptococcus gattii* in the United States: clinical aspects of infection with an emerging pathogen. Clin Infect Dis 2011;53:1188–95.
11. Chen S, Meyer W, Sorrell T. *Cryptococcus gattii* infections. Clin Microbiol Rev 2014;27(4):980–1024.
12. Phillips P, Galanis E, MacDougall L, et al. Longitudinal clinical findings and outcome among patients with *Cryptococcus gattii* infection in British Columbia. Clin Infect Dis 2015;60(9):1368–76.
13. Hagen F, Khayhan K, Theelen B, et al. Recognition of seven species in the *Cryptococcus gatti/Cryptococcus neoformans* species complex. Fungal Genet Biol 2015;78:16–48.
14. Chen S, Sorrell T, Nimmo G, et al. Epidemiology and host- and variety-dependent characteristics of infection due to *Cryptococcus neoformans* in Australia and New Zealand. Australasian Cryptococcal Study Group. Clin Infect Dis 2000;31:499–508.
15. Chen Y, Litvintseva A, Frazzitta A, et al. Comparative analyses of clinical and environmental populations of Cryptococcus neoformans in Botswana. Mol Ecol 2015;24(14):3559–71.
16. Emmons C. Saprophytic sources of Cryptococcus neoformans associated with the pigeon (*Columba livia*). Am J Hyg 1955;62(3):227–32.
17. Steenbergen J, Shuman H, Casadevall A. *Cryptococcus neoformans* interactions with amoebae suggest an explanation for its virulence and intracellular pathogenic strategy in macrophages. Proc Natl Acad Sci U S A 2001;98:15245.

18. Ruiz A, Neilson J, Bulmer G. Control of *Cryptococcus neoformans* in nature by biotic factors. Sabouraudia 1982;20(1):21–9.
19. Ellis D, Pfeiffer T. Natural habitat of *Cryptococcus neoformans* var gattii. J Clin Microbiol 1990;28:1642–4.
20. Hoang L, Maguire J, Doyle P, et al. Cryptococcus neoformans infections at Vancouver Hospital and Health Sciences Centre (1997-2002): epidemiology, microbiology and histopathology. J Med Microbiol 2004;53(Pt 9):935.
21. Datta K, Bartlett K, Baer R, et al. Spread of *Cryptococcus gattii* into Pacific Northwest region of the United States. Emerg Infect Dis 2009;15(8):1185–91.
22. Springer D, Chaturvedi V. Projecting global occurrence of *Cryptococcus gattii.* Emerg Infect Dis 2010;16(1):14–20.
23. Hull CM, Heitman J. Genetics of *Cryptococcus neoformans*. Annu Rev Genet 2002;36:557–615.
24. Lin X, Hull C, Heitman J. Sexual reproduction between partners of the same mating type in Cryptococcus neoformans. Nature 2005;434:1017–21.
25. Sukroongreung S, Kitiniyom K, Nilakul X, et al. Pathogenicity of basidiospores of *Filobasidiella neoformans* var. *neoformans*. Med Mycol 1998;36(6):419–24.
26. Fraser J, Giles S, Wenink E, et al. Same-sex mating and the origin of the Vancouver Island *Cryptococcus gattii* outbreak. Nature 2005;437:1360–4.
27. Byrnes E, Li W, Lewit Y, et al. Emergence and pathogenicity of highly virulent *Cryptococcus gattii* genotypes in the Northwest United States. PLoS Pathog 2010;6(4):e1000850.
28. Litvintseva A, Marra R, Nielsen K, et al. Evidence of sexual recombination among *Cryptococcus neoformans* serotype A isolates in sub-Saharan Africa. Eukaryot Cell 2003;2(6):1162–8.
29. Hajjeh RA, Conn LA, Stephens DS, et al. Cryptococcosis: population-based multistate active surveillance and risk factors in human immunodeficiency virus-infected persons. Cryptococcal Active Surveillance Group. J Infect Dis 1999;179:449–54.
30. Perfect JR, Casadevall A. Cryptococcosis. Infect Dis Clin North Am 2002;16: 837–74.
31. Perfect JR. Cryptococcus neoformans and *Cryptococcus gattii*. In: Bennett JE, Dolin R, Blaser MJ, editors. Mandell, Douglas, and Bennett's principles and practice of infectious diseases. 8th edition. Philadelphia: Elsevier Saunders; 2015. p. 2934–48.
32. Bratton E, El Husseini N, Chastain C, et al. Comparison and temporal trends of three groups with Cryptococcosis: HIV-infected, solid organ transplant, and HIV-negative/non-transplant. PLoS One 2012;7(8):e43582.
33. Christianson J, Engber W, Andes D. Primary cutaneous cryptococcosis in immunocompetent and immunocompromised hosts. Med Mycol 2003;41(3):177–88.
34. Goldman D, Khine H, Abadi J, et al. Pediatrics 2001;107(5):E66.
35. Shao X, Mednick A, Alvarez M, et al. An innate immune system cell is a major determinant in species-related susceptibility to fungal pneumonia. J Immunol 2005;175:3244–51.
36. Perfect JR. *Cryptococcus neoformans*: a sugar-coated killer with designer genes. FEMS Immunol Med Microbiol 2005;45:395–404.
37. Sun H, Alexander B, Lortholary O, et al. Unrecognized pretransplant and donor-derived cryptococcal disease in organ transplant recipients. Clin Infect Dis 2010;51(9):1062–9.
38. Krockenberger M, Malik R, Ngamskulrungroj P, et al. Pathogenesis of pulmonary *Cryptococcus gattii* infection: a rat model. Mycopathologia 2010;170(5):315–30.

39. Santangelo R, Zoellner H, Sorrell T, et al. Role of extracellular phospholipases and mononuclear phagocytes in dissemination of cryptococcosis in a murine model. Infect Immun 2004;72:1693–9.
40. Maruvada R, Zhu L, Pearce D, et al. Cryptococcus neoformans phospholipase B1 activates host cell Rac1 for traversal across the blood-brain barrier. Cell Microbiol 2012;14(10):1544–53.
41. Ahi M, Li S, Zheng C, et al. Real-time imaging of trapping and urease-dependent transmigration of *Cryptococcus neoformans* in mouse brain. J Clin Invest 2010;120(5):1683–93.
42. Charlier C, Nielsen K, Daou S, et al. Evidence of a role for monocytes in dissemination and brain invasion by Cryptococcus neoformans. Infect Immun 2009;77(1):120–7.
43. Casadevall A. Cryptococci at the brain gate: break and enter or use a Trojan horse? J Clin Invest 2010;120(5):1389–92.
44. Coelho C, Bocca A, Casadevall A. The tools for virulence of Cryptococcus neoformans. Adv Appl Microbiol 2014;87:1–41.
45. Okagaki L, Strain A, Nielsen J, et al. Cryptococcal cell morphology affects host cell interactions and pathogenicity. PLoS Pathog 2010;6:e1000953.
46. Zaragoza O, Garcia-Rodas R, Nosanchuk J, et al. Fungal cell gigantism during mammalian infection. PLoS Pathog 2010;6:e1000945.
47. Tucker S, Casadevall A. Replication of *Cryptococcus neoformans* in macrophages is accompanied by phagosomal permeabilization and accumulation of vesicles containing polysaccharide in the cytoplasm. Proc Natl Acad Sci U S A 2002;99(5):3165–70.
48. Alvarez M, Casadevall A. Phagosome extrusion and host-cell survival after *Cryptococcus neoformans* phagocytosis by macrophages. Curr Biol 2006;16:2161–5.
49. Geunes-Boyer S, Beers M, Perfect J, et al. Surfactant protein D facilitates Cryptococcus neoformans infection. Infect Immun 2012;80(7):2444–53.
50. Warr W, Bates JH, Stone A. The spectrum of pulmonary cryptococcosis. Ann Intern Med 1968;69:1109–16.
51. Brizendine K, Baddley J, Pappas P. Pulmonary cryptococcosis. Semin Respir Crit Care Med 2011;32(6):727–34.
52. Chen S, Korman T, Slavin M, et al. Antifungal therapy and management of complications of cryptococcosis due to *Cryptococcus Gattii*. Clin Infect Dis 2013; 57(4):543–51.
53. Franco-Paredes C, Womack T, Bohlmeyer T, et al. Management of *Cryptococcus gattii* meningoencephalitis. Lancet Infect Dis 2015;15:348–55.
54. Speed B, Dunt D. Clinical and host differences between infections with the two varieties of Cryptococcus neoformans. Clin Infect Dis 1995;21:28–34.
55. Singh N, Gayowski T, Wagener MM, et al. Clinical spectrum of invasive cryptococcosis in liver transplant recipients receiving tacrolimus. Clin Transplant 1997; 11:66–70.
56. Odom A, Muir S, Lim E, et al. Calcineurin is required for virulence of Crytptococcus neoformans. EMBO J 2007;16:2576–89.
57. Allen R, Barter CE, Cachou LL, et al. Disseminated cryptococcosis after transurethral resection of the prostate. Aust N Z J Med 1982;12:296–9.
58. Larsen RA, Bozzette S, McCutchan JA, et al. Persistent Cryptococcus neoformans infection of the prostate after successful treatment of meningitis. California Collaborative Treatment Group. Ann Intern Med 1989;111:125–8.
59. Staib F, Seibold M, L'Age M. Persistence of *Cryptococcus neoformans* in seminal fluid and urine under itraconazole treatment. The urogenital tract (prostate) as a niche for *Cryptococcus neoformans*. Mycoses 1990;33:369–73.

60. Okun E, Butler WT. Ophthalmologic complications of cryptococcal meningitis. Arch Ophthalmol 1964;71:52–7.
61. Rex JH, Larsen RA, Dismukes WE, et al. Catastrophic visual loss due to *Cryptococcus neoformans* meningitis. Medicine (Baltimore) 1993;72:207–24.
62. Liu PY. Cryptococcal osteomyelitis: case report and review. Diagn Microbiol Infect Dis 1998;30(1):33–5.
63. Albert-Braun S, Venema F, Bausch J, et al. *Cryptococcus neoformans* peritonitis in a patient with alcoholic cirrhosis: case report and review of the literature. Infection 2005;33:282–8.
64. Shelburne SA, Visnegarwala F, Darcourt J, et al. Incidence and risk factors for immune reconstitution inflammatory syndrome during HAART. AIDS 2005; 19(4):399–406.
65. Lortholary O, Fontanet A, Memain N, et al. Incidence and risk factors of immune reconstitution inflammatory syndrome complicating HIV-associated cryptococcosis in France. AIDS 2005;19(10):1043–9.
66. Bicanic T, Meintjes G, Rebe K, et al. Immune reconstitution inflammatory syndrome in HIV-associated cryptococcal meningitis: a prospective study. J Acquir Immune Defic Syndr 2009;51(2):130–4.
67. Sungkanuparph S, Filler SG, Chetchotisakd P, et al. Cryptococcal immune reconstitution inflammatory syndrome after HAART in AIDS patients with cryptococcal meningitis: a prospective multicenter study. Clin Infect Dis 2009;49(6):931–4.
68. Boulware DR, Meya DB, Bergemann TL, et al. Clinical features and serum biomarkers in HIV immune reconstitution inflammatory syndrome after cryptococcal meningitis: a prospective cohort study. PLoS Med 2010;7(12):e1000384.
69. Haddow LJ, Easterbrook PJ, Mosam A, et al. Defining immune reconstitution inflammatory syndrome: evaluation of expert opinion versus 2 case definitions in a South African cohort. Clin Infect Dis 2009;49(9):1424–32.
70. Shelburne SA 3rd, Darcourt J, White AC Jr, et al. The role of immune reconstitution inflammatory syndrome in AIDS-related *Cryptococcus neoformans* disease in the era of HAART. Clin Infect Dis 2005;40(7):1049–52.
71. Sungkanuparph S, Jongwutiwes U, Kiertiburanakul S. Timing of cryptococcal immune reconstitution inflammatory syndrome after HAART in patients with AIDS and cryptococcal meningitis. J Acquir Immune Defic Syndr 2007;45(5):595–6.
72. Kambugu A, Meya DB, Rhein J, et al. Outcomes of cryptococcal meningitis in Uganda before and after the availability of HAART. Clin Infect Dis 2008; 46(11):1694–701.
73. Boulware DR, Bonham SC, Meya DB, et al. Paucity of initial cerebrospinal fluid inflammation in cryptococcal meningitis is associated with subsequent immune reconstitution inflammatory syndrome. J Infect Dis 2010;202(6):962–70.
74. da Cunha Colombo ER, Mora DJ, Silva-Vergara ML. Immune reconstitution inflammatory syndrome (IRIS) associated with *Cryptococcus neoformans* infection in AIDS patients. Mycoses 2011;54(4):e178–82.
75. Rambeloarisoa J, Batisse D, Thiebaut JB, et al. Intramedullary abscess resulting from disseminated cryptococcosis despite immune restoration in a patient with AIDS. J Infect 2002;44(3):185–8.
76. Skiest DJ, Hester LJ, Hardy RD. Cryptococcal immune reconstitution inflammatory syndrome: report of four cases in three patients and review of the literature. J Infect 2005;51(5):e289–97.
77. Singh N, Lortholary O, Alexander BD, et al. Allograft loss in renal transplant recipients with *Cryptococcus neoformans* associated immune reconstitution syndrome. Transplantation 2005;80(8):1131–3.

78. Conti HR, Shen F, Nayyar N, et al. Th17 cells and IL-17 receptor signaling are essential for mucosal host defense against oral candidiasis. J Exp Med 2009; 206(2):299–311.

79. Sun HY, Singh N. Opportunistic infection-associated immune reconstitution syndrome in transplant recipients. Clin Infect Dis 2011;53(2):168–76.

80. Lanternier F, Chandesris MO, Poiree S, et al. Cellulitis revealing a cryptococcosis-related immune reconstitution inflammatory syndrome in a renal allograft recipient. Am J Transplant 2007;7(12):2826–8.

81. Crespo G, Cervera C, Michelena J, et al. Immune reconstitution syndrome after voriconazole treatment for cryptococcal meningitis in a liver transplant recipient. Liver Transplant 2008;14(11):1671–4.

82. Singh N. Novel immune regulatory pathways and their role in immune reconstitution syndrome in organ transplant recipients with invasive mycoses. Eur J Clin Microbiol Infect Dis 2008;27(6):403–8.

83. Sun H, Alexander B, Huprikar S, et al. Predictors of immune reconstitution syndrome in organ transplant recipients with cryptococcosis: implications for the management of immunosuppression. Clin Infect Dis 2015;60(1):36–44.

84. Ecevit IZ, Clancy CJ, Scmalfuss IM, et al. The poor prognosis of central nervous system cryptococcosis among nonimmunosuppressed patients: a call for better disease recognition and evaluation of adjuncts to antifungal therapy. Clin Infect Dis 2006;42:1443–7.

85. Haddow LJ, Colebunders R, Meintjes G, et al. Cryptococcal immune reconstitution inflammatory syndrome in HIV-1-infected individuals: proposed clinical case definitions. Lancet Infect Dis 2010;10(11):791–802.

86. Tan DB, Yong YK, Tan HY, et al. Immunological profiles of immune restoration disease presenting as mycobacterial lymphadenitis and cryptococcal meningitis. HIV Med 2008;9(5):307–16.

87. Scriven J, Rhein J, Hullsiek K, et al. Early ART after cryptococcal meningitis is associated with cerebrospinal fluid pleocytosis and macrophage activation in a multisite randomized trial. J Infect Dis 2015;212(5):769–78.

88. Jarvis J, Meintjes G, Bicanic T, et al. Cerebrospinal fluid cytokine profiles predict risk of early mortality and immune reconstitution inflammatory syndrome in HIV-associated cryptococcal meningitis. PLoS Pathog 2014;11(4):e1004754.

89. Chang C, Omarjee S, Lim A, et al. Chemokine levels and chemokine receptor expression in the blood and the cerebrospinal fluid of HIV-infected patients with cryptococcal meningitis and cryptococcosis-associated immune reconstitution syndrome. J Infect Dis 2013;208:1604–12.

90. Trevenzoli M, Cattelan AM, Rea F, et al. Mediastinitis due to cryptococcal infection: a new clinical entity in the HAART era. J Infect 2002;45(3):173–9.

91. Blanche P, Gombert B, Ginsburg C, et al. HIV combination therapy: immune restitution causing cryptococcal lymphadenitis dramatically improved by anti-inflammatory therapy. Scand J Infect Dis 1998;30(6):615–6.

92. Meintjes G, Lawn SD, Scano F, et al. Tuberculosis-associated immune reconstitution inflammatory syndrome: case definitions for use in resource-limited settings. Lancet Infect Dis 2008;8(8):516–23.

93. Perfect JR, Dismukes WE, Dromer F, et al. Clinical Practice Guide lines for the Management of Cryptococcal Disease: 2010 update by the Infectious Disease Society of America. Clin Infect Dis 2010;50:291–322.

94. Bicanic T, Harrison T, Niepieklo A, et al. Symptomatic relapse of HIV-associated cryptococcal meningitis after initial fluconazole monotherapy: the role of fluconazole resistance and immune reconstitution. Clin Infect Dis 2006;43(8):1069–73.

95. Bicanic T, Muzoora C, Brouwer AE, et al. Independent association between rate of clearance of infection and clinical outcome of HIV-associated cryptococcal meningitis: analysis of a combined cohort of 262 patients. Clin Infect Dis 2009;49(5):702–9.
96. Meintjes G, Wilkinson RJ, Morroni C, et al. Randomized placebo-controlled trial of prednisone for paradoxical tuberculosis-associated immune reconstitution inflammatory syndrome. AIDS 2010;24(15):2381–90.
97. Graybill JR, Sobel J, Saag M, et al. Diagnosis and management of increased intracranial pressure in patients with AIDS and cryptococcal meningitis. The NIAID Mycoses Study Group and AIDS Cooperative Treatment Groups. Clin Infect Dis 2000;30(1):47–54.
98. Narayanan S, Banerjee C, Holt PA. Cryptococcal immune reconstitution syndrome during steroid withdrawal treated with hydroxychloroquine. Int J Infect Dis 2011;15(1):e70–3.
99. Sitapati AM, Kao CL, Cachay ER, et al. Treatment of HIV-related inflammatory cerebral cryptococcoma with adalimumab. Clin Infect Dis 2010;50(2):e7–10.
100. Scemla A, Gerber S, Duquesne A, et al. Dramatic improvement of severe cryptococcosis-induced immune reconstitution syndrome with adalimumab in a renal transplant recipient. Am J Transplant 2015;15:560–4.
101. Brunel A, Reynes J, Tuaillon E, et al. Thalidomide for steroid-dependent immune reconstitution inflammatory syndromes during AIDS. AIDS 2012;26(16):2110–2.
102. Biagetti C, Nicola M, Borderi M, et al. Paradoxical immune reconstitution inflammatory syndrome associated with previous *Cryptococcus neoformans* infection in an HIV-positive patient requiring neurosurgical intervention. New Microbiol 2009;32(2):209–12.
103. Zolopa A, Andersen J, Powderly W, et al. Early HAART reduces AIDS progression/death in individuals with acute opportunistic infections: a multicenter randomized strategy trial. PLoS One 2009;4(5):e5575.
104. French MA. HIV/AIDS: immune reconstitution inflammatory syndrome: a reappraisal. Clin Infect Dis 2009;48(1):101–7.
105. Diamond RD, Bennett JE. Prognostic factors in cryptococcal meningitis. A study in 111 cases. Ann Intern Med 1974;80:176–81.
106. Antinori S. New Insights into HIV/AIDS-Associated Cryptococcosis. ISRN AIDS 2013;2013:471363.
107. Shibuya K, Coulson WF, Wollman JS, et al. Histopathology of cryptococcosis and other fungal infections in patients with acquired immunodeficiency syndrome. Int J Infect Dis 2001;5:78–85.
108. Sato Y, Osabe S, Kuno H, et al. Rapid diagnosis of cryptococcal meningitis by microscopic examination of centrifuged cerebrospinal fluid sediment. J Neurol Sci 1999;164:72–5.
109. Kanjanavirojkul N, Sripa C, Puapairoj A. Cytologic diagnosis of *Cryptococcus neoformans* in HIV-positive patients. Acta Cytol 1997;41:493–6.
110. Malabonga VM, Basti J, Kamholz SL. Utility of bronchoscopic sampling techniques for cryptococcal disease in AIDS. Chest 1991;99:370–2.
111. Lee LN, Yang PC, Kuo SH, et al. Diagnosis of pulmonary cryptococcosis by ultrasound guided percutaneous aspiration. Thorax 1993;48:75–8.
112. Tanner DC, Weinstein MP, Fedorciw B, et al. Comparison of commercial kits for detection of cryptococcal antigen. J Clin Microbiol 1994;32:1680–4.
113. Wu TC, Koo SY. Comparison of three commercial cryptococcal latex kits for detection of cryptococcal antigen. J Clin Microbiol 1983;18:1127–30.
114. Stamm AM, Polt SS. False-negative cryptococcal antigen test. JAMA 1980;244:1359.

115. Bloomfield N, Gordon MA, Elmendorf DF. Detection of *Cryptococcus neoformans* antigen in body fluids by latex particle agglutination. Proc Soc Exp Biol Med 1963;114:64–7.

116. Jarvis JN, Percival A, Bauman S, et al. Evaluation of a novel point-of-care cryptococcal antigen test on serum, plasma and urine from patients with HIV-associated cryptococcal meningitis. Clin Infect Dis 2011;53:1019–23.

117. Lindsley MD, Mekha N, Baggett HC, et al. Evaluation of a newly developed lateral flow immunoassay for the diagnosis of Cryptococcus. Clin Infect Dis 2011;53:321–5.

118. McMullan BJ, Halliday C, Sorrell TC, et al. Clinical utility of the cryptococcal antigen lateral flow assay in a diagnostic mycology laboratory. PLoS One 2012;7:e49451.

119. Binnicker MJ, Jespersen DJ, Bestrom JE, et al. Comparison of four assays for the detection of cryptococcal antigen. Clin Vaccine Immunol 2012;19:1988–90.

120. Hansen J, Slechta ES, Gates-Hollingsworth MA, et al. Large-scale evaluation of the Immuno-Mycologics lateral flow and Enzyme-Linked immunoassays for detection of cryptococcal antigen in serum and cerebrospinal fluid. Clin Vaccine Immunol 2013;20:52–5.

121. Huang H, Fan L, Rajbanshi B, et al. Evaluation of a new cryptococcal antigen lateral flow immunoassay in serum, cerebrospinal fluid and urine for the diagnosis of cryptococcosis: a meta-analysis and systematic review. PLoS One 2015;10(5):e0127117.

122. Kabanda T, Siedner M, Klausner J, et al. Point-of-care diagnosis and prognostication of cryptococcal meningitis with the cryptococcal lateral flow assay on cerebrospinal fluid. Clin Infect Dis 2014;58(1):113–6.

123. Williams D, Kiiza T, Kwizera R, et al. Evaluation of fingerstick cryptococcal antigen lateral flow assay in HIV-infected persons: a diagnostic accuracy study. Clin Infect Dis 2015;61(3):464–7.

124. Jarvis JN, Harrison TS, Lawn SD, et al. Cost effectiveness of cryptococcal antigen screening as a strategy to prevent cryptococcal meningitis in South Africa. PLoS One 2013;8:e69288.

125. Bindschadler DD, Bennett JE. Serology of human cryptococcosis. Ann Intern Med 1968;69:45–52.

126. Saag MS, Powderly WG, Cloud GA, et al. Comparison of amphotericin B with fluconazole in the treatment of acute AIDS-associated cryptococcal meningitis. The NIAID Mycoses Study Group and the AIDS Clinical Trials Group. N Engl J Med 1992;326(8):3–89.

127. Powderly WG, Cloud GA, Dismukes WE, et al. Measurement of cryptococcal antigen in serum and cerebrospinal fluid: value in the management of AIDS-associated cryptococcal meningitis. Clin Infect Dis 1994;18:789–92.

128. Bicanic T, Meintjes G, Wood R, et al. Fungal burden, early fungicidal activity, and outcome in cryptococcal meningitis in antiretroviral-naive or antiretroviral-experienced patients treated with amphotericin B or fluconazole. Clin Infect Dis 2007;45(1):76–80.

129. Jarvis J, Bicanic T, Loyse A, et al. Determinants of mortality in a combined cohort of 501 patients With HIV-associated cryptococcal meningitis: implications for improving outcomes. Clin Infect Dis 2014;58(5):736–45.

130. Perfect J, Bicanic T. Cryptococcosis diagnosis and treatment: what do we know now. Fungal Genet Biol 2015;78:49–54.

131. Leenders AC, Reiss P, Portegies P, et al. Liposomal amphotericin B (AmBisome) compared with amphotericin B both followed by oral fluconazole in the treatment of AIDS-associated cryptococcal meningitis. AIDS 1997;11:1463–71.

132. Hamill RJ, Sobel JD, El-Sadr W, et al. Comparison of 2 doses of liposomal amphotericin B and conventional amphotericin B deoxycholate for treatment of AIDS-associated acute cryptococcal meningitis: a randomized, double-blind clinical trial of efficacy and safety. Clin Infect Dis 2010;51(2):225–32.

133. van der Horst CM, Saag MS, Cloud GA, et al. Treatment of cryptococcal meningitis associated with the acquired immunodeficiency syndrome. National Institute of Allergy and Infectious Diseases Mycoses Study Group and AIDS Clinical Trials Group. N Engl J Med 1997;337:15–21.

134. Dismukes WE, Cloud G, Gallis HA, et al. Treatment of cryptococcal meningitis with combination amphotericin B and flucytosine for four as compared with six weeks. N Engl J Med 1987;317:334–41.

135. Day JN, Chau T, Wolbers M, et al. Combination antifungal therapy for cryptococcal meningitis. N Engl J Med 2013;368:1291–302.

136. Brouwer AE, Rajanuwong A, Chieraku W, et al. Combination antifungal therapies for HIV-associated cryptococcal meningitis: a randomised trial. Lancet 2004; 363:1764–7.

137. Dromer F, Bernede-Bauduin C, Guillemot D, et al. Major role for amphotericin-flucytosine combination in severe cryptococcosis. PLoS One 2008;3(8):e2870.

138. O'Connor L, Livermore J, Sharp A, et al. Pharmacodynamics of liposomal amphotericin B and flucytosine for cryptococcal meningoencephalitis: safe and effective regimens for immunocompromised patients. J Infect Dis 2013;208:351–61.

139. Bratton E, El Husseini N, Chastain C, et al. Approaches to antifungal therapies and their effectiveness among patients with cryptococcosis. Antimicrob Agents Chemother 2013;57(6):2485–95.

140. Robinson PA, Bauer M, Leal MAE, et al. Early mycological treatment failure in AIDS-associated cryptococcal meningitis. Clin Infect Dis 1999;28:82–92.

141. Dromer F, Mathoulin-Pelissier S, Launay O, et al. Determinants of disease presentation and outcome during cryptococcosis: The Crypto A/D Study. PLoS Med 2007;4:e21.

142. Drew RH, Perfect JR. Flucytosine. In: Yu V, Weber R, Raoult D, editors. Antimicrobial therapy and vaccines. New York: Apple Trees Productions; 1997. p. 656–7.

143. Pappas PG, Chetchotisakd P, Larsen RA, et al. A phase II randomized trial of amphotericin B alone or combined with fluconazole in the treatment of HIV-associated cryptococcal meningitis. Clin Infect Dis 2009;48:1775–83.

144. Loyse A, Wilson D, Meintjes G, et al. Comparison of the early fungicidal activity of high-dose fluconazole, voriconazole, and flucytosine as second-line drugs given in combination with amphotericin B for the treatment of HIV-associated cryptococcal meningitis. Clin Infect Dis 2012;54:121–8.

145. Bahr N, Rolfes M, Musubire A, et al. Standardized electrolyte supplementation and fluid management improves survival during amphotericin therapy for cryptococcal meningitis in resource-limited settings. Open Forum Infect Dis 2014;1(2):ofu070.

146. Muzoora C, Kabanda T, Ortu G, et al. Short course amphotericin B with high dose fluconazole for HIV-associated cryptococcal meningitis. J Infect 2012; 64:76–81.

147. Jackson A, Nussbaum J, Phulusa J, et al. A phase II randomized controlled trial adding oral flucytosine to high-dose fluconazole with short-course amphotericin B for cryptococcal meningitis. AIDS 2012;26:1363–70.

148. Nussbaum JC, Jackson A, Namarika D, et al. Combination flucytosine and high-dose fluconazole compared with fluconazole monotherapy for the treatment of cryptococcal meningitis: a randomized trial in Malawi. Clin Infect Dis 2010;50: 338–44.

149. Bozette SA, Larsen RA, Chiu J, et al. A placebo-controlled trial of maintenance therapy with fluconazole after treatment for cryptococcal meningitis in the Acquired Immunodeficiency Syndrome. N Engl J Med 1991;324:580–4.
150. Vibhagool A, Sungkanuparph S, Mootsikapun P, et al. Discontinuation of secondary prophylaxis for cryptococcal meningitis in human immunodeficiency virus-infected patients treated with HAART: a prospective, multicenter, randomized study. Clin Infect Dis 2003;36:1329–31.
151. Mussini C, Pezzotti P, Miro JM, et al. Discontinuation of maintenance therapy for cryptococcal meningitis in patients with AIDS treated with HAART: an international observational study. Clin Infect Dis 2004;38:565–71.
152. Denning DW, Tucker RM, Hanson LH, et al. Itraconazole therapy for cryptococcal meningitis and cryptococcosis. Arch Intern Med 1989;149:2301–8.
153. Saag MS, Cloud GA, Graybill JR, et al. A comparison of itraconazole versus fluconazole as maintenance therapy for AIDS-associated cryptococcal meningitis. National Institute of Allergy and Infectious Diseases Mycoses Study Group. Clin Infect Dis 1999;28:291–6.
154. Perfect JR, Marr KA, Walsh TJ, et al. Voriconazole treatment for less-common, emerging or refractory fungal infections. Clin Infect Dis 2003;36(9):1122–31.
155. Pitisuttithum P, Negroni R, Graybill JR, et al. Activity of posaconazole in the treatment of central nervous system fungal infections. J Antimicrob Chemother 2005; 56:745–55.
156. Bisson G, Molefi M, Bellamy S, et al. Early versus delayed antiretroviral therapy and cerebrospinal fluid fungal clearance in adults with HIV and cryptococcal meningitis. Clin Infect Dis 2013;56(8):1165–73.
157. Njei B, Kongnyuy EJ, Kumar S, et al. Optimal timing for HAART initiation in patients with HIV infection and concurrent cryptococcal meningitis. Cochrane Database Syst Rev 2013;(2):CD009012.
158. Makadzange AT, Ndhlovu CE, Takarinda K, et al. Early versus delayed initiation of HAART for concurrent HIV infection and cryptococcal meningitis in sub-Saharan Africa. Clin Infect Dis 2010;50(11):1532–8.
159. Abdool Karim S, Naidoo K, Grobler A, et al. Integration of antiretroviral therapy with tuberculosis treatment. N Engl J Med 2011;365(16):1492.
160. Blanc F, Sok T, Laureillard D, et al. Earlier versus later start of antiretroviral therapy in HIV-infected adults with tuberculosis. N Engl J Med 2011;365(16):1471.
161. Boulware D, Meya D, Muzoora C, et al. Timing of antiretroviral therapy after cryptococcal meningitis. N Engl J Med 2014;370:2487–98.
162. Singh N, Lortholary O, Alexander BD, et al. Antifungal management practices and evolution of infection in organ transplant recipients with *Cryptococcus neoformans* infection. Transplantation 2005;80:1033–9.
163. Singh N, Lortholary O, Alexander BD, et al. An immune reconstitution syndrome-like illness associated with *Cryptococcus neoformans* infection in organ transplant recipients. Clin Infect Dis 2005;40:1756–61.
164. Bennett JE, Dismukes WE, Duma RJ, et al. A comparison of amphotericin B alone and combined with flucytosine in the treatment of cryptococcal meningitis. N Engl J Med 1970;301(3):126–31.
165. Denning DW, Armstrong RW, Lewis BH, et al. Elevated cerebrospinal fluid pressures in patients with cryptococcal meningitis and acquired immunodeficiency syndrome. Am J Med 1991;91:267–72.
166. Rolfes M, Hullsiek K, Rhein J, et al. The effect of therapeutic lumbar punctures on acute mortality from cryptococcal meningitis. Clin Infect Dis 2014;59(11): 1607–14.

167. Newton PN, Thai le H, Tip NQ, et al. A randomized, double-blind, placebo-controlled trial of acetazolamide for the treatment of elevated intracranial pressure in cryptococcal meningitis. Clin Infect Dis 2002;35:769–72.

168. Park MK, Hospenthal DR, Bennett JE. Treatment of hydrocephalus secondary to cryptococcal meningitis by use of shunting. Clin Infect Dis 1999;28:629–33.

169. Velez JD, Allendorfer R, Luther M, et al. Correlation of in vitro azole susceptibility testing with in vivo response in a murine model of cryptococcal meningitis. J Infect Dis 1993;168:508–10.

170. Aller AI, Martin-Mazuelos E, Lozano F, et al. Correlation of fluconazole MICs with clinical outcome in cryptococcal infection. Antimicrob Agents Chemother 2000; 44:1544–8.

171. Smith R, Mba-Jonas A, Tourdjman M, et al. Treatment and outcomes among patients with *Cryptococcus gattii* infections in the United States Pacific Northwest. PLoS One 2014;9(2):e88875.

172. Nightingale SD, Cal SX, Peterson DM, et al. Primary prophylaxis with fluconazole against systemic fungal infections in HIV-positive patients. AIDS 1992;6:191–4.

173. Chetchotisakd P, Sungkanuparph S, Thinkhamrop B, et al. A multicentre, randomized, double-blind, placebo-controlled trial of primary cryptococcal meningitis prophylaxis in HIV-infected patients with severe immune deficiency. HIV Med 2004;5(3):140–3.

174. Chang L, Phipps W, Kennedy G, et al. Antifungal interventions for the primary prevention of cryptococcal disease in adults with HIV. Cochrane Database Syst Rev 2005;(3):CD004773.

175. French N, Gray K, Watera C, et al. Cryptococcal infection in a cohort of HIV-1 infected Ugandan adults. AIDS 2002;16:1031–8.

176. McKenney J, Bauman S, Neary B, et al. Prevalence, correlates and outcomes of cryptococcal antigen positivity among patients with AIDS, United States, 1986-2012. Clin Infect Dis 2015;60(6):959–65.

177. Jarvis JN, Lawn SD, Vogt M, et al. Screening for cryptococcal antigenemia in patients accessing an antiretroviral treatment program in South Africa. Clin Infect Dis 2009;48:856–62.

178. Meya D, Manabe Y, Castelnuovo B, et al. Cost-effectiveness of serum cryptococcal antigen screening to prevent deaths among HIV-infected persons with a CD4$^+$ cell count of < 100 cells/μL who start HIV therapy in resource-limited settings. Clin Infect Dis 2010;51(4):448–55.

179. Kaplan J, Vallabhaneni S, Smith R, et al. Cryptococcal antigen screening and early antifungal treatment to prevent cryptococcal meningitis: a review of the literature. J Acquir Immune Defic Syndr 2015;68:S331–9.

180. Smith R, Nguyen T, Ha H, et al. Prevalence of cryptococcal antigenemia and cost-effectiveness of a cryptococcal antigen screening program – Vietnam. PLoS One 2013;8(4):e62213.

181. World Health Organization. Rapid advice: diagnosis, prevention and management of Cryptococcal disease in HIV-infected adults, adolescents and children. Geneva (Switzerland): World Health Organization; 2011.

182. Rajasinham R, Boulware D. Reconsidering cryptococcal antigen screening in the US among persons with CD4 < 100 cells/mcl. Clin Infect Dis 2012;55:1742–4.

183. Singh N, Dromer F, Perfect JR, et al. Cryptococcosis in solid organ transplant recipients: current state of the science. Clin Infect Dis 2008;47:1321–7.

184. Devi SJ, Scheerson R, Egan W, et al. *Cryptococcus neoformans* serotype A glucuronoxylomannan protein conjugate vaccines: synthesis, characterization, and immunogenicity. Infect Immun 1991;59:3700–7.

185. Mukherjee J, Zuckier LS, Scharff MD, et al. Therapeutic efficacy of monoclonal antibodies to *Cryptococcus neoformans* glucuronoxylomannan alone and in combination with amphotericin B. Antimicrob Agents Chemother 1994;38:580–7.

186. Wormley F, Perfect J, Steele C, et al. Protection against cryptococcosis by using a murine gamma interferon-producing *Cryptococcus neoformans* strain. Infect Immun 2007;75:1453–63.

187. Jarvis J, Meintjes G, Rebe K, et al. Adjunctive interferon-γ immunotherapy for the treatment of HIV-associated cryptococcal meningitis: a randomized controlled trial. AIDS 2012;26(9):1105–13.

188. Pappas P, Bustamante B, Ticona E, et al. Recombinant interferon-gamma 1b as adjunctive therapy for AIDS-related acute cryptococcal meningitis. J Infect Dis 2004;1889(12):2185–91.

189. Isiodras S, Samonis G, Boumpas D, et al. Fungal infections complicating tumor necrosis factorα blockade therapy. Mayo Clin Proc 2008;83(2):181–94.

190. Lin Y, Shiau S, Fang C. Risk factors for invasive Cryptococcus neoformans diseases: a case-control study. PLoS One 2015;10(3):e0119090.

191. Singh N, Perfect JR. Immune reconstitution syndrome associated with opportunistic mycoses. Lancet Infect Dis 2007;7(6):395–401.

Histoplasmosis

Lawrence J. Wheat, MD[a],*, Marwan M. Azar, MD[b],
Nathan C. Bahr, MD[c], Andrej Spec, MD[d],
Ryan F. Relich, MD, PhD, D(ABMM), MLS(ASCP)CMSM[CM][e], Chadi Hage, MD[f]

KEYWORDS

- Histoplasmosis • Histoplasma • Disseminated • Pulmonary
- Central nervous system • Serology • Antigen • Antibody

KEY POINTS

- Although histoplasmosis is highly endemic in certain regions of the Americas, disease may be seen globally and should not be overlooked in patients with unexplained pulmonary or systemic illnesses.
- Most patients exhibit pulmonary signs and symptoms, accompanied by radiographic abnormalities, which often are mistaken for community-acquired pneumonia caused by bacterial or viral agents.
- Once a diagnosis is considered, a panel of mycologic and non–culture-based assays is adequate to establish a diagnosis in a few days to a week in most patients.
- Once diagnosed, the treatment is highly effective even in immunocompromised patients.

INTRODUCTION

Histoplasmosis is the most common endemic mycosis in the United States and in certain areas of Mexico and Central and South America. In the United States, of the endemic mycoses, histoplasmosis was the most common cause for hospitalization and death.[1] Hammerman[2] cited Centers for Disease Control and Prevention surveillance records that estimated approximately 500,000 infections yearly. Analysis of skin test data suggests a higher infection rate. For example, 20% of recruits were positive for histoplasmin skin test reactivity in a landmark US Navy study.[3] Assuming an average age of 20 years, the yearly infection rate is 1%, representing approximately 3 million infections per year based on the 2010 US census.

[a] MiraVista Diagnostics, 4705 Decatur Boulevard, Indianapolis, IN 46241, USA; [b] Section of Infectious Diseases, Yale School of Medicine, New Haven, CT, USA; [c] Division of Infectious Diseases, University of Kansas, 3901 Rainbow Boulevard, Mailstop 1028, Kansas City, KS 66160, USA; [d] Washington University School of Medicine, 660 South Euclid Avenue, Box 8051, Saint Louis, MO 63110, USA; [e] Division of Clinical Microbiology, Department of Pathology and Laboratory Medicine, IU Health Pathology Laboratory, Indiana University School of Medicine, 350 West 11th Street, Indianapolis, IN 46202, USA; [f] Methodist Professional Center-1, Suite 230, 1801 N Senate Boulevard, Indianapolis, IN 46202, USA
* Corresponding author.
E-mail address: jwheat@miravistalabs.com

Infect Dis Clin N Am 30 (2016) 207–227
http://dx.doi.org/10.1016/j.idc.2015.10.009
0891-5520/16/$ – see front matter © 2016 Elsevier Inc. All rights reserved.

EPIDEMIOLOGY

Histoplasmosis is most commonly understood as intensely endemic in the Ohio and Mississippi River Valleys in the United States and much of Latin America (**Fig. 1**),[3,4] although it has been known for some time that other areas around the world saw cases as well.[5] The HIV pandemic and the increasing use of other immunosuppressive medications, such as calcineurin and tumor necrosis factor inhibitors, has resulted in more cases of histoplasmosis and thus improved understanding of the distribution of this fungus.[6–8] Factors accounting for the geographic distribution of histoplasmosis are poorly understood but include moderate temperature and bird or bat guano containing soil.

Histoplasma may be found in so-called microfoci inside and outside the endemic areas for histoplasmosis. The characteristic of these microfoci is contamination with bird/or bat guano. The activities that have been most commonly identified as sources for exposure to *Histoplasma capsulatum* include farming, exposure to chicken coops or caves, remodeling or demolition of old buildings, and cutting down trees or clearing brush from sites in which blackbirds have roosted.[9–11]

These microfoci challenge the perception of where histoplasmosis might occur in the United States, as evidenced by recent reports from Idaho and Montana.[12] Outside the United States, histoplasmosis incidence is best understood and highest in parts of Mexico and South and Central America and is largely driven by the AIDS pandemic.[13–18] In French Guiana, progressive disseminated histoplasmosis (PDH) is the most common AIDS-defining illness, where this condition was detected by 1 retrospective in approximately 41% of HIV-positive hospitalized patients with fever and a CD4[+] count less than 200.[13,14,16,19] In Columbia, more than 70% of patients with histoplasmosis included in a survey conducted from 1992 to 2008 had HIV/AIDS,[20] and in Brazil, histoplasmosis is highly endemic in several regions; histoplasmin positivity may be up to approximately 90% in some areas.[4]

Histoplasmosis also is endemic in parts of Asia, Southeast Asia, and India. In China, 75% of cases occur along the Yangtze River, most in association with AIDS,[21] and histoplasmin skin test positivity ranges from 6% to 50%. More than 1200 cases of PDH have been reported in Thailand[22] and recent cases have been reported in South Korea as well.[23] In India, cases have been recognized since the 1950s and histoplasmin sensitivity rates have been reported from 4.7% to 12.3%.[24,25] Information is more limited in Africa, but cases have been reported in patients with AIDS in Zimbabwe, South Africa, Uganda, and Tanzania,[9,26,27] and many cases were diagnosed in Europe after travel.[25,28,29] Histoplasmosis in Europe without travel to endemic areas is rare but cases have been reported in Spain.[30] The newly recognized worldwide distribution clearly has an effect on histoplasmosis management.[31]

PATHOGENESIS

Infection with *H capsulatum* occurs by inhaling microconidia after disturbance of environmental sites containing the organism.[32] Infection is usually asymptomatic in healthy individuals unless a large inoculum has been inhaled.[25] In the absence of immunocompromising conditions, acute infection resolves with the development of cell-mediated immunity.[33] As a consequence of production of T lymphocytes that recognize the organism, tumor necrosis factor α and interferon gamma are induced, activating macrophages to inhibit the growth of the organism and to provide protection against reinfection.[32,33] Depletion of T cells resulting in lower levels of these cytokines results in increased mortality and fungal burden.[32]

Although organisms persist in granulomas for life in most healthy individuals, the organisms are typically not viable and consequently latent infection, as seen in

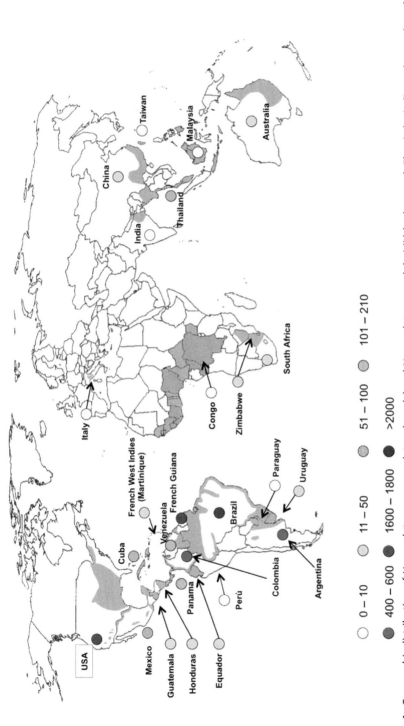

Fig. 1. Geographic distribution of *H capsulatum* var. *capsulatum* (*purple*) and *H capsulatum* var. *duboisii* (*shadow area*). The circles indicate the number of published cases of autochthonous AIDS-associated histoplasmosis (via Scopus query). The majority of African cases has been observed outside Africa. (*From* Bahr NC, Antinori S, Wheat LJ, et al. Histoplasmosis infections worldwide: thinking outside of the Ohio River Valley. Curr Trop Med Rep 2015;2(2):70–80; with permission.)

tuberculosis, is rare in histoplasmosis in a normal host.[32] Cellular immunity may not develop in individuals who are immunocompromised, however, permitting progression of the infection and death, if untreated; and immunity may wane in previously infected individuals who become immunocompromised, causing PDH after reinfection.[25,32]

CLINICAL
Acute Pulmonary Histoplasmosis

After inhalation of *Histoplasma* microconidia, a majority (90%) of patients develop subclinical, self-limited, and most often unrecognized disease (**Table 1**). Symptoms are more likely to manifest after high-inoculum exposures, in immunocompromised patients, in those at the extremes of age, and possibly with more intrinsically virulent strains.[34,35] The overt acute pulmonary syndrome occurs after a median incubation period of 14 days and is characterized by fever, chills, dyspnea, and cough. Although not a pathognomonic feature, substernal chest pain can result from enlarged mediastinal or hilar lymph nodes compressing on nearby structures. A minority of patients (6%) may exhibit rheumatologic (arthralgias, arthritis, and erythema nodosum) manifestations.[36] The illness is not readily distinguishable from other more common causes of community-acquired viral or bacterial pneumonia,[37] but nonresponse to antibiotics or antivirals is suggestive. Chest imaging typically demonstrates diffuse bilateral patchy opacities with conspicuous hilar and mediastinal adenopathy (**Fig. 2**). The illness usually resolves within 1 to 2 weeks, but in severe cases, prolonged symptoms, acute respiratory distress syndrome (ARDS), or disseminated disease can ensue.

Subacute Pulmonary Histoplasmosis

In contrast to acute pulmonary histoplasmosis, the subacute form is characterized by a more attenuated and insidious course of several months' duration and is the result of a lower-inoculum exposure. Chest radiographs commonly reveal hilar and mediastinal adenopathy but airspace disease is more likely to be focal or patchy than diffuse (see **Fig. 2**).[38] Patients often receive multiple courses of antibiotics for presumed bacterial pneumonia without improvement.

Chronic Pulmonary Histoplasmosis

Chronic pulmonary histoplasmosis occurs classically in older male patients (>50 years) with lungs damaged by years of smoking.[39] Symptoms of productive cough, dyspnea, fever, chest pain, night sweats, and weight loss can persist but typically recur in bouts of exacerbation, accompanied by radiographic worsening. Chest radiographs first show patchy infiltrates, most often in the upper lobes that consolidate and eventually progress to areas resembling cavitation representing inflammation surrounding preexisting bullae (see **Fig. 2**). Over time, inflammation spreads to surrounding tissues, leading to fibrosis, volume loss with compensatory enlargement of cavities, and pleural thickening. As opposed to the acute and subacute forms, hilar and mediastinal lymph nodes do not enlarge but are often calcified. In many ways, the syndrome closely resembles pulmonary tuberculosis. A form of chronic noncavitary pulmonary histoplasmosis has been described in which patients were more likely to have nontraditional risk factors (no underlying lung disease, nonsmokers, and female) and negative cultures.[40]

Pulmonary Nodules

In endemic areas, pulmonary nodules are frequently noted on imaging performed for other purposes. Although incidentally found, biopsies are often sought to rule out

Table 1
Key features of pulmonary histoplasmosis

Risk Factors	Symptoms	Symptom Duration	Chest Imaging	Hilar and Mediastinal Lymph Nodes	Mimicked Disease		Treatment Indicated?	Antifungal	Treatment Duration
High-inoculum exposure <2 y or >50 y old Immunocompromised Virulent strain	Fever, chills, dyspnea, cough, chest pain, arthritis, arthralgia, erythema nodosum	1–2 wk	Diffuse bilateral patchy opacities	Enlarged	Community-acquired viral or bacterial pneumonia	Acute pulmonary histoplasmosis	Mild – no Moderate – yes Severe – yes	X Itraconazole AMB for 1–2 wk followed by itraconazole	X 12 wk 12 wk (total)
Same as acute except for low-inoculum exposure	Same as acute but symptoms are milder	Weeks to months	Focal or patchy opacities	Enlarged	Community-acquired bacterial pneumonia	Subacute pulmonary histoplasmosis	<1 mo – no ≥1 mo – yes	X Itraconazole	X 6–12 wk
Male >50 y old Structural lung disease Smoking	Fever, dyspnea, cough, chest pain, night sweats, and weight loss	Months to years	Cavitation, fibrosis, volume loss, pleural thickening Upper lobes most commonly affected	Not enlarged Calcified	Pulmonary tuberculosis	Chronic pulmonary histoplasmosis	Yes	Itraconazole	12–24 mo and until there is no further radiographic improvement

AMB, amphotericin B; X, non-.

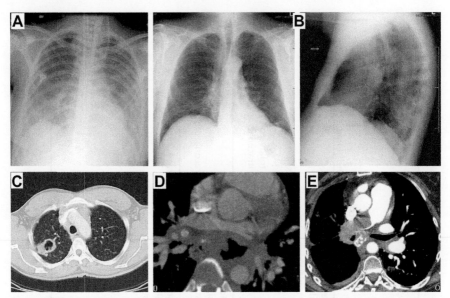

Fig. 2. Representative radiographs of various manifestations of histoplasmosis. (*A*) Acute pulmonary histoplasmosis with bilateral lower lobe airspace disease, hilar adenopathy, and hypoxic respiratory failure after a large inoculum exposure at a construction site in an otherwise healthy middle-aged man. (*B*) Subacute pulmonary histoplasmosis presenting as persistent community-acquired pneumonia despite standard antibiotic treatment. Chest radiograph showing right lower lobe infiltrates and right hilar adenopathy. (*C*) Chronic pulmonary histoplasmosis presenting with productive cough, low-grade fever, weight loss, and night sweats in an older man with emphysema. CT chest showing right upper lobe thick walled cavity with surrounding airspace disease. Sputum culture grew *H capsulatum*. (*D*) MG presenting with chronic cough and chest pain. No airspace disease but bulky mediastinal lymphadenopathy. (*E*) FM, CT scan showing mediastinal soft tissue density with extrinsic compression of the pulmonary artery and calcified mediastinal adenopathy in a patient with worsening dyspnea and intermittent chest pain (**Table 2**). FM, fibrosing mediastinitis; GM, granulomatous mediastinitis.

malignancy. Pathology reveals necrotizing or non-necrotizing granulomas and organisms are usually seen on stains but cultures are usually negative. The nodules represent healed or sequestered infection and may persist indefinitely, calcify, or cavitate. Rarely, nodules can gradually enlarge and appear mass-like, forming a histoplasmoma.

Mediastinal Lymphadenopathy (or Mediastinal Adenitis)

Enlarged mediastinal lymph nodes commonly accompany pulmonary infiltrates in the setting of acute and subacute pulmonary histoplasmosis. The inflamed nodes may compress nearby anatomic structures, characteristically leading to chest pain from mediastinal distention, chronic cough or atelectasis from bronchial impingement, dysphagia from esophageal compression or venous congestion from superior vena cava obstruction.[41] Due to smaller and more pliable airways, children are higher risk of airway compression. Moreover, mediastinal adenitis tends to affect younger populations (age <20 years). A majority of patients with mediastinal lymphadenopathy, however, are asymptomatic, the findings being reflective of previous unrecognized disease and discovered incidentally on chest imaging for other purposes. PET scans do not readily distinguish neoplastic versus histoplasmosis-derived mediastinal lymphadenopathy.[42] Biopsies often ensue to rule out malignancy, with pathology showing

Table 2
Key features of mediastinal histoplasmosis

	Timing	Compressive Symptoms Incidence	Compressive Symptoms Severity	CT Chest	Granulomas	Necrosis	Fistula	Calcifications	Treatment Indicated?	Treatment
Mediastinal adenitis	Early complication	Most often, not present	Mild Rarely moderate to severe	Homogenous mediastinal mass	Yes	No	No	No	If compressive symptoms present or if patient is immune suppressed	Steroid taper and itraconazole for 6–12 wk
MG	Early or late complication	Most often, not present	Mild Rarely moderate to severe	Heterogeneous mediastinal mass	Yes	Yes	Yes	No if early Yes if late	If compressive symptoms or fistula present	Partial resection, necrosis débridement and/or fistula repair and itraconazole for 6–12 wk
MF	Late complication	Always present	Moderate to severe	Homogenous mediastinal mass obstructing surrounding structures	May or may not be present	No	No	Yes	If compressive symptoms present	Bronchial artery Embolization, vascular stents Surgery (high mortality) No antifungals

granulomas with or without calcification, but a positive histoplasmosis serum or urine antigen or serum antibody may obviate invasive sampling. CT scans are helpful to distinguish mediastinal adenitis—homogenous density of a solid lymph node—from mediastinal granuloma (MG)—heterogenous density of necrotic lymph node (see **Fig. 2**).

Mediastinal Granuloma

An MG is an amalgamated mass of necrotic mediastinal lymph nodes encased in a thin fibrotic capsule, often paratracheal or subcarinal in location, which can be up to 10 cm in size (see **Fig. 2**).[43] As with mediastinal adenitis, MG is often asymptomatic but may also compress surrounding tissues, leading to symptoms specific to the impinged structure. Additionally, fistulae can burrow from necrotic lymph nodes into the nearby airways, esophagus, or surgical tracts if mediastinoscopy was performed.[44] All or part of the necrotic contents may then empty into the recipient organ. Flares of MG manifested by fever, constitutional symptoms, and chest pain may occur as a result of new fistulization, further enlargement of the granuloma, or superinfection of the necrotic tissues.[45] On CT scans, the necrotic contents of MG appear heterogenous but biopsies may be needed to differentiate MG from other necrotizing granulomatous disorders. There is no evidence to suggest that MG evolves into mediastinal fibrosis (MF), as previously thought.

Mediastinal Fibrosis (or Fibrosing Mediastinitis)

MF is a rare and sometimes devastating complication in which an abnormal and exuberant fibrotic response to past infection occurs. This leads to encasement of mediastinal structures and impingement of the esophagus, airways, and great vessels, including the pulmonary artery and superior vena cava.[46] The ensuing symptoms and signs are the result of obstruction of the aforementioned structures; recurrent hemoptysis is the most common symptom whereas airway and vascular occlusion are the most dreaded complications.[47] The underlying mechanism has not been elucidated, but an aberrant inflammatory response to residual *H capsulatum* antigens within mediastinal tissues has been postulated. Chest radiographs may show a widened mediastinum but are often normal. CT scans characteristically reveal an infiltrative mediastinal mass encasing or encroaching on surrounding structures, intermixed with calcified lymph nodes (see **Fig. 2**).[48] Antibodies to *H capsulatum* are often present and indicate past infection but antigen testing is usually negative. The diagnostic feature of MF is evidence of obstruction of mediastinal structures on imaging in the presence of dense calcification. Histopathologic evidence of fibrosis is not specific enough to be diagnostic; therefore, a tissue diagnosis is not warranted and procedures to obtain tissues may cause serious complications involving vascular or airway structures trapped in the fibrotic tissue. Moreover, although yeast forms may sometimes be seen in tissues, cultures tend to be negative. In contrast to MG, which may be an early or late complication, MF always develops many years after the initial infection.

Histoplasmoma

Rarely, patients may develop a slowly enlarging pulmonary nodule, which has been called an enlarging histoplasmoma,[49] causing concern about neoplasia. Lesions range in diameter from 8 mm to 35 mm and enlarge slowly (2 mm/y). Histologically, they are characterized by a necrotic center surrounded by a fibrous-like capsule. Organisms may be seen in the necrotic center but usually cannot be isolated in culture.

Broncholithiasis

As mediastinal nodes calcify, they may erode into adjacent bronchi causing broncholithiasis.[50] Patients may experience recurrent hemoptysis and expectorate small gravel-like particles of tissue. Bronchial obstruction or tracheoesophageal fistula may also complicate broncholithiasis.

Presumed Ocular Histoplasmosis

A finding of presumed ocular histoplasmosis is usually diagnosed in individuals residing in endemic areas with retinal lesions that have been attributed to histoplasmosis. Evidence that histoplasmosis causes this syndrome is weak,[51] however, and antifungal therapy does not affect the clinical course and outcome. The eye also may be rarely involved in patients with disseminated histoplasmosis (Specht and colleagues, 1991).

Disseminated Histoplasmosis

Hematogenous spread outside the lungs occurs during the acute infection but is rarely recognized clinically.[52] These patients recover with the development of cellular immunity to *H capsulatum*,[52] and patients who are unable to control the dissemination are at an increased risk for developing PDH. This occurs in approximately 1 in 2000 acute infections,[17] with a 10-fold higher risk in patients who are immunosuppressed or at the extremes of age (younger children and older adults).[53] If no cause for immune dysfunction is readily apparent, investigations should be undertaken to look for less apparent causes of immunocompromise,[54,55] such as CD4 lymphopenia,[56] common variable immunodeficiency,[54] hyper-IgE (Job) syndrome,[57] and defects in the interleukin 12 or interferon gamma pathways.[58] Work identifying other causes of immunocompromise is ongoing.

Common clinical manifestations include fever, fatigue, malaise, anorexia, weight loss, and respiratory symptoms.[52] Physical examination frequently reveals lymphadenopathy, hepatomegaly, and/or splenomegaly, with skin and oral lesions less common.[59] Skin lesions seem more common in cases in Latin America.[60] Laboratory tests usually show anemia, leukopenia, thrombocytopenia, and elevated hepatic enzymes and bilirubin[52]; elevated lactate dehydrogenase[61] and ferritin[62] are nonspecific but suggestive of PDH. Shock with hepatic, renal, and respiratory failure (including ARDS) and coagulopathy may complicate severe cases and may be mistaken for bacterial sepsis.[63] Most common sites of involvement are liver, spleen, gastrointestinal tract, and bone marrow.[13] Dissemination can also be seen in skin, adrenal glands, central nervous system, and endocardium.[64] Adrenal insufficiency and reactive hemophagocytic syndrome can complicate the course.[65–67] Meningitis, cerebritis, and focal brain or spinal cord lesions occur in 5% to 10% of cases, as either manifestations of widely disseminated infection or isolated findings.[68] Pulmonary imaging is characterized by diffuse reticulonodular, interstitial, or miliary infiltrates but may be unrevealing in 10% to 50% of the cases.[69]

DIAGNOSIS
Pathology

Rapid identification of *H capsulatum* var. *capsulatum* is facilitated by visualization of ovoid yeast cells measuring 2 μm to 4 μm in greatest dimension in tissue and/or body fluid specimens. The average size of *H capsulatum* var. *duboisii* (range, approximately 6–12 μm or greater), however, is often much larger than that of *H capsulatum* var. *capsulatum*, so presumptive identification should not rely solely on microscopic morphology. Budding yeast is connected at a narrow base, which helps distinguish

H capsulatum from other microorganisms, including smaller forms of *Blastomyces dermatitidis*. Most often, *H capsulatum* yeast is localized within mononuclear phagocytic cells, such as macrophages and monocytes; however, in many preparations, extracellular yeast can also be observed. Additional attributes that are helpful for rendering a presumptive identification in stained microscopic preparations are its tinctorial properties and the presence of a pseudocapsule. **Fig. 3** shows the microscopic appearance of *H capsulatum* var. *capsulatum* stained by 8 different methods. Romanowsky-type stains, including Diff-Quik (Baxter [Siemens Healthcare, Malvern, PA]), Giemsa, and Wright-Giemsa stains (see **Fig. 3**A, B, and H), impart a dark blue hue to the fungal nuclear compartment. A thin blue rim of stained yeast sacculus and a zone of pallor near a cell pole are also readily observable. Special stains, such as the Grocott-Gömöri methenamine–silver (GMS), mucicarmine, and periodic acid–Schiff (PAS) stains (see **Fig. 3**C, F, and G), can provide contrast to yeast cells, in cases of GMS and PAS stains, but may obscure the observation of *H capsulatum* in the case of mucin stains, such as mucicarmine. In the latter method, however, this observations facilitates the discrimination of *H capsulatum* from encapsulated varieties of *Cryptococcus neoformans* and *C gattii*, which both stain red. The Gram stain can also provide useful insight into the identification of yeast within clinical specimens, including blood cultures that grow yeast forms of consistent size, shape, and budding characteristics as *H capsulatum*. In properly stained specimens, *H capsulatum* stains red or fuchsia, depending on the counterstain used.

The highest yield may be achieved in respiratory specimens or bone marrow biopsy in patients with PDH.[70] Less commonly, organisms may be seen in respiratory specimens, mediastinal lymph nodes, or lung tissue from patients with pulmonary histoplasmosis. Demonstration of organisms in mediastinal lymph nodes or lung tissue does not, however, distinguish active from healed histoplasmosis, because nonviable

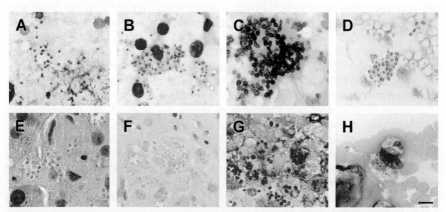

Fig. 3. Tinctorial and morphologic attributes of *H capsulatum* in stained clinical specimens. (*A*) Diff-Quik: BAL fluid smear showing extracellular yeast forms. (*B*) Giemsa stain: tissue touch preparation demonstrating numerous yeast within a histiocyte and in the surrounding space. (*C*) GMS stain: abundant black-colored yeast cells in a tissue touch preparation. Both extracellular and intrahistiocytic forms are seen. (*D*) Gram stain: red-colored yeast cells in a blood culture smear. (*E*) Hematoxylin-eosin stain: liver biopsy containing numerous intracellular and extracellular yeast forms. Note the presence of colorless halos surrounding yeast. (*F*) Mucicarmine stain: yeast forms are barely visible without the aid of increased contrast. (*G*) PAS stain: magenta-colored yeast are evident scattered throughout the epidermis of a skin biopsy specimen. (*H*) Wright-Giemsa: yeast forms evident within a monocyte in a peripheral blood smear. Scale bar, 10 μm; original magnification, ×1000.

organisms persist in these tissues indefinitely. It is not uncommon to observe nonviable *H capsulatum* within old granulomas, a finding that can sometimes confound an inexperienced pathologist when the clinical history is inconsistent with histoplasmosis. In immunocompetent individuals, *H capsulatum* infection elicits granuloma formation in which yeast is often present within histiocytes. Granulomas eventually under caseation and the presence of cavitary lesions are also observable. Lesions associated with *H capsulatum* infection resemble those of other infectious diseases, especially tuberculosis and sarcoidosis. In cases of disseminated histoplasmosis in immunocompromised hosts, yeast forms are often found within histiocytes scattered throughout infected organs rather than in granulomas.

Other fungi and microorganisms may be mistaken for *H capsulatum*. Fungi, including *Candida glabrata*, *B dermatitidis*, capsule-deficient strains of *C neoformans* and *C gattii*, *Talaromyces marneffei*, and *Pneumocystis jirovecii* and the protozoa *Leishmania* spp, *Toxoplasma gondii*, and *Trypanosoma cruzi* are common examples. Mucicarmine staining for capsular material may be used to distinguish pathogenic cryptococci from *H capsulatum*, but capsule-deficient strains may be misidentified by this technique. Fungal stains, such as GMS and PAS, can be used to distinguish protozoa. **Table 3** shows examples and contrasts morphologic features, respectively, of microorganisms that are often confused with *H capsulatum*. Furthermore, *H capsulatum* yeast forms may be present in small numbers and are occasionally overlooked by a pathologist experienced with morphologic identification of *H capsulatum*.

Culture

Cultures are most useful in patients with disseminated or chronic pulmonary histoplasmosis, positive in 50% to 85% of cases. In disseminated disease, the highest culture yield is from bone marrow or blood, positive in more than 75% of cases.[70] Organisms can be isolated from sputum or bronchoscopy specimens from 75% of patients with chronic pulmonary histoplasmosis.[70] Up to 4 weeks is required to isolate the organism in culture. The mold form of *H capsulatum* usually grows as a white or buff and suede-like or cottony mycelium. Microscopic examination of mold growth reveals characteristic large, rounded tuberculate macroconidia originating from short, hyaline conidiophores. *Sepedonium* spp produce similar-appearing conidia, so definitive identification should not be based on microscopic analysis alone (see **Table 3**). The highly infectious microconidia may or may not be observable, however. For definitive identification, DNA probes are commonly used, but nucleic acid sequencing and other laboratory-developed molecular methods can be used. Mold cultures of *H capsulatum* should always be manipulated in a certified biological safety cabinet by trained technologists, and manipulations other than presumptive identification should be conducted in a biosafety level-3 laboratory by employees wearing respiratory protection and appropriate personal protective equipment.

Antigen Testing

A galactomannan antigen may be detected in the body fluids in patients with histoplasmosis, offering another method for rapid diagnosis. The highest yield for antigen detection occurs in patients with PDH or APH, in whom antigen may be detected in 80% to 95% of cases. Less often, antigen may be detected in patients with subacute or chronic pulmonary histoplasmosis.[70] The highest yield for antigen detection is achieved by testing both urine and serum. For example, in APH, antigen was detected in 83% of patients by testing both urine and serum, of which more than

Table 3							
Attributes of *Histoplasma capsulatum* and microorganisms commonly confused for *Histoplasma capsulatum*							
Organism	Size (μm)	Shape	Attachment of Buds	Cell Wall Thickness	Grocott-Gömöri Methenamine–Silver	Periodic Acid–Schiff	Mucin
H capsulatum var. capsulatum	2–4	Globose or ovoid	Narrow base	Thin	Positive	Positive	Negative
H capsulatum var. duboisii	~6–12 or larger	Ovoid	Narrow base	Thick, refractile	Positive	Positive	Negative
B dermatitidis	5–15 or larger	Globose	Broad base	Thick	Positive	Positive	Negative
C glabrata	2–5	Ovoid	Narrow base	Thin	Positive	Positive	Positive
C neoformans and C gattii	3–8	Globose or ovoid	Narrow base	Thin	Positive	Positive	Positive[a]
Leishmania spp (amastigotes)	<4	Ovoid	N/A	N/A	Negative	Negative	Negative
P jirovecii (cyst forms)	5–8	Rounded, irregular	N/A	Thin	Positive	Positive	Negative
T gondii (bradyzoites)	<4	Ovoid	N/A	N/A	Negative	Negative	Negative
Trypanosoma cruzi (asmastigotes)	<4	Ovoid	N/A	N/A	Negative	Negative	Negative

[a] Unencapsulated variants stains negative.

a third were positive only in serum.[71] Antigen may be found in the CSF of 75% of patients with meningitis caused by histoplasmosis (anecdotal experience of the authors) and BAL fluid in 90% of patients with chronic pulmonary histoplasmosis or diffuse pulmonary histoplasmosis, complicating PDH.[72] Cross-reactions occur most often in patients with blastomycosis, penicilliosis marneffei, and paracoccidioidomycosis[70]; in 10% of patients with coccidioidomycosis[73,74]; and rarely in aspergillosis.[72,75]

Antibody Testing

The immunodiffusion (ID), complement fixation (CF), and enzyme immunoassay are commonly used for detection of antibodies for diagnosis of histoplasmosis. H and/ or M precipitin bands are demonstrated by the ID test. H precipitins, present in less than 25% of patients, usually clear within the first 6 months after infection.[76,77] M precipitins are present in 75% individuals and may persist for several years. CF titers of 1:8 or higher are found in most patients with histoplasmosis, whereas titers of 1:32 or higher are more suggestive of active infection. CF titers may persist for several years after acute infection. Both the ID and CF should be performed to obtain the highest sensitivity for diagnosis. Cross-reactions occur in some patients with blastomycosis or coccidioidomycosis.

Many physicians are unfamiliar with use these tests, believing them positive in a majority of patients from endemic areas for histoplasmosis. Positivity rates in healthy individuals who reside in highly endemic areas are low. M precipitins were present in healthy subjects in 0.5% by ID, 5% by CF, at titers of 1:8 or 1:16, and 10% by enzyme immunoassay.[76,77]

Antibodies require 4 to 8 weeks to develop after acute infection[77] and may be negative when a patient is first seen but positive when repeated 1 to 2 months later. Antibodies also may be negative in immunocompromised patients, especially those who have undergone solid organ transplantation.[8,70]

Molecular

Although publications suggest that polymerase chain reaction (PCR) is useful for diagnosis of histoplasmosis,[78–80] and assays are commercially available,[81] their role is uncertain. The assay reported by authors at the Mayo Clinic was positive in only 2 of 6 culture positive bronchoalveolar lavage (BAL) specimens.[81] In another study, fewer than 10% of antigen-positive urine specimens were PCR positive, and those were from patients with positive urine cultures.[82] PCR also was negative in serum (n = 10) and cerebrospinal fluid (CSF) (n = 10) and positive in 2 of 9 (22%) antigen-positive BAL specimens.[83]

TREATMENT

Histoplasmosis resolves without treatment in most healthy individuals, in whom treatment is usually not recommended. The main exception is healthy individuals with recent exposure to a site contaminated with the organism, in whom early treatment is usually recommended to shorten the duration of illness and prevent the rare occurrence of PDH. In contrast, histoplasmosis is progressive in most immunocompromised patients, in whom PDH is highly likely and treatment is always recommended. Rare exceptions occur in immunocompromised patients in whom immunosuppression is reduced or eliminated before the diagnosis of histoplasmosis is established, in which spontaneous recovery may occur.[17,84,85]

Manifestations That Are Usually or Always Treated

Acute pulmonary histoplasmosis (usually treated)

In patients with mild acute pulmonary histoplasmosis, treatment is not warranted, because the illness is self-limited.[86] On the other hand, patients with moderate to severe disease, diffuse bilateral infiltrates on chest imaging, or immunosuppression usually require treatment. Amphotericin B, preferably a lipid formulation, is the drug of choice for hospitalized patients and those with respiratory distress or disseminated disease. It should be administered for 1 to 2 weeks followed by itraconazole for a total of at least 12 weeks.[87] In the setting of respiratory compromise, there is some clinical experience to suggest that systemic corticosteroids may alleviate the hypoxemia by reducing parenchymal inflammation.[88] In milder cases, itraconazole alone for 12 weeks can suffice.

Chronic pulmonary histoplasmosis (always treated)

In the setting of chronic pulmonary histoplasmosis, antifungal therapy has been shown to induce clinical and radiographic remission, lead to fungal clearance from sputum cultures, and improve survival.[89–91] Patients should be treated with itraconazole for 12 to 24 months but also as long as there is continued radiologic improvement on serial chest imaging (CT or chest radiograph) done at 4-month to 6-month intervals. To ensure adequate itraconazole serum concentration, drug levels should be checked after 2 weeks of therapy and subsequently as needed in follow-up of dosage change, initiation of other medications that may affect itraconazole metabolism, or suspected adverse drug effects. Patients should be monitored for 1 year after discontinuation of therapy because of high rates of relapses (approximately 15%).[92] These patients also are at high risk for lung cancer, which should be considered if new lesions appear during or after therapy.

Progressive disseminated histoplasmosis (always treated)

Disseminated histoplasmosis is usually fatal if untreated[90] and treatment is recommended in all cases.[87] Treatments should focus on 2 objectives: administration of effective antifungal therapy and reversal or improvement of the underlying immunodeficiency. Immunocompromised patients without concrete evidence of dissemination should be treated as if they have PDH with at least 12 months of itraconazole, and they may need to be treated lifelong if immunosuppression cannot be reduced.[87]

Liposomal amphotericin B, given for 1 to 2 weeks followed by itraconazole for 1 year is recommended in hospitalized patients.[87,93,94] Liposomal amphotericin B is preferred to deoxycholate due to improved response (88% vs 64%) and a trend toward improved mortality (2% vs 13%).[95] Itraconazole alone administered for at least a year is effective in milder cases. Alternatives agents with activity against histoplasma that can be used for salvage therapy include fluconazole,[87,96] voriconazole,[97] posaconazole,[98] and isavuconazole.[99] Fluconazole is known to have higher treatment failures than itraconazole,[96] and increased minimum inhibitory concentrations to voriconazole have been observed, which was not true of posaconazole.[100] Furthermore, isavuconazole is structurally more similar to fluconazole and voriconazole than it is to posaconazole and itraconazole, and the experience with its use in histoplasmosis is limited. Therefore, posaconazole has emerged as the preferred alternative therapy.[93]

Treatment should be continued for at least 12 months and until antigenemia and antigenuria have resolved.[87] During the treatment period, therapeutic drug monitoring should be used to overcome absorption difficulties encountered with itraconazole. Lifelong maintenance treatment may be needed in immunocompromised patients who do not achieve a reduction in immunosuppression. Antigen levels should be checked in the blood and urine at the time of diagnosis and at 2 weeks, 1 month, and every 3 to 4 months afterward, up to 6 months after therapy is discontinued.[87,93] Any increase in antigens or clinical worsening during or after treatment should be investigated by evaluating drug levels, adherence, and immune status. Clinical worsening during therapy may represent treatment failure, immune reconstitution inflammatory syndrome (IRIS),[7,8,84] or an unrelated condition. Evidence that IRIS is the cause for clinical worsening includes adherence to therapy, adequate triazole blood levels, declining antigenuria and/or antigenemia, negative cultures despite demonstration of yeast in the tissues, failure to improve after intensification or change of antifungal therapy, and improvement after immunosuppressive therapy for IRIS.

The response to therapy in patients with meningitis is inferior to that in other types of histoplasmosis: 20% to 40% of patients with meningitis die and up to half of responders relapse after therapy is stopped.[87] Accordingly, liposomal amphotericin B for 4 to 6 weeks followed by itraconazole for at least 1 year and until CSF abnormalities, including antigen concentration, have resolved is recommended.[87] Lifelong therapy may be needed in patients who relapse or in those whose CSF findings do not return to normal. Although itraconazole fails to achieve detectable levels in CSF whereas fluconazole achieves excellent levels in CSF, fluconazole is less active against *Histoplasma* than itraconazole and was less effective in treating experimental *Histoplasma* meningitis.[101] The role of voriconazole and posaconazole for treatment of *Histoplasma* meningitis remains unknown.

Finally, immunosuppression should be reduced. This includes treatment with antiretroviral medications in patients with HIV, decreased dose of glucocorticoids, discontinuation of tumor necrosis factor inhibitors, and decrease in antirejection medications in transplant patients. Furthermore, interferon gamma may prove a useful adjunct therapy in patients with defects in the interferon gamma interleukin 12 pathway.[102,103]

Manifestations That Usually Are Not Treated

Subacute pulmonary histoplasmosis
As with acute pulmonary histoplasmosis, the subacute form is usually self-limited and does not require therapy. If the illness persists for more than 1 month, experts recommend initiating treatment with itraconazole, for a total of 6 to 12 weeks, with the intent of hastening recovery and preventing development of PDH, for which evidence is lacking.[87]

Pulmonary nodules
Exclusion of malignancy is the most important aspect in management. Patients in whom pulmonary nodules caused by histoplasmosis are diagnosed incidentally do not warrant treatment. Nodules may appear concomitantly with diffuse or localized infiltrates in acute and subacute pulmonary histoplasmosis, in which case antifungal therapy is appropriate.

Mediastinal lymphadenopathy (or mediastinal adenitis)
Asymptomatic mediastinal lymphadenopathy should not be treated. Most cases of symptomatic disease are self-limited but in patients with symptoms of airway or esophageal compression, a course of steroids may induce regression of lymph nodes and relieve symptoms. Antifungal therapy with itraconazole is indicated for patients receiving steroids, due to their ensuing immunosuppression and if symptoms do not improve after 1 month of observation, with the intent of reducing the risk of progressive disseminated disease.

Mediastinal granuloma

In symptomatic patients, surgery for resection of overhanging portions, fistula repair, and evacuation of necrotic contents may be helpful. Because fungal organisms are often present within the nodes, itraconazole for 6 to 12 weeks can be administered in conjunction with surgeries, although there is no evidence that antifungal therapy alters the course in patients with MG. In some instances, the MG silently discharges the totality of its contents into the esophagus or and airway and resolves. Treatment of asymptomatic MG is not indicated.[87]

Mediastinal fibrosis

Antifungal treatment of MF is not recommended because the underlying pathogenesis is likely an exaggerated immune response rather than progressive infection. In a majority of reports, there was no benefit to extended antifungal therapy[46,47,104] but therapies targeting the immune system, such as rituximab, may have a role and deserve further study.[105] Interventions should be targeted at the specific complications of MF, including vascular or airway stenting for obstructions and bronchial artery embolization for recurrent or severe hemoptysis.[106] Due to distorted tissue planes and a concentration of collateral vessels in the fibrosed mediastinum, surgery is high risk (mortality >20%) and should be reserved for patients with severe manifestations.[107]

Presumed ocular histoplasmosis

There is no solid evidence that presumed ocular histoplasmosis is caused by *H capsulatum*.[51] The diagnostic tests for histoplasmosis are negative in such patients. Furthermore, treatment of histoplasmosis does not alter the outcome in patients with this condition.

REFERENCES

1. Chu JH, Feudtner C, Heydon K, et al. Hospitalizations for endemic mycoses: a population-based national study. Clin Infect Dis 2006;42(6):822–5.
2. Hammerman KJ, Powell KE, Tosh FE. The incidence of hospitalized cases of systemic mycotic infections. Sabouraudia 1974;12:33–45.
3. Edwards LB, Acquaviva FA, Livesay VT, et al. An atlas of sensitivity to tuberculin, PPD-B and histoplasmin in the United States. Am Rev Respir Dis 1969;99:1–18.
4. Colombo AL, Tobon A, Restrepo A, et al. Epidemiology of endemic systemic fungal infections in Latin America. Med Mycol 2011;49(8):785–98.
5. Klugman HB, Lurie H. Systemic histoplasmosis in South Africa. A review of the previous cases and a report of an additional case–the first successfully treated. S Afr Med J 1963;37:29–31.
6. Nacher M, Adenis A, Mc DS, et al. Disseminated histoplasmosis in HIV-infected patients in South America: a neglected killer continues on its rampage. PLoS Negl Trop Dis 2013;7(11):e2319.
7. Vergidis P, Hage CA, Assi MA, et al. Histoplasmosis complicating tumor necrosis factor (TNF) blocker therapy. 49th Annual Meeting of the Infectious Diseases Society of America. Boston, October 20–23, 2011.
8. Assi M, Martin S, Wheat LJ, et al. Histoplasmosis after solid organ transplant. Clin Infect Dis 2013;57(11):1542–9.
9. Cottle LE, Gkrania-Klotsas E, Williams HJ, et al. A multinational outbreak of histoplasmosis following a biology field trip in the ugandan rainforest. J Travel Med 2013;20(2):83–7.

10. Medeiros AA, Marty SD, Tosh FE, et al. Erythema nodosum and erythema multiforme as clinical manifestations of histoplasmosis in a community outbreak. N Engl J Med 1966;274:415–20.
11. Leads from the MMWR. Cave-associated histoplasmosis–Costa Rica. JAMA 1988;259(24):3535–6.
12. Nett RJ, Skillman D, Riek L, et al. Histoplasmosis in idaho and montana, USA, 2012-2013. Emerg Infect Dis 2015;21(6):1071–2.
13. Assi MA, Sandid MS, Baddour LM, et al. Systemic histoplasmosis: a 15-year retrospective institutional review of 111 patients. Medicine (Baltimore) 2007; 86(3):162–9.
14. Jones PG, Cohen RL, Batts DH, et al. Disseminated histoplasmosis, invasive pulmonary aspergillosis, and other opportunistic infection in a homosexual patient with acquired immune deficiency syndrome. Sex Transm Dis 1983;10:202–4.
15. Kaur J, Myers AM. Homosexuality, steroid therapy, and histoplasmosis. Ann Intern Med 1983;99:567.
16. Pasternak J, Bolivar R. Bone marrow examination and culture in the diagnosis of acquired immunodeficiency syndrome (AIDS). Arch Intern Med 1983;143:1495.
17. Sathapatayavongs B, Batteiger BE, Wheat J, et al. Clinical and laboratory features of disseminated histoplasmosis during two large urban outbreaks. Medicine (Baltimore) 1983;62(5):263–70.
18. Bartholomew C, Raju C, Patrick A, et al. AIDS on Trinidad. Lancet 1984;1(8368):103.
19. Kohler RB, Wilde CI, Johnson W, et al. Immunologic diversity among serogroup 1 Legionella pneumophila urinary antigens demonstrated by monoclonal antibody enzyme-linked immunosorbent assays. J Clin Microbiol 1988;26:2059–63.
20. Arango M, Castaneda E, Agudelo CI, et al. Histoplasmosis: results of the Colombian national survey, 1992-2008. Biomedica 2011;31(3):344–56.
21. Pan B, Chen M, Pan W, et al. Histoplasmosis: a new endemic fungal infection in China? Review and analysis of cases. Mycoses 2013;56(3):212–21.
22. Norkaew T, Ohno H, Sriburee P, et al. Detection of environmental sources of histoplasma capsulatum in Chiang Mai, Thailand, by nested PCR. Myco 2013; 176(5–6):395–402.
23. Jung EJ, Park DW, Choi JW, et al. Chronic cavitary pulmonary histoplasmosis in a non-HIV and immunocompromised patient without overseas travel history. Yonsei Med J 2015;56(3):871–4.
24. Randhawa HS. Occurrence of histoplasmosis in Asia. Mycopathol Mycol Appl 1970;41(1):75–89.
25. Loulergue P, Bastides F, Baudouin V, et al. Literature review and case histories of Histoplasma capsulatum var. duboisii infections in HIV-infected patients. Emerg Infect Dis 2007;13(11):1647–52.
26. Gumbo T, Just-Nübling G, Robertson V, et al. Clinicopathological features of cutaneous histoplasmosis in human immunodeficiency virus-infected patients in Zimbabwe. Trans R Soc Trop Med Hyg 2001;95(6):635–6.
27. Lofgren SM, Kirsch EJ, Maro VP, et al. Histoplasmosis among hospitalized febrile patients in northern Tanzania. Trans R Soc Trop Med Hyg 2012;106(8): 504–7.
28. Inojosa W, Rossi MC, Laurino L, et al. Progressive disseminated histoplasmosis among human immunodeficiency virus-infected patients from West-Africa: report of four imported cases in Italy. Infez Med 2011;19(1):49–55.
29. Antinori S, Magni C, Nebuloni M, et al. Histoplasmosis among human immunodeficiency virus-infected people in Europe: report of 4 cases and review of the literature. Medicine (Baltimore) 2006;85(1):22–36.

30. Rodriguez-Tudela JL, Alastruey-Izquierdo A, Gago S, et al. Burden of serious fungal infections in Spain. Clin Microbiol Infect 2015;21(2):183–9.
31. Murphy RA, Gounder L, Manzini TC, et al. Challenges in the management of disseminated progressive histoplasmosis in human immunodeficiency virus-infected patients in resource-limited settings. Open Forum Infect Dis 2015; 2(1):ofv025.
32. Horwath MC, Fecher RA, Deepe GS Jr. Histoplasma capsulatum, lung infection and immunity. Future Microbiol 2015;10:967–75.
33. Knox KS, Hage CA. Histoplasmosis. Proc Am Thorac Soc 2010;7(3):169–72.
34. Medoff G, Maresca B, Lambowitz AM, et al. Correlation between pathogenicity and temperature sensitivity in different strains of Histoplasma capsulatum. J Clin Invest 1986;78(6):1638–47.
35. Sepulveda VE, Williams CL, Goldman WE. Comparison of phylogenetically distinct histoplasma strains reveals evolutionarily divergent virulence strategies. MBio 2014;5(4):e01376–14.
36. Rosenthal J, Brandt KD, Wheat LJ, et al. Rheumatologic manifestations of histo-plasmosis in the recent Indianapolis epidemic. Arthritis Rheum 1983;26(9): 1065–70.
37. Hage CA, Knox KS, Wheat LJ. Endemic mycoses: overlooked causes of com-munity acquired pneumonia. Respir Med 2012;106(6):769–76.
38. Wheat LJ. Histoplasmosis: a review for clinicians from non-endemic areas. Mycoses 2006;49(4):274–82.
39. Wheat LJ, Wass J, Norton J, et al. Cavitary histoplasmosis occurring during two large urban outbreaks. Analysis of clinical, epidemiologic, roentgenographic, and laboratory features. Medicine (Baltimore) 1984;63(4):201–9.
40. Kennedy CC, Limper AH. Redefining the clinical spectrum of chronic pulmonary histoplasmosis: a retrospective case series of 46 patients. Medicine (Baltimore) 2007;86(4):252–8.
41. Goodwin RA, Alcorn GL. Histoplasmosis with symptomatic lymphadenopathy. Chest 1980;77(2):213–5.
42. Croft DR, Trapp J, Kernstine K, et al. FDG-PET imaging and the diagnosis of non-small cell lung cancer in a region of high histoplasmosis prevalence. Lung Cancer 2002;36(3):297–301.
43. Schwarz J, Schaen MD, Picardi JL. Complications of the arrested primary histo-plasmic complex. JAMA 1976;236:1157–61.
44. Parish JM, Rosenow EC III. Mediastinal granuloma and mediastinal fibrosis. Semin Respir Crit Care Med 2002;23(2):135–43.
45. Scully RE, Mark EJ, McNeely WF, et al. Case records of the Massachusetts gen-eral hospital: Case 39-1991 presentation of case. N Engl J Med 1991;325: 949–56.
46. Goodwin RA, Nickell JA, des Prez RM. Mediastinal fibrosis complicating healed primary histoplasmosis and tuberculosis. Medicine (Baltimore) 1972;51(3):227–46.
47. Loyd JE, Tillman BF, Atkinson JB, et al. Mediastinal fibrosis complicating histo-plasmosis. Medicine (Baltimore) 1988;67(5):295–310.
48. Rossi SE, McAdams HP, Rosado-de-Christenson ML, et al. Fibrosing mediasti-nitis. Radiographics 2001;21(3):737–57.
49. Goodwin RA Jr, Snell JD Jr. The enlarging histoplasmoma. Concept of a tumor-like phenomenon encompassing the tuberculoma and coccidioidoma. Am Rev Respir Dis 1969;100(1):1–12.
50. Arrigoni MG, Bernatz PE, Donoghue FE. Broncholithiasis. J Thorac Cardiovasc Surg 1971;62:231–7.

51. Ciulla TA, Piper HC, Xiao M, et al. Presumed ocular histoplasmosis syndrome: update on epidemiology, pathogenesis, and photodynamic, antiangiogenic, and surgical therapies. Curr Opin Ophthalmol 2001;12(6):442–9.
52. Kauffman CA. Histoplasmosis: a clinical and laboratory update. Clin Microbiol Rev 2007;20(1):115–32.
53. Wheat LJ, Slama TG, Norton JA, et al. Risk factors for disseminated or fatal histoplasmosis. Analysis of a large urban outbreak. Ann Intern Med 1982;96(2):159–63.
54. Antachopoulos C, Walsh TJ, Roilides E. Fungal infections in primary immunodeficiencies. Eur J Pediatr 2007;166(11):1099–117.
55. Lionakis MS, Holland SM. Human invasive mycoses: immunogenetics on the rise. J Infect Dis 2015;211(8):1205–7.
56. Kortsik C, Elmer A, Tamm I. Pleural effusion due to *Histoplasma capsulatum* and idiopathic CD4 lymphocytopenia. Respiration 2003;70(1):118–22.
57. Alberti-Flor JJ, Granda A. Ileocecal histoplasmosis mimicking Crohn's disease in a patient with Job's syndrome. Digestion 1986;33(3):176–80.
58. Zerbe CS, Holland SM. Disseminated histoplasmosis in persons with interferon-gamma receptor 1 deficiency. Clin Infect Dis 2005;41(4):e38–41.
59. Goodwin RA Jr, Shapiro JL, Thurman GH, et al. Disseminated histoplasmosis: clinical and pathologic correlations. Medicine (Baltimore) 1980;59(1):1–33.
60. Karimi K, Wheat LJ, Connolly P, et al. Differences in histoplasmosis in patients with acquired immunodeficiency syndrome in the United States and Brazil. J Infect Dis 2002;186(11):1655–60.
61. Corcoran GR, Al-Abdely H, Flanders CD, et al. Markedly elevated serum lactate dehydrogenase levels are a clue to the diagnosis of disseminated histoplasmosis in patients with AIDS. Clin Infect Dis 1997;24(5):942–4.
62. Kirn DH, Fredericks D, McCutchan JA, et al. Serum ferritin levels correlate with disease activity in patients with AIDS and disseminated histoplasmosis. Clin Infect Dis 1995;21(4):1048–9.
63. Wheat LJ, Connolly-Stringfield PA, Baker RL, et al. Disseminated histoplasmosis in the acquired immune deficiency syndrome: clinical findings, diagnosis and treatment, and review of the literature. Medicine (Baltimore) 1990;69(6):361–74.
64. Riddell J, Kauffman CA, Smith JA, et al. Histoplasma capsulatum endocarditis: multicenter case series with review of current diagnostic techniques and treatment. Medicine (Baltimore) 2014;93(5):186–93.
65. Sarosi GA, Voth DW, Dahl BA, et al. Disseminated histoplasmosis: Results of long-term follow-up. Ann Intern Med 1971;75:511–6.
66. Tiab M, Mechinaud F, Harousseau JL. Haemophagocytic syndrome associated with infections. Baillieres Best Pract Res Clin Haematol 2000;13(2):163–78.
67. Rouphael NG, Talati NJ, Vaughan C, et al. Infections associated with haemophagocytic syndrome. Lancet Infect Dis 2007;7(12):814–22.
68. Wheat LJ, Batteiger BE, Sathapatayavongs B. Histoplasma capsulatum infections of the central nervous system. A clinical review. Medicine (Baltimore) 1990;69(4):244–60.
69. Conces DJ Jr, Stockberger SM, Tarver RD, et al. Disseminated histoplasmosis in AIDS: findings on chest radiographs. AJR Am J Roentgenol 1993;160(1):15–9.
70. Hage CA, Ribes JA, Wengenack NL, et al. A multicenter evaluation of tests for diagnosis of histoplasmosis. Clin Infect Dis 2011;53(5):448–54.
71. Swartzentruber S, Rhodes L, Kurkjian K, et al. Diagnosis of acute pulmonary histoplasmosis by antigen detection. Clin Infect Dis 2009;49(12):1878–82.

72. Hage CA, Davis TE, Fuller D, et al. Diagnosis of histoplasmosis by antigen detection in BAL fluid. Chest 2010;137(3):623–8.
73. Durkin M, Connolly P, Kuberski T, et al. Diagnosis of coccidioidomycosis with use of the coccidioides antigen enzyme immunoassay. Clin Infect Dis 2008;47(8):e69–73.
74. Durkin M, Estok L, Hospenthal D, et al. Detection of coccidioides antigenemia following dissociation of immune complexes. Clin Vaccine Immunol 2009;16(10): 1453–6.
75. Wheat LJ, Hackett E, Durkin M, et al. Histoplasmosis-associated cross-reactivity in the BioRad platelia aspergillus enzyme immunoassay. Clin Vaccine Immunol 2007;14(5):638–40.
76. Wheat J, French ML, Kohler RB, et al. The diagnostic laboratory tests for histo-plasmosis: analysis of experience in a large urban outbreak. Ann Intern Med 1982;97(5):680–5.
77. Wheat LJ. Histoplasmosis in Indianapolis. Clin Infect Dis 1992;14(Suppl 1):S91–9.
78. Bialek R, Cirera AC, Herrmann T, et al. Nested PCR assays for detection of Blas-tomyces dermatitidis DNA in paraffin-embedded canine tissue. J Clin Microbiol 2003;41(1):205–8.
79. Simon S, Veron V, Boukhari R, et al. Detection of Histoplasma capsulatum DNA in human samples by real-time polymerase chain reaction. Diagn Microbiol Infect Dis 2010;66(3):268–73.
80. Cordeiro RA, Brilhante RS, Rocha MF, et al. Twelve years of coccidioidomycosis in Ceara State, Northeast Brazil: epidemiologic and diagnostic aspects. Diagn Microbiol Infect Dis 2010;66(1):65–72.
81. Babady NE, Buckwalter SP, Hall L, et al. Detection of Blastomyces dermatitidis and Histoplasma capsulatum from Culture Isolates and Clinical Specimens by Use of Real-Time PCR. J Clin Microbiol 2011;49(9):3204–8.
82. Tang YW, Li H, Durkin MM, et al. Urine polymerase chain reaction is not as sen-sitive as urine antigen for the diagnosis of disseminated histoplasmosis. Diagn Microbiol Infect Dis 2006;54(4):283–7.
83. Wheat LJ. Improvements in diagnosis of histoplasmosis. Expert Opin Biol Ther 2006;6(11):1207–21.
84. Myint T, Anderson AM, Sanchez A, et al. Histoplasmosis in patients with human Immunodeficiency virus/acquired immunodeficiency syndrome (HIV/AIDS): multicenter study of outcomes and factors associated with relapse. Medicine (Baltimore) 2014;93(1):11–8.
85. Stewart A, Wheat LJ, Madura J. Occurrence of pulmonary histoplasmosis after jejunoileal bypass for obesity. Am Rev Respir Dis 1978;118(1):155.
86. Chamany S, Mirza SA, Fleming JW, et al. A large histoplasmosis outbreak among high school students in Indiana, 2001. Pediatr Infect Dis J 2004;23(10):909–14.
87. Wheat LJ, Freifeld AG, Kleiman MB, et al. Clinical practice guidelines for the management of patients with histoplasmosis: 2007 update by the Infectious Dis-eases Society of America. Clin Infect Dis 2007;45(7):807–25.
88. Wynne JW, Olsen GN. Acute histoplasmosis presenting as the adult respiratory distress syndrome. Chest 1974;66:158–61.
89. Dismukes WE, Bradsher RW Jr, Cloud GC, et al. Itraconazole therapy for blas-tomycosis and histoplasmosis. Am J Med 1992;93:489–97.
90. Furcolow ML. Comparison of treated and untreated severe histoplasmosis. JAMA 1963;183:121–7.
91. Putnam LR, Sutliff WD, Larkin JC, et al. Histoplasmosis cooperative study: Chronic pulmonary histoplasmosis treated with amphotericin B alone and with amphotericin B and triple sulfonamide. Am Rev Respir Dis 1968;97:96–102.

92. Baum GL, Larkin JC Jr, Sutliff WD. Follow-up of patients with chronic pulmonary histoplasmosis treated with amphotericin B. Chest 1970;58(6):562–5.
93. La Hoz RM, Loyd JE, Wheat LJ, et al. How I Treat Histoplasmosis. Curr Fungal Infect Rep 2014.
94. Carlos WG, Rose AS, Wheat LJ, et al. Blastomycosis in indiana: digging up more cases. Chest 2010;138(6):1377–82.
95. Johnson PC, Wheat LJ, Cloud GA, et al. Safety and efficacy of liposomal amphotericin B compared with conventional amphotericin B for induction therapy of histoplasmosis in patients with AIDS. Ann Intern Med 2002;137(2):105–9.
96. Wheat J, MaWhinney S, Hafner R, et al. Treatment of histoplasmosis with fluconazole in patients with acquired immunodeficiency syndrome. National Institute of Allergy and Infectious Diseases Acquired Immunodeficiency Syndrome Clinical Trials Group and Mycoses Study Group. Am J Med 1997;103(3):223–32.
97. Freifeld A, Proia L, Andes D, et al. Voriconazole use for endemic fungal infections. Antimicrob Agents Chemother 2009;53(4):1648–51.
98. Restrepo A, Tobon A, Clark B, et al. Salvage treatment of histoplasmosis with posaconazole. J Infect 2007;54(4):319–27.
99. Thompson GR III, Wiederhold NP. Isavuconazole: a comprehensive review of spectrum of activity of a new triazole. Myco 2010;170(5):291–313.
100. Wheat LJ, Connolly P, Smedema M, et al. Activity of newer triazoles against Histoplasma capsulatum from patients with AIDS who failed fluconazole. J Antimicrob Chemother 2006;57:1235–9.
101. Haynes RR, Connolly PA, Durkin MM, et al. Antifungal therapy for central nervous system histoplasmosis, using a newly developed intracranial model of infection. J Infect Dis 2002;185(12):1830–2.
102. Duplessis CA, Tilley D, Bavaro M, et al. Two cases illustrating successful adjunctive interferon-gamma immunotherapy in refractory disseminated coccidioidomycosis. J Infect 2011;63(3):223–8.
103. Vinh DC. Insights into human antifungal immunity from primary immunodeficiencies. Lancet Infect Dis 2011;11(10):780–92.
104. Davis A, Pierson D, Loyd JE. Mediastinal fibrosis. Semin Respir Infect 2001; 16(2):119–30.
105. Westerly BD, Johnson GB, Maldonado F, et al. Targeting B lymphocytes in progressive fibrosing mediastinitis. Am J Respir Crit Care Med 2014;190(9):1069–71.
106. Albers EL, Pugh ME, Hill KD, et al. Percutaneous vascular stent implantation as treatment for central vascular obstruction due to fibrosing mediastinitis. Circulation 2011;123(13):1391–9.
107. Mathisen DJ, Grillo HC. Clinical manifestations of mediastinal fibrosis and histoplasmosis. Ann Thorac Surg 1992;54:1053–8.

Coccidioidomycosis

Nathan W. Stockamp, MD[a], George R. Thompson III, MD[b,c],*

KEYWORDS

- Coccidioidomycosis • Coccidioides • Epidemiology • Treatment • Meningitis
- Primary infection

KEY POINTS

- The incidence and geographic range of coccidioidomycosis continues to expand.
- Coccidioidomycosis is responsible for up to 25% of all community-acquired pneumonia within the endemic region.
- Pulmonary nodules secondary to prior coccidioidal infection represent a significant problem within the endemic region and are not easily distinguishable from malignancy.
- Disseminated coccidioidal infection requires long courses of antifungal therapy increasing toxicity concerns.

INTRODUCTION

Coccidioidomycosis is a fungal disease caused by *Coccidioides immitis* and *C posadasii*. These dimorphic saprophytic fungi lay latent as a mycelial form in dry desert soil developing into arthroconidia. The organism seems to survive well in areas with lower amounts of rainfall (12–50 cm per year), few winter freezes, and alkaline soils. Initial human infection occurs primarily by inhalation of aerosolized spores and in rare cases through direct cutaneous inoculation.[1,2] The inoculum needed for infection can be quite small, even a few arthroconidia.[3] Following inhalation, arthroconidia undergo morphologic change and turn into spherules (large structures containing endospores).[4] This structure can rupture, leading to the spread of endospores hematogenously or through the lymphatics into virtually any organ, which in turn may develop into a new spherule. Human disease can range from asymptomatic to severe,

No conflicts of interest.

[a] Division of Infectious Disease, Department of Internal Medicine, University of California, San Francisco, Fresno, San Francisco, CA, USA; [b] Division of Infectious Diseases, Department of Internal Medicine, University of California, Davis, Davis, CA, USA; [c] Department of Medical Microbiology and Immunology, University of California, Davis, Davis, CA, USA
* Corresponding author. Division of Infectious Diseases, Department of Medicine, University of California, Davis, 4150 V Street, Suite G500, Sacramento, CA 95817.
E-mail address: grthompson@ucdavis.edu

Infect Dis Clin N Am 30 (2016) 229–246
http://dx.doi.org/10.1016/j.idc.2015.10.008
id.theclinics.com

disseminated disease, and death. Individual control of disease depends greatly on that host's immune response.

EPIDEMIOLOGY

The geographic range of *Coccidioides* has been derived from clinical cases, soil testing, and from skin testing performed in 1957 throughout the Southwestern United States.[5,6] The exact ecologic niche remains to be determined. Endemic areas where disease is prevalent include Arizona, California, New Mexico, Nevada, Utah, Washington, Texas, Mexico, and some areas in Guatemala, Honduras, Venezuela, Brazil, Argentina, and Paraguay.[7,8] In the United States, the annual incidence of coccidioidomycosis is variable but overall is increasing, from a rate of 5.3 per 100,000 in 1998 to a rate of 42.6 in 2011.[9] Of these cases reported to the Centers for Disease Control and Prevention, 66% were from Arizona and 31% from California. Despite the increased incidence, from an analysis of death certificates, the age-adjusted mortality rate from 1990 to 2008 has remained stable at approximately 0.59 per million person years.[10] There were 1451 coccidioidomycosis-related deaths in California compared with 1010 in Arizona despite its higher annual reported case rate.

The incidence of coccidioidomycosis in California and Arizona can vary greatly by geographic region and may be seasonal in pattern. In a yearly summary by the California Department of Health, the overall incidence of coccidioidal infection in the state increased from 4.3 to 11.6 per 100,000 population between 2001 and 2010.[11] In Kern County, however, the rate reported in 2011 was much higher, 241 per 100,000 population.[12] Similar increases have been observed in Arizona.[13,14] The reasons for the overall increase are not fully clear and have been attributed to changing environmental conditions, human activities in endemic areas, changing surveillance methods and definitions, increased numbers of immunosuppressed individuals, and even improved awareness and diagnostic testing rates.[15] In endemic regions, the people most affected are construction and farm workers, military personnel, archaeologists, excavators, inmates, and officers in correctional facilities.

Epidemics in endemic regions have occurred after dust storms, earthquakes, and earth excavation where dispersion of arthroconidia is facilitated.[2,13] In Washington State, 3 cases were recently reported, an area not previously considered endemic; follow-up soil testing showed the presence of *Coccidioides immitis*, suggesting the geographic range of this organism is larger than previously thought.[16,17] After coccidioidomycosis became a reportable condition, the case rate even in nonendemic regions (eg, recent report in Missouri) increased substantially; but many cases were among people who never previously traveled to an endemic region and were diagnosed serologically rather than by culture, polymerase chain reaction (PCR), or histopathologically.[18] Clinical cases of coccidioidomycosis in patients from nonendemic regions are often reported; but frequently a link is established, however brief the transit, to an endemic region.[19] There is even a case report of coccidioidomycosis in Hong Kong in a patient who is thought to have contracted the disease by sweeping shipping containers from the United States with no other link to the endemic region.[20]

DIAGNOSTIC TESTING

Currently, diagnosis can be established using immunologic assays, culture, or histopathology of tissues involved.[21] In mammalian tissues, coccidioidomycosis exists nearly exclusively as a characteristic spherule with endospores (**Fig. 1**). Spherules are approximately 60 to 100 μm in diameter and can contain hundreds of variable-sized daughter endospores, each capable of propagating infection. Rarely, hyphae

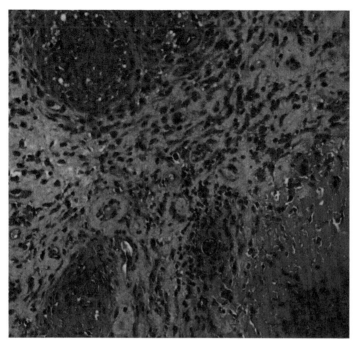

Fig. 1. *Coccidioides* spherules with associated granuloma obtained from a hip fluid collection (hematoxylin-eosin, magnification ×40).

and other atypical forms have been identified in tissues, such as lung cavities or bone.[22–25] In addition to histopathology, culture of the fungus isolated from a clinical specimen (ie, bronchoalveolar lavage, cerebrospinal fluid [CSF] culture, tissue culture) confirms the diagnosis.[21] Nucleic acid amplification is still being evaluated and developed for use in clinical diagnosis, with several centers using novel primers.[26–30] Its potential ability to effectively detect organism in culture-negative samples would be welcome but is as yet unproven. Skin testing to identify the presence of cellular immunity to *Coccidioides* species is also being redeveloped after a multi-decade absence; the reader is referred to the excellent review by Wack and colleagues.[31] Its use is anticipated in both clinical and epidemiologic scenarios and for screening of at-risk populations.

Currently, most clinical infections are diagnosed serologically in the setting of a compatible clinical syndrome. Immunodiffusion (ID) for the detection of immunoglobulin G–(IgG) and IgM-specific antibodies is a preferred test for detection of exposure to *C immitis*, with high specificity. Complement fixation (CF) tests for IgG-specific antibody are most useful in immunocompetent patients, both for diagnosis and long-term disease assessment.[32] The CF titer can be useful in monitoring disease activity and may revert to negative with long-term disease control. CF titers greater than 1:16 increase the possibility of disseminated disease. Very early in a patient's infection, serologic results may be negative. Most frequently performed on blood samples, serology may also be performed on CSF and other samples, such as joint or pleural fluid. Serologic assays are less reliable in immunocompromised patients with 20% to 50% of patients testing negative with these methods. In forms of disease with a more benign clinical course, such as patients with isolated pulmonary nodules confirmed by culture or histopathology, serologic testing may often be negative.

Other assays, such as latex agglutination and enzyme-linked immunosorbent assay, have been used in the endemic region as well, though with mixed results and often with a high false-positive rate.[33,34] *Coccidioides* galactomannan antigen testing and serum $(1 \rightarrow 3)$-β-D-glucan are available in some reference laboratories and undergoing further evaluation for their role in patient diagnosis or management.[35] Identification may also be possible through the use of commercially available ribosomal RNA probes.[36]

CLINICAL MANIFESTATIONS AND MANAGEMENT

Coccidioidomycosis is a highly variable illness. On inhalation of the spores, 60% of people may develop an asymptomatic infection or a mild respiratory illness and the rest will develop the disease in a variable manner.[37] Disseminated infection or progressive pulmonary infection occurs in 1% to 3% of people infected with *Coccidioides* spp. Dissemination is often an early clinical event; the most common extrapulmonary (EP) sites include skin, lymph nodes, bones, joints, and the most severe being the central nervous system.

Although coccidioidomycosis manifests primarily as a respiratory illness, in certain groups the chance of dissemination or development of a chronic infection remains high. Individuals with human immunodeficiency virus (HIV)/AIDS and recipients of immune-modulating drugs or immunosuppressive drugs or high-dose corticosteroids are at high risk for dissemination and chronic infection.[38] Diabetes mellitus is a significant risk factor for severe pulmonary infection as well as chronic structural lung disease or cardiopulmonary disease. Dissemination is more common in women in the third trimester of pregnancy or immediately post-partum.[39,40] There is also a several-fold higher relative risk of dissemination in individuals of African American and Filipino decent.[37] Accordingly, mortality rates are observed to be higher in persons greater than 65 years of age, men, Native Americans, and Hispanics as well as those with conditions such as vasculitis, rheumatoid arthritis, systemic lupus erythematosus, HIV infection, tuberculosis, diabetes mellitus, chronic obstructive pulmonary disease, and non-Hodgkin lymphoma.[10] Treatment and/or monitoring of such groups should be approached carefully and with diligence.

Management entails careful periodic assessment. Limited pulmonary infections may not require treatment, whereas other patients may require short-course, prolonged, or lifetime antifungal therapy, which is determined by comorbidities, risk of dissemination, and persistent systemic signs and symptoms, such as fever, night sweats, weight loss of more than 10%, fatigue, radiographic findings of extensive infiltrates involving multiple lobes or effusion, and CF of 1:16 or higher.[38]

Primary Pulmonary Infection

In endemic regions, primary coccidioidal pneumonia may account for approximately 25% of all community-acquired pneumonia.[41] It occurs 1 to 3 weeks after the exposure to arthroconidia. The presence of erythema nodosum or erythema multiforme is considered a favorable prognostic sign and is due to robust immune response rather than dissemination.[42] Radiographic findings are usually consistent with segmental or lobar consolidations and may have hilar or mediastinal adenopathy.[15] Before the advent of advanced imaging, mediastinal adenopathy was thought to be a risk factor for disseminated disease; however, more recent evidence has not demonstrated such an association.[43] Pleural effusion has been estimated to occur in 5% to 15% of primary pulmonary coccidioidomycosis.[30,44] In a recent series, pleural effusions were diagnosed more often in those with primary pulmonary infection than those with disseminated disease (*P*<.001).[44] Pleural effusions are exudative, often with a lympho-cytic predominance, and may have eosinophilia. Empyema occurred in a quarter of pleural effusions, and resolution required thoracotomy in one series.[44] However, in a recent series of pediatric cases, McCarty and colleagues[45] found that of 13 patients with pleural effusion and 4 with empyema, none required decortication and only 2 were in need of chest tube drainage.

Whether to treat or to observe acute pneumonia is an unresolved matter because of the lack of prospective randomized trials. Indeed, current guidelines depend heavily on expert opinion and clinical experience. It is estimated that approximately 95% of symptomatic primary coccidioidomycosis may resolve spontaneously.[38,46] Although many clinicians may elect to treat diagnosed primary coccidioidomycosis, the use of empirical antifungals for community-acquired pneumonia in endemic regions is un-proven; in fact, very early administration may abrogate the development of IgG anti-bodies (although the clinical significance of this is unclear).[47] Factors that do influence the decision to treat are prolonged infection, radiographic findings, CF titers, immunosuppression, and comorbidities. If antifungal therapy is determined neces-sary, fluconazole or itraconazole are recommended for 3 to 6 months and possibly longer depending on the clinical response. Pregnant patients have significant risk for dissemination and can be treated with amphotericin B (AmB) or immediately post-partum with fluconazole.[38] Some experts suggest the use of azoles during the second and third trimester and an AmB-based regimen during the first trimester.[39]

Diffuse Pneumonia

Diffuse pneumonia is a more severe form of the disease that can happen in a setting of high inoculum exposure or with accompanying immunosuppression and is often seen in patients with the risk factors mentioned earlier (**Box 1**). Patients are ill appearing in mild to moderate respiratory distress often with fever. Radiographic finding are usually consistent with multilobar diffuse infiltrates and adenopathy. Serious complications, such as pleural effusions, empyema, and acute respiratory distress syndrome (ARDS), are often seen.[15] Even with antifungal therapy, clinical improvement in such disease may be slow and patients often require significant and prolonged supportive care.

Box 1
Risk factors for severe or disseminated coccidioidomycosis

Filipino or African ethnicity

HIV/AIDS

Immunosuppressive medications
  Prednisone
  TNF-α inhibitors
  Chemotherapy
  Organ transplantation (tacrolimus, and so forth)

Diabetes mellitus

Pregnancy

Cardiopulmonary disease

CF titer of 1:16 or greater

Abbreviation: TNF, tumor necrosis factor.

ARDS as a consequence of coccidioidal infection carries a very high mortality rate. AmB is frequently used until clinical improvement occurs, followed by an azole for at least 1 year or longer. In selected individuals with ongoing immunosuppression or irreversible conditions, long-term maintenance therapy with an azole is suggested. The role of adjunctive corticosteroid therapy in coccidioidomycosis-associated ARDS has not been defined, and considerable debate exists between different clinicians.

Residual Nodule, Cavity, and Chronic Infiltrates

Approximately 5% of patient with resolution of primary pneumonic infiltrate can develop a pulmonary nodule or cavity. The initial identification of a coccidioidal infection could be a pulmonary nodule or cavity found incidentally on imaging studies. Nodules due to *Coccidioides* are often difficult to differentiate from malignancy, especially in persons who have not been diagnosed with coccidioidomycosis previously (**Fig. 2**). PET/ computed tomography has been used but is not always able to differentiate malignancy from coccidioidal pulmonary nodules. In an endemic region of California with a lung nodule program, approximately one-third of nodules are attributable to *Coccidioides*. Certain factors may have increased association with a coccidioidal nodule rather than malignancy, including male sex, age less than 55 years, lack of underlying pulmonary disease, farm labor or construction occupations, a nodule less than 2 cm in size, and a nodule described as diffuse or smooth in appearance.[48] Immunologic assays may be less reliable in this setting; often a bronchoscopy or biopsy is required to establish the diagnoses via histopathology, culture, and possibly PCR. Asymptomatic nodules attributed to coccidioidomycosis do not require treatment. When such lesions are stable over time with repeated radiographic imaging over 2 years in combination with a benign clinical course, no intervention is necessary.[19] Any treatment decision should take into account patient risk factors, serologic studies, and characteristics of the lesion.

Coccidioidomycosis is also known to cause cavitary disease in the lung, ranging from asymptomatic to symptomatic and/or ruptured. Although cavities are characteristically described as thin-walled and solitary, the morphology can be variable. Asymptomatic cavities can often be monitored radiographically, and the use of azole therapy is unproven. Symptomatic cavities may cause local discomfort or hemoptysis, and bacterial superinfection is possible. For symptomatic cavities or in those with elevated CF titers, a course of oral antifungals may be considered in order to improve symptoms but may not result in cavity closure. A more serious complication is a rupture of a cavity into the pleural space causing hydropneumothorax. In such cases,

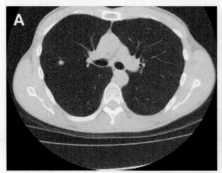 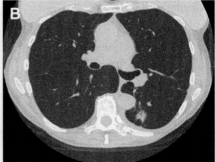

Fig. 2. Panel (*A*) coccidioidal nodule in a male, 40-pack-year smoker. Panel (*B*) adenocarcinoma of the lung in an asymptomatic, nonsmoking woman who recalls a respiratory infection 3 months prior. (*Courtesy of* Dr Michael Peterson, UCSF-Fresno, CA, USA.)

antifungal therapy along with surgical closure by lobectomy with decortication should be considered, especially in younger healthy patients. Initial antifungal therapy can include AmB or azole therapy.

A small percentage of patients may develop chronic fibrocavitary disease, which encompasses persistent ongoing symptoms of cough, fever, weight loss, and fatigue lasting for several months. Radiographic findings may show multifocal consolidations with cavitary lesions. Fluconazole or itraconazole are often prescribed for longer durations (a year or longer). If the response is suboptimal despite prolonged therapy, options include increased dosing or changing agents to AmB or an alternative azole. Newer azoles can be tried and have been used successfully.[49] Surgical options should be explored in those not responsive to therapy with persistent hemoptysis.

Extrapulmonary Disease

EP disease often develops through hematogenous or lymphatic spread and can involve one or multiple sites. Patients in certain risk groups or with impaired immunity as previously discussed are also at higher risk of dissemination. Depending on the anatomic site of infection, patients invariably require prolonged antifungals, with some needing concomitant surgical intervention for debridement and stabilization. Surgical treatment is especially important with vertebral column involvement with associated neurologic deficits. Surgical intervention can be essential where there is formation of abscesses, clinical evidence of worsening or incomplete disease control, persisting focal symptoms, and neurologic or physiologic compromise.[38,50] Dissemination to a wide range of tissues has been described. Common sites of dissemination include the meninges, skeleton, skin, and joints; but there are reports of involvement in glandular tissue, peritoneum, visceral organs the including liver and pancreas, the pericardium, bone marrow, kidney and bladder, and male and female reproductive organs.[51,52]

The initial antifungal therapy recommended is fluconazole or itraconazole. However, the preferred treatment of osseous coccidioidomycosis is itraconazole.[53] For patients with disseminated infections that seem to be worsening rapidly or who do not respond to initial oral azole therapy, strategies include switching therapy to another azole, or to AmB deoxycholate (AmB-d), or a lipid-based AmB, or even an azole in combination with AmB. These choices are frequently based on case reports and the clinical experience of the treating physician. Treatment duration is prolonged; often several years until disease is inactive both clinically and serologically with close follow-up for relapses.

Coccidioidal Meningitis

The most deleterious EP dissemination is the spread of *Coccidioides* spp to the central nervous system (CNS) causing meningitis. A lumbar puncture with analysis of CSF should be done in any patient with suspected or previously diagnosed coccidioidomycosis presenting with a headache, blurry vision, photophobia, meningismus, decline in cognition, hearing changes, and focal neurologic deficit. As illustrated in a recent retrospective study, there is no evidence to support routine CSF analysis in patients in at-risk groups (age, ethnicity, CF titer, and so forth) if they do not have CNS symptoms.[54] The diagnosis of coccidioidal meningitis (CM) is based on a positive serologic testing (ID/CF) or culture of CSF. CSF analysis typically shows an elevated white blood cell count with a mixed or lymphocytic pleocytosis, a high level of protein (sometimes measurable in grams per deciliter rather than milligrams per deciliter), and a low level of glucose. Imaging studies are helpful in evaluating complications associated with meningitis. Initial features of illness may be difficult to distinguish from other causes without detailed testing, notably tuberculosis and even autoimmune illnesses.

When left untreated, CM is uniformly fatal.[55] In a historical series reported by Vincent and colleagues,[55] before the availability of antifungals, 17 patients with CM were followed, all of whom died within 31 months. This review also commented on the combined survival statistics described in 5 reports of 117 patients whereby 91% of patients with CM died within 1 year and all died within 2 years. Although the fatality has improved with the use of AmB and azoles, morbidity is still substantial because of complications from the disease, devices used for treatment management, and side effects of the medications, as much higher recommended doses are necessary for a prolonged period of time.[56]

The most common life-threatening complications of meningitis include hydrocephalus, CNS vasculitis, cerebral ischemia, infarction, vasospasm, and hemorrhage. Basilar meningitis and spinal cord involvement may also be encountered. In patients with hydrocephalus, a ventricular shunt is necessary for decompression. Such shunts, often placed distally into the abdominal cavity, may develop secondary infections, obstruction due to persistent coccidioidomycosis, and/or abdominal pseudocysts.[57] It is not uncommon for patients to require multiple shunt revisions. As illustrated in several case reports, repeated obstruction of the shunt and isolation of fungus should alert one to seek alternate antifungal therapy. Some clinicians have used steroids for vasculitis, though this is considered anecdotal.

For the treatment of CM, most clinicians prefer therapy with oral fluconazole.[38] Although the dose studied in an uncontrolled clinical trial was 400 mg, it is common to begin therapy with 800 to 1200 mg per day of fluconazole.[56,58] Before the advent of azoles, AmB was the only drug of choice but was ineffective when given intravenously and required frequent administrations via the intrathecal (IT) route. Because of challenges of administration, toxicity associated with this route, and lack of experience in using this method, current practitioners seldom resort to recommending AmB as initial therapy, although lipid formulations have been used in the salvage setting successfully.[59] Although there are no trials comparing IT AmB and fluconazole, the response rate of IT AmB has ranged from 51% to 100% in studies published before 1986 and with fluconazole the rate is near 79%.[58,60] With fluconazole symptoms resolve within 4 to 8 months, though there is a delay in normalization of CSF abnormalities, which may persist in the presence of a shunt. Based on clinical experience and because of an extremely high relapse of 78% noted in a small series when therapy is discontinued, lifelong treatment with azoles is recommended.[61]

Assessing a patient's response to therapy is primarily a matter of serial evaluation and clinical judgment. Favorable signs include return to premorbid functioning, decreasing CF titers, and excellent adherence to medical care and therapy. Some patients with chronic meningitis have refractory illness with poor recovery or exceptionally slow improvement. A combination of serology and repeated CSF evaluation may be necessary to assess microbiologic and serologic improvement. Adherence counseling, assessment of drug-drug interactions, therapeutic drug monitoring, and consideration of alternative antifungal therapy may be necessary. For patients with CM who are failing treatment and/or have refractory coccidioidal disease, salvage regimens may be necessary. Both voriconazole and posaconazole have been used in this situation, with a growing body of case series and clinical experience to support their use.

Coccidioidomycosis in Immunocompromised Patients

Patients with impaired immune function are at risk for both symptomatic infection as well as reactivation of latent disease. The risks of novel infection are often presumed higher in such a group, but definitive incidence data are limited. In a study of 2246 solid organ transplant (SOT) recipients in Arizona, 239 (10.6%) had positive serologic testing with nearly all (212 of 239) showing evidence of coccidioidomycosis before transplantation.[62] Posttransplant, an additional 27 of the 2246 patients (1.2%) developed newly acquired, active disease. In a study of allogeneic hematopoietic stem-cell transplant (allo-HSCT) patients, 11 of 426 (2.6%) developed active coccidioidomycosis after transplant.[63] In these groups, the rates of dissemination and mortality are higher than in the general population, with up to 55% mortality observed in allo-HCT recipients and 28% in SOT recipients.[62–64] Observation of such outcomes has led many clinicians to recommend prophylaxis in high-risk transplant recipients. Because of the suboptimal testing sensitivities, achieving a diagnosis can be challenging and may require multiple testing modalities.[62]

Further studies have demonstrated that patients with serologic evidence of prior coccidioidomycosis before organ transplantation have higher rates of posttransplant coccidioidomycosis than others, suggesting that Coccidioides may reactivate from latency, with some risk factors including high-dose prednisone, and treatment of rejection.[65] In the aforementioned study of allo-HSCT patients, 8 of 426 (1.9%) had asymptomatic positive serologic tests before transplantation, and 2 (25%) had reactivation following transplantation. Although antifungal prophylaxis has been evaluated and seems effective in some studies, it may not be a panacea. In a study of 100 patients with coccidioidomycosis who underwent SOT, 94% received antifungal prophylaxis; of this group, 5 patients experienced reactivated infection.[66] Notably, all patients survived with modified ongoing antifungal therapies.

It should also be noted that donor-derived coccidioidomycosis is possible.[67] Transmission rates are difficult to determine, but onset of disease has a high mortality in these patients. Pretransplant recipient and donor screening in endemic areas or with a history of travel to endemic areas is recommended. Multiple testing modalities may be considered depending on clinical presentation and may include serology, pathology, culture, PCR, and, in the future, skin-testing. An excellent review has been recently published.[62] In patients with HIV, coccidioidomycosis may be considered an opportunistic infection. Although primary prophylaxis has not been demonstrated to be effective, treatment of primary pulmonary coccidioidomycosis is warranted, especially if CD4+ lymphocyte counts are less than 250 cells per microliter.[68] Secondary prophylaxis may be considered until counts increase greater than 250 cells per microliter.

The advent of biological therapies and targeted chemotherapeutics has resulted in further questions regarding their use in endemic areas. At present, the exact risks of acquiring coccidioidomycosis on any given biological agent are unknown. In a convenience sample in an endemic area, 1.9% of patients in a rheumatology center had evidence of coccidioidomycosis.[69] The prevalence in patients with rheumatoid arthritis (RA) was approximately 3.1%, but use of tumor necrosis factor α inhibitors could not be proven to have association in this study. In contrast, a prior study of patients receiving infliximab and etanercept found 13 cases of coccidioidomycosis (7 of 247 in the infliximab group vs 4 of 738 treated with other modalities, relative risk 5.23, $P<.01$).[70] Screening may be used, but the benefit is unclear. Antifungal prophylaxis is not currently recommended.

ANTIFUNGAL THERAPY
Amphotericin

In severe or refractory coccidioidal disease, intravenous AmB is considered the drug of choice. AmB is a polyene antifungal agent that binds to sterols in the fungal cell membrane causing intracellular components to leak resulting in cell death. Its use came into practice in the mid-1950s; recognition of the poor CNS penetration led to the development of administering IT AmB via lumbar, cisternal, or ventricular routes in salvage settings.[71] IT treatment changed the outcome of CM; however, numerous surgical, mechanical, and infectious complications along with headaches, paresthesia, nerve palsies, myelopathy, arachnoiditis, hemorrhage, transverse myelitis, and more have led to its use only for those with refractory disease and also with consultation with experienced physicians who have pioneered these techniques.

Data on the use of lipid preparations of AmB are scant and are largely derived from animal models. Clemons and colleagues[72] compared the efficacy of intravenous liposomal AmB with those of oral fluconazole and intravenous AmB-d for the treatment of experimental CM. All regimens reduced the numbers of colony forming units (CFU) in the brain and spinal cord; however, liposomal AmB–treated animals had 3 to 11 fold lower numbers of CFU than fluconazole and 6 to 35 fold lower numbers of CFU than AmB-d-treated rabbits. Another animal model that compared intravenous AmB lipid complex (ABLC), AmB-d, and oral fluconazole showed that ABLC cleared CFU from CSF faster than AmB-d or fluconazole.[73] Although no formal guidelines exist regarding the use of these agents, the data discussed earlier indicate that lipid formulations of AmB may be of benefit, as it can be administered at higher doses with less toxicity.

Azoles

The introduction of azoles was a significant breakthrough in the treatment of coccidioidomycosis for both meningeal and nonmeningeal disease. These agents act by inhibiting the synthesis of ergosterol in the fungal cell membrane.[74] The first trials with azoles included clotrimazole, then miconazole whose use quickly faded because of toxicity, frequency of dosing, ineffectiveness, and lack of oral availability. Ketoconazole was the first oral agent to be used in the treatment of coccidioidomycosis, although only 20% to 30% of patients demonstrated a clinical response to 200 to 400 mg/d. Dose escalation was attempted to increase drug efficacy; however, gastrointestinal intolerance, adrenal insufficiency, and gynecomastia ultimately limited the use of this agent.[75,76]

Third-generation azoles, the triazoles, were introduced in the 1980s and showed promising efficacy with less toxicity, especially with higher dosing and prolonged use. First was itraconazole with excellent in vitro activity against *Coccidioides* spp.[77] The Mycosis Study Group documented its tolerance and efficacy in which 57% of the 47 patients with nonmeningeal coccidioidomycosis achieved remission.[78] In one randomized double-blind placebo-controlled trial for nonmeningeal coccidioidomycosis, patients with skeletal infections responded twice as frequently to itraconazole than fluconazole, though the study dose of fluconazole was lower than is currently used.[53] Itraconazole CSF penetration is not optimal; but it does concentrate in fatty tissues, including the brain, and has demonstrated efficacy in the treatment of CM.[79] Among its different formulations, itraconazole solution has greater bioavailability than capsules and is maximally absorbed in the fasting state.[74] For the maximum absorption of the capsular form, an acidic environment with intake of a high-fat meal is preferred. At doses of 800 mg and higher, adverse effects included adrenal insufficiency, hypertension, hypokalemia, and edema. Negative inotropic effects have also been reported,[80] but this is uncommon in clinical practice.

Fluconazole was the next to be developed, and it still remains the preferred triazole because of its excellent bioavailability, tolerability, CNS penetration, slow clearance (24- to 30-hour half-life), little hepatotoxicity, renal clearance, no endocrine side effects, reasonable response rates in prior reports, and generally lower costs. In a multicenter, open-label, single-arm study, among 75 evaluable patients, a satisfactory response was observed in 12 (86%) of the 14 patients with skeletal, 22 (55%) of the 40 patients with chronic pulmonary, and 16 (76%) of the 21 patients with soft tissue disease.[81] Forty-one patients who responded were followed off the drug, and 15 (37%) of them experienced reactivation of infection. Tucker and colleagues[82,83] identified fluconazole to have potential use in coccidioidal meningitis. This study was followed by the landmark study by Galgiani and colleagues[58] that showed fluconazole to achieve the same response rate for CM as its historical counterpart IT AmB. Thus, because of its favorable activity and minimal toxicity, current guidelines recommend fluconazole (800–1200 mg) as the preferred agent for meningeal infection. Daily doses up to 2000 mg have been used in some cases. With improving host control of the infection, fluconazole doses may be decreased slowly over time; but a specific effective maintenance dose for meningeal and/or disseminated disease is not well established.

The disadvantage of azole therapy is the inability to eradicate the fungus, which seems to be a class effect; thus, treatment is continued indefinitely as a suppressive rather than curative therapy for CM, although newer formulations and agents may offer mean fungicidal concentrations achievable in clinical care. Therapeutic drug monitoring of fluconazole can be done in patients with complicated courses of illness or who are not responding clinically. Commonly encountered adverse effects with higher doses ($\geq$400 mg) of fluconazole include dry mouth, dry skin, nausea, reversible alopecia, and abnormal liver function tests.

Newer Triazoles

Voriconazole and posaconazole are newer triazoles and are primarily used in patients whose coccidioidal infection is refractory to first-line azole therapy. They both have excellent activity in vitro against *Coccidioides* spp (**Table 1**).[84] In vitro concentration studies are frequently based on mycelial phase fungal growth, and extrapolation to human disease is the subject of ongoing evaluation. Similar to fluconazole, voriconazole is an attractive choice because of its favorable pharmacokinetic/pharmacodynamics in the CSF. Voriconazole is available in parenteral and oral formulations with excellent oral bioavailability. Therapeutic drug monitoring should be considered, as voriconazole serum concentrations can vary between individuals.[74] Administration of voriconazole may be complicated by drug-drug interactions as a result of its inhibition of CYP2C9, CYP2C19, and CYP3A4 enzymes. Adverse effects may also limit use; besides the visual disturbance, neurotoxicity, hepatotoxicity, photopsia, and QTc prolongation, concerns have been raised with long-term use of voriconazole for the

Table 1				
In vitro susceptibility of *Coccidioides* isolates to selected antifungal agents				
***Coccidioides* spp 30 Isolates**	**MIC Range**	**Geometric Mean MIC**	**MIC$_{50}$**	**MIC$_{90}$**
Amphotericin B	0.03–0.125	0.056	0.06	0.125
Itraconazole	0.03–0.5	0.149	0.125	0.5
Fluconazole	2–64	8.774	8	32
Voriconazole	0.06–1.0	0.193	0.125	0.5
Posaconazole	0.06–1.0	0.183	0.125	0.5
Isavuconazole	0.125–1.0	0.28	0.25	0.5

Abbreviation: MIC, minimal inhibitory concentration.

Data from Gonzalez GM. In vitro activities of isavuconazole against opportunistic filamentous and dimorphic fungi. Medical Mycol 2009;47(1):74.

development of periostitis because of hyperfluorosis and melanoma in situ.[85–87] However, a small study of nontransplant patients with chronic coccidioidomycosis on long-term fluorinated triazole therapies did not identify significant long-term osseous effects despite elevated plasma fluoride levels.[85]

Posaconazole has also been shown to have potent in vitro and in vivo activity against *Coccidioides* spp. It has been tested in murine models and shown to be 200 fold or greater as potent as fluconazole and 50 fold or greater potent as itraconazole along with having fungicidal activity in vivo against *C immitis*.[88] Posaconazole is available in liquid, capsule, and intravenous formulations. Historically, it was available in liquid form only, requiring it be taken with a fatty meal and acidic beverage, which limited optimal absorption in severely ill patients. Most reported studies on the use of posaconazole were done before the advent of capsule and intravenous formulations. Adverse events include gastrointestinal effects, rash, and elevated transaminases.[89] Drug cost remains a significant problem for many patients.

Isavuconazole is a newly available extended-spectrum triazole with in vitro activity against *Coccidioides* spp.[84] Limited clinical data have been presented to date regarding the in vivo efficacy, and thus far it has been prescribed only to patients with primary coccidioidal pneumonia. It has been effectively used for other invasive fungal infections, including *Aspergillus*, Mucorales, and other endemic fungi as well; a clinical trial for the treatment of nonmeningeal disseminated and chronic coccidioidomycosis is currently underway.

Echinocandins

The echinocandins have little inherent activity against *Coccidioides* spp in the mycelial phase; however, the potential efficacy has been demonstrated in murine models of infection.[90] There are case reports of caspofungin being used in combination with azole- or amphotericin-based therapies. In a series of 9 pediatric patients, Levy and colleagues[91] have reported clinical improvement in 8 cases in which a salvage regimen of caspofungin plus voriconazole was used following treatment failures. As publications describing the potential efficacy of these agents are limited, this class should not be used as monotherapy in the treatment of coccidioidomycosis at this time.

Interferon Gamma Therapy

In vitro studies have demonstrated interferon (IFN)-γ production by peripheral blood mononuclear cells is reduced in patients with chronic coccidioidomycosis,[92–94] and defects within interleukin 12/IFN-γ have been reported in several patients with disseminated coccidioidal infection.[95,96] These findings have encouraged the use of adjunctive exogenous IFN-γ along with antifungal use in patients with refractory disseminated coccidioidomycosis, although its use is limited by patient tolerability, expense, and a lack of a clear benefit in the absence of compelling clinical data.[97]

Future Therapies

Future innovative ways to target this disease are in development. Nikkomycin Z has shown promise with a possibility of cure in murine models of infection. Safety trials have been conducted, and clinical trials are anticipated in 2016 or shortly thereafter.

As this organism is capable of eliciting a wide range of immunologic reactions, further research in the areas of immunotherapy and vaccination will be of great importance. It is well known that some hosts are able to effectively control infection, whereas others develop severe complications. The current knowledge of host risk factors and immunogenetics is in the early stages, and a better understanding of the mechanisms for effective host control of disease may allow the possibility of intervention.[46,98]

SUMMARY

The management of coccidioidomycosis depends on the last 6 decades of clinical experience. For most human infections, the disease is relatively benign. However, for others, the outcome is one of severe debility and even death. Even in cases of relatively benign disease, the possibility of recurrence is problematic. For clinicians both in endemic areas and elsewhere, knowledge of the identification and management of this illness will continue to be necessary. Although there is an increasing experience with several highly active antifungal therapies, it is still not possible to reliably eradicate infection and prevent relapses with chronic disseminated coccidioidomycosis. CM is one of a few infectious diseases that require lifetime suppressive therapy for CM because of its devastating results. Although newer and more effective treatments are needed and in development, for now fluconazole and itraconazole remain the predominant therapy along with AmB formulations. The correlation of failures with reliable susceptibility data may also enable better treatment decisions, keeping in consideration the newer triazoles for refractory disease.

REFERENCES

1. Hector RF, Laniado-Laborin R. Coccidioidomycosis–a fungal disease of the Americas. PLoS Med 2005;2(1):e2.
2. Schneider E, Hajjeh RA, Spiegel RA, et al. A coccidioidomycosis outbreak following the Northridge, Calif, earthquake. JAMA 1997;277(11):904–8.
3. Kong YC, Levine HB, Madin SH, et al. Fungal multiplication and histopathologic changes in vaccinated mice infected with Coccidioides immitis. J Immunol 1964; 92:779–90.
4. Lee CY, Thompson 3rd GR, Hastey CJ, et al. Coccidioides endospores and spherules draw strong chemotactic, adhesive, and phagocytic responses by individual human neutrophils. PLoS One 2015;10(6):e0129522.
5. Brown J, Benedict K, Park BJ, et al. Coccidioidomycosis: epidemiology. Clin Epidemiol 2013;5:185–97.
6. Edwards PQ, Palmer CE. Prevalence of sensitivity to coccidioidin, with special reference to specific and nonspecific reactions to coccidioidin and to histoplasmin. Dis Chest 1957;31(1):35–60.
7. Talamantes J, Behseta S, Zender CS. Statistical modeling of valley fever data in Kern County, California. Int J Biometeorology 2007;51(4):307–13.
8. Stevens DA. Coccidioidomycosis. N Engl J Med 1995;332(16):1077–82.
9. Centers for Disease Control and Prevention. Increase in reported coccidioidomycosis–United States, 1998-2011. MMWR Morb Mortal Wkly Rep 2013;62(12): 217–21.
10. Huang JY, Bristow B, Shafir S, et al. Coccidioidomycosis-associated Deaths, United States, 1990-2008. Emerg Infect Dis 2012;18(11):1723–8.
11. California Department of Public Health. Coccidioidomycosis yearly summary report, 2001 – 2010. Available at: http://www.cdph.ca.gov/healthinfo/discond/Pages/Coccidioidomycosis.aspx. Accessed March 3, 2015.
12. Emery K, Lancaster M, Oubsuntia V, et al. Coccidioidomycosis cases continue to rise in Kern County during 2011. Presented at Coccidioidomycosis Study Group 56th Annual Meeting. University of Arizona. Tucson, March 24, 2012.

13. Ampel NM. Coccidioidomycosis: a review of recent advances. Clin Chest Med 2009;30(2):241–51.
14. Parish JM, Blair JE. Coccidioidomycosis. Mayo Clin Proc 2008;83(3):343–8 [quiz: 8–9].
15. Thompson GR 3rd. Pulmonary coccidioidomycosis. Semin Respir Crit Care Med 2011;32(6):754–63.
16. Litvintseva AP, Marsden-Haug N, Hurst S, et al. Valley fever: finding new places for an old disease: coccidioides immitis found in Washington State soil associated with recent human infection. Clin Infect Dis 2015;60(1):e1–3.
17. Marsden-Haug N, Goldoft M, Ralston C, et al. Coccidioidomycosis acquired in Washington State. Clin Infect Dis 2013;56(6):847–50.
18. Turabelidze G, Aggu-Sher RK, Jahanpour E, et al. Coccidioidomycosis in a state where it is not known to be endemic - Missouri, 2004-2013. MMWR Morbidity mortality weekly Rep 2015;64(23):636–9.
19. Baddley JW, Winthrop KL, Patkar NM, et al. Geographic distribution of endemic fungal infections among older persons, United States. Emerg Infect Dis 2011; 17(9):1664–9.
20. Tang TH, Tsang OT. Images in clinical medicine. Fungal infection from sweeping in the wrong place. N Engl J Med 2011;364(2):e3.
21. De Pauw B, Walsh TJ, Donnelly JP, et al. Revised definitions of invasive fungal disease from the European Organization for Research and Treatment of Cancer/Invasive Fungal Infections Cooperative Group and the National Institute of Allergy and Infectious Diseases Mycoses Study Group (EORTC/MSG) Consensus Group. Clin Infect Dis 2008;46(12):1813–21.
22. Schuetz AN, Pisapia D, Yan J, et al. An atypical morphologic presentation of Coccidioides spp. in fine-needle aspiration of lung. Diagn Cytopathol 2012;40(2): 163–7.
23. Kaufman L, Valero G, Padhye AA. Misleading manifestations of Coccidioides immitis in vivo. J Clin Microbiol 1998;36(12):3721–3.
24. Ke Y, Smith CW, Salaru G, et al. Unusual forms of immature sporulating Coccidioides immitis diagnosed by fine-needle aspiration biopsy. Arch Pathol Lab Med 2006;130(1):97–100.
25. Raab SS, Silverman JF, Zimmerman KG. Fine-needle aspiration biopsy of pulmonary coccidioidomycosis. Spectrum of cytologic findings in 73 patients. Am J Clin Pathol 1993;99(5):582–7.
26. Mitchell M, Dizon D, Libke R, et al. Development of a real-time PCR Assay for identification of Coccidioides immitis by use of the BD Max system. J Clin Microbiol 2015;53(3):926–9.
27. Gago S, Buitrago MJ, Clemons KV, et al. Development and validation of a quantitative real-time PCR assay for the early diagnosis of coccidioidomycosis. Diagn Microbiol Infect Dis 2014;79(2):214–21.
28. Johnson SM, Simmons KA, Pappagianis D. Amplification of coccidioidal DNA in clinical specimens by PCR. J Clin Microbiol 2004;42(5):1982–5.
29. Binnicker MJ, Buckwalter SP, Eisberner JJ, et al. Detection of Coccidioides species in clinical specimens by real-time PCR. J Clin Microbiol 2007;45(1): 173–8.
30. Thompson GR, Sharma S, Bays DJ, et al. Coccidioidomycosis: adenosine deaminase levels, serologic parameters, culture results, and polymerase chain reaction testing in pleural fluid. Chest 2013;143(3):776–81.
31. Wack EE, Ampel NM, Sunenshine RH, et al. The return of delayed-type hypersensitivity skin testing for Coccidioidomycosis. Clin Infect Dis 2015;61(5):787–91.

32. Pappagianis D. Serologic studies in coccidioidomycosis. Semin Respir Infect 2001;16(4):242–50.
33. Kuberski T, Herrig J, Pappagianis D. False-positive IgM serology in coccidioidomycosis. J Clin Microbiol 2010;48(6):2047–9.
34. Blair JE, Mendoza N, Force S, et al. Clinical specificity of the enzyme immunoassay test for coccidioidomycosis varies according to the reason for its performance. Clin Vaccine Immunol 2013;20(1):95–8.
35. Thompson GR 3rd, Bays DJ, Johnson SM, et al. Serum (1->3)-beta-D-glucan measurement in coccidioidomycosis. J Clin Microbiol 2012;50(9):3060–2.
36. Sandhu GS, Kline BC, Stockman L, et al. Molecular probes for diagnosis of fungal infections. J Clin Microbiol 1995;33(11):2913–9.
37. Smith CE, Beard RR. Varieties of coccidioidal infection in relation to the epidemiology and control of the diseases. Am J Public Health Nations Health 1946; 36(12):1394–402.
38. Galgiani JN, Ampel NM, Blair JE, et al. Coccidioidomycosis. Clin Infect Dis 2005; 41(9):1217–23.
39. Bercovitch RS, Catanzaro A, Schwartz BS, et al. Coccidioidomycosis during pregnancy: a review and recommendations for management. Clin Infect Dis 2011;53(4):363–8.
40. Powell BL, Drutz DJ, Huppert M, et al. Relationship of progesterone- and estradiol-binding proteins in Coccidioides immitis to coccidioidal dissemination in pregnancy. Infect Immun 1983;40(2):478–85.
41. Valdivia L, Nix D, Wright M, et al. Coccidioidomycosis as a common cause of community-acquired pneumonia. Emerg Infect Dis 2006;12(6):958–62.
42. Eldridge ML, Chambers CJ, Sharon VR, et al. Fungal infections of the skin and nail: new treatment options. Expert Rev Anti Infect Ther 2014;12(11): 1389–405.
43. Mayer AP, Morris MF, Panse PM, et al. Does the presence of mediastinal adenopathy confer a risk for disseminated infection in immunocompetent persons with pulmonary coccidioidomycosis? Mycoses 2013;56(2):145–9.
44. Merchant M, Romero AO, Libke RD, et al. Pleural effusion in hospitalized patients with Coccidioidomycosis. Respir Med 2008;102(4):537–40.
45. McCarty JM, Demetral LC, Dabrowski L, et al. Pediatric coccidioidomycosis in central California: a retrospective case series. Clin Infect Dis 2013;56(11): 1579–85.
46. Thompson GR 3rd, Stevens DA, Clemons KV, et al. Call for a California coccidioidomycosis consortium to face the top ten challenges posed by a recalcitrant regional disease. Mycopathologia 2015;179(1–2):1–9.
47. Thompson GR 3rd, Lunetta JM, Johnson SM, et al. Early treatment with fluconazole may abrogate the development of IgG antibodies in coccidioidomycosis. Clin Infect Dis 2011;53(6):e20–4.
48. Ronaghi R, Rashidian A, Peterson M, et al. Central valley lung nodule calculator: development and prospective analysis of a newly developed calculator in a Coccidiodomycosis endemic area. Presented at 59th Annual Coccidioidomycosis Study Group. San Diego, April 11, 2015.
49. Kim MM, Vikram HR, Kusne S, et al. Treatment of refractory coccidioidomycosis with voriconazole or posaconazole. Clin Infect Dis 2011;53(11):1060–6.
50. Szeyko LA, Taljanovic MS, Dzioba RB, et al. Vertebral coccidioidomycosis: presentation and multidisciplinary management. Am J Med 2012;125(3):304–14.
51. Nelson EC, Thompson GR 3rd, Vidovszky TJ. Image of the month. Disseminated coccidioidomycosis. Arch Surg 2012;147(1):95–6.

52. Nguyen C, Barker BM, Hoover S, et al. Recent advances in our understanding of the environmental, epidemiological, immunological, and clinical dimensions of coccidioidomycosis. Clin Microbiol Rev 2013;26(3):505–25.
53. Galgiani JN, Catanzaro A, Cloud GA, et al. Comparison of oral fluconazole and itraconazole for progressive, nonmeningeal coccidioidomycosis. A randomized, double-blind trial. Mycoses Study Group. Ann Intern Med 2000;133(9):676–86.
54. Thompson G 3rd, Wang S, Bercovitch R, et al. Routine CSF analysis in coccidioidomycosis is not required. PLoS One 2013;8(5):e64249.
55. Vincent T, Galgiani JN, Huppert M, et al. The natural history of coccidioidal meningitis: VA-Armed Forces cooperative studies, 1955-1958. Clin Infect Dis 1993; 16(2):247–54.
56. Johnson RH, Einstein HE. Coccidioidal meningitis. Clin Infect Dis 2006;42(1):103–7.
57. Narasimhan A, Rashidian A, Faiad G, et al. Study of prevalence, risk factors and outcomes of abdominal pseudocyst (APC) in patients with coccidioidal meningitis (CM) and ventriculoperitoneal shunts (VPS). Presented Infectious Diseases of America 49th Annual meeting. Boston, October 22, 2011.
58. Galgiani JN, Catanzaro A, Cloud GA, et al. Fluconazole therapy for coccidioidal meningitis. The NIAID-Mycoses Study Group. Ann Intern Med 1993;119(1): 28–35.
59. Mathisen G, Shelub A, Truong J, et al. Coccidioidal meningitis: clinical presentation and management in the fluconazole era. Medicine 2010;89(5):251–84.
60. Bouza E, Dreyer JS, Hewitt WL, et al. Coccidioidal meningitis. An analysis of thirty-one cases and review of the literature. Medicine 1981;60(3):139–72.
61. Dewsnup DH, Galgiani JN, Graybill JR, et al. Is it ever safe to stop azole therapy for *Coccidioides immitis* meningitis? Ann Intern Med 1996;124(3):305–10.
62. Mendoza N, Blair JE. The utility of diagnostic testing for active coccidioidomycosis in solid organ transplant recipients. Am J Transplant 2013;13(4):1034–9.
63. Mendoza N, Noel P, Blair JE. Diagnosis, treatment, and outcomes of coccidioidomycosis in allogeneic stem cell transplantation. Transpl Infect Dis 2015;17(3):380–8.
64. Vucicevic D, Carey EJ, Blair JE. Coccidioidomycosis in liver transplant recipients in an endemic area. Am J Transplant 2011;11(1):111–9.
65. Blair JE, Kusne S, Carey EJ, et al. The prevention of recrudescent coccidioidomycosis after solid organ transplantation. Transplantation 2007;83(9):1182–7.
66. Keckich DW, Blair JE, Vikram HR, et al. Reactivation of coccidioidomycosis despite antifungal prophylaxis in solid organ transplant recipients. Transplantation 2011;92(1):88–93.
67. Engelthaler DM, Chiller T, Schupp JA, et al. Next-generation sequencing of *Coccidioides immitis* isolated during cluster investigation. Emerg Infect Dis 2011; 17(2):227–32.
68. Masannat FY, Ampel NM. Coccidioidomycosis in patients with HIV-1 infection in the era of potent antiretroviral therapy. Clin Infect Dis 2010;50(1):1–7.
69. Mertz LE, Blair JE. Coccidioidomycosis in rheumatology patients: incidence and potential risk factors. Ann N Y Acad Sci 2007;1111:343–57.
70. Bergstrom L, Yocum DE, Ampel NM, et al. Increased risk of coccidioidomycosis in patients treated with tumor necrosis factor alpha antagonists. Arthritis Rheum 2004;50(6):1959–66.
71. Stevens DA, Shatsky SA. Intrathecal amphotericin in the management of coccidioidal meningitis. Semin Respir Infect 2001;16(4):263–9.
72. Clemons KV, Sobel RA, Williams PL, et al. Efficacy of intravenous liposomal amphotericin B (AmBisome) against coccidioidal meningitis in rabbits. Antimicrob Agents Chemother 2002;46(8):2420–6.

73. Capilla J, Clemons KV, Sobel RA, et al. Efficacy of amphotericin B lipid complex in a rabbit model of coccidioidal meningitis. J Antimicrob Chemother 2007;60(3): 673–6.

74. Thompson GR 3rd, Cadena J, Patterson TF. Overview of antifungal agents. Clin Chest Med 2009;30(2):203–15.

75. Pont A, Graybill JR, Craven PC, et al. High-dose ketoconazole therapy and adrenal and testicular function in humans. Arch Intern Med 1984;144(11):2150–3.

76. Galgiani JN, Stevens DA, Graybill JR, et al. Ketoconazole therapy of progressive coccidioidomycosis. Comparison of 400- and 800-mg doses and observations at higher doses. Am J Med 1988;84(3 Pt 2):603–10.

77. Stevens DA, Clemons KV. Azole therapy of clinical and experimental coccidioidomycosis. Ann N Y Acad Sci 2007;1111:442–54.

78. Graybill JR, Stevens DA, Galgiani JN, et al. Itraconazole treatment of coccidioidomycosis. NAIAD Mycoses Study Group. Am J Med 1990;89(3):282–90.

79. Tucker RM, Denning DW, Dupont B, et al. Itraconazole therapy for chronic coccidioidal meningitis. Ann Intern Med 1990;112(2):108–12.

80. Qu Y, Fang M, Gao B, et al. Itraconazole decreases left ventricular contractility in isolated rabbit heart: mechanism of action. Toxicol Appl Pharmacol 2013;268(2): 113–22.

81. Catanzaro A, Galgiani JN, Levine BE, et al. Fluconazole in the treatment of chronic pulmonary and nonmeningeal disseminated coccidioidomycosis. NIAID Mycoses Study Group. Am J Med 1995;98(3):249–56.

82. Tucker RM, Williams PL, Arathoon EG, et al. Pharmacokinetics of fluconazole in cerebrospinal fluid and serum in human coccidioidal meningitis. Antimicrob Agents Chemother 1988;32(3):369–73.

83. Tucker RM, Galgiani JN, Denning DW, et al. Treatment of coccidioidal meningitis with fluconazole. Rev Infect Dis 1990;12(Suppl 3):S380–9.

84. Gonzalez GM. In vitro activities of isavuconazole against opportunistic filamentous and dimorphic fungi. Med Mycol 2009;47(1):71–6.

85. Thompson GR 3rd, Bays D, Cohen SH, et al. Fluoride excess in coccidioidomycosis patients receiving long-term antifungal therapy: an assessment of currently available triazoles. Antimicrob Agents Chemother 2012;56(1):563–4.

86. Miller DD, Cowen EW, Nguyen JC, et al. Melanoma associated with long-term voriconazole therapy: a new manifestation of chronic photosensitivity. Arch Dermatol 2010;146(3):300–4.

87. Wermers RA, Cooper K, Razonable RR, et al. Fluoride excess and periostitis in transplant patients receiving long-term voriconazole therapy. Clin Infect Dis 2011;52(5):604–11.

88. Lutz JE, Clemons KV, Aristizabal BH, et al. Activity of the triazole SCH 56592 against disseminated murine coccidioidomycosis. Antimicrob Agents Chemother 1997;41(7):1558–61.

89. Stevens DA, Rendon A, Gaona-Flores V, et al. Posaconazole therapy for chronic refractory coccidioidomycosis. Chest 2007;132(3):952–8.

90. Gonzalez GM, Gonzalez G, Najvar LK, et al. Therapeutic efficacy of caspofungin alone and in combination with amphotericin B deoxycholate for coccidioidomycosis in a mouse model. J Antimicrob Chemother 2007;60(6):1341–6.

91. Levy ER, McCarty JM, Shane AL, et al. Treatment of pediatric refractory coccidioidomycosis with combination voriconazole and caspofungin: a retrospective case series. Clin Infect Dis 2013;56(11):1573–8.

92. Ampel NM, Kramer LA. In vitro modulation of cytokine production by lymphocytes in human coccidioidomycosis. Cell Immunol 2003;221(2):115–21.

93. Ampel NM, Christian L. In vitro modulation of proliferation and cytokine production by human peripheral blood mononuclear cells from subjects with various forms of coccidioidomycosis. Infect Immun 1997;65(11):4483–7.
94. Corry DB, Ampel NM, Christian L, et al. Cytokine production by peripheral blood mononuclear cells in human coccidioidomycosis. J Infect Dis 1996;174(2):440–3.
95. Vinh DC, Masannat F, Dzioba RB, et al. Refractory disseminated coccidioidomycosis and mycobacteriosis in interferon-gamma receptor 1 deficiency. Clin Infect Dis 2009;49(6):e62–5.
96. Vinh DC. Coccidioidal meningitis: disseminated disease in patients without HIV/AIDS. Medicine (Baltimore) 2011;90(1):87.
97. Kuberski TT, Servi RJ, Rubin PJ. Successful treatment of a critically ill patient with disseminated coccidioidomycosis, using adjunctive interferon-gamma. Clin Infect Dis 2004;38(6):910–2.
98. Thompson GR 3rd, Bays D, Taylor SL, et al. Association between serum 25-hydroxyvitamin D level and type of coccidioidal infection. Med Mycol 2013;51(3):319–23.

Blastomycosis

Caroline G. Castillo, MD[a], Carol A. Kauffman, MD[a,b],
Marisa H. Miceli, MD[a,*]

KEYWORDS

- Endemic mycoses • *B dermatitidis* • Blastomycosis • Fungal pneumonia
- Amphotericin B • Itraconazole

KEY POINTS

- *Blastomyces dermatitidis* is endemic to the shore of lakes and rivers in Central and Southern North America.
- Infection can occur in any host but is more severe in immunocompromised patients.
- Acute respiratory distress syndrome and central nervous system involvement are the two most serious complications of blastomycosis.
- Early diagnosis of blastomycosis can be made by demonstrating distinctive yeast forms in tissue biopsy and by antigen detection using enzyme immunoassay techniques.
- Mild to moderate blastomycosis is treated with itraconazole, and moderate to severe blastomycosis with lipid formulations of amphotericin B followed by itraconazole.

INTRODUCTION

Blastomycosis is one of 3 major dimorphic endemic mycoses that occur predominantly in North America. Infection is acquired by inhalation of organisms that exist as molds in the environment; conversion to the yeast phase occurs in the lungs.[1–3] Most cases of infection with *Blastomyces dermatitidis* are asymptomatic or manifest as an undiagnosed, self-limited illness. Symptomatic blastomycosis can present as acute or chronic pulmonary infection; a small number of patients progress to severe lung involvement manifested as acute respiratory distress syndrome (ARDS).[4] Hematogenous dissemination can involve many organs; but skin lesions are most commonly seen, followed by involvement of the genitourinary tract in men and osteoarticular structures. Diagnosis has improved with the use of antigen detection assays,[5] and

All authors declare that they have no financial or commercial conflicts of interest.
^a Division of Infectious Diseases, University of Michigan Health System, 3119 Taubman Center, Ann Arbor, MI 48109, USA; ^b Division of Infectious Diseases, Veterans Affairs Ann Arbor Healthcare System, 2215 Fuller Road, Ann Arbor, MI 48105, USA
* Corresponding author.
E-mail address: mmiceli@med.umich.edu

Infect Dis Clin N Am 30 (2016) 247–264
http://dx.doi.org/10.1016/j.idc.2015.10.002
0891-5520/16/$ – see front matter © 2016 Elsevier Inc. All rights reserved.

id.theclinics.com

new azole antifungal agents have increased the available armamentarium for treatment of this infection.[6]

EPIDEMIOLOGY

Blastomycosis is seen most frequently in the Mississippi and Ohio River valleys, Midwestern states and Canadian provinces that border the Great Lakes, and areas adjacent to the Saint Lawrence Seaway[1,7–14] (**Fig. 1**). However, occasional cases have been reported from Florida, Colorado, Hawaii, Israel, India, Africa, and Central and South America.[2,15,16] Within areas known to be endemic for blastomycosis, the disease occurs in certain areas much more frequently than in others.[7,8,13] A survey in Wisconsin found that the mean annual incidence was 40.4 per 100,000 persons in one county, and for a specific area within that county it was 101.3 per 100,000 persons.[8] Within endemic areas, the specific environmental niche for *B dermatitidis* is likely soil and decaying vegetation, especially in proximity to lakes and rivers.[7] It is difficult to isolate *B dermatitidis* from soil samples, delaying firm identification of the specific environmental requirements for this organism.

Mandatory public health reporting of blastomycosis is required in only 6 states and 2 Canadian provinces, so the true occurrence of this infection in humans is unknown. More cases are reported in men than women, which is most likely related to having greater risk for exposure in the environment. In some but not all instances, a history of activities that led to disruption of soil or decaying wood can be elicited.[7] In some reports, the incidence has been reported to be higher among African American populations in the United States and aboriginal populations in Canada.[10,11] One report described an outbreak of blastomycosis that clustered in certain neighborhoods in north central Wisconsin in which the rate of infection was 12 times higher among Asian residents, most of whom were immigrants of Hmong ethnicity.[17] Typical environmental exposures usually associated with blastomycosis were absent, raising speculation of genetic factors predisposing to disease among this group of individuals.

B dermatitidis also infects animals, especially dogs.[1] In areas of north central Wisconsin with many human cases, the incidence in canine cases is correspondingly high.[18] In one report as many as a third of patients who had blastomycosis and who

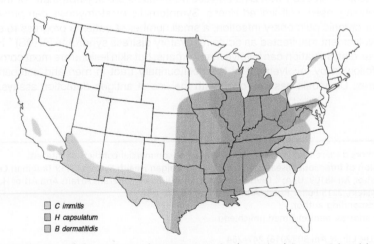

Fig. 1. Distribution of the major endemic mycoses in the United States. *C immitis, Coccidioides immitis; H capsulatum, Histoplasma capsulatum.*

- ☐ *C immitis*
- ▨ *H capsulatum*
- ☐ *B dermatitidis*

owned a dog reported that their dog was diagnosed with blastomycosis, often before the patients were found to have blastomycosis.[8]

PATHOGENESIS

B dermatitidis is a thermally dimorphic fungus that grows as a mold in the environment, as yeast in tissues, and at 35°C to 37°C in the laboratory. The environmental mold phase is typically observed in the laboratory at 25°C as white colonies that slowly turn a light brown color. The colonies consist of branching septate hyphae that produce conidia. Yeast cells are 8 to 20 μm in diameter and are characterized by a doubly thick, refractile cell wall and broad-based budding, with the daughter cell often as large as the mother cell before detachment. These characteristic features are useful for the identification of B dermatitidis (**Fig. 2**).

In the environment, conidia are aerosolized during activities that involve disruption of soil or decaying wood. Inhalation of aerosolized conidia represents the primary mechanism of infection of B dermatitidis, although rarely B dermatitidis can be directly inoculated by trauma and cause infection.[19] Key features in the pathogenesis of blastomycosis are summarized in **Fig. 3**.

Conidia are vulnerable to phagocytosis by macrophages and neutrophils.[1] Conidia that escape the innate immune host defenses convert to the yeast form. Conversion to the yeast form induces yeast-phase specific virulence factors that are critical for pathogenicity, immune evasion, and proliferation.[3] For example, changes in the composition of the cell wall that occur during this transition, including reduction in beta (1,3)-D-glucan, impede recognition of the yeast by dectin-1 receptors on innate immune cells.[20] This change might explain why beta (1,3)-D-glucan testing is not useful for the diagnosis of blastomycosis and may relate to the poor activity of echinocandins against B dermatitidis.[21] Important phase-specific genes for virulence factors of B dermatitidis have been described.[3] Molecular manipulation of these genes has been instrumental in our understanding of the pathogenesis of B dermatitidis infection.

The initial neutrophilic response and the subsequent cell-mediated immune response are manifested as a pyogranulomatous tissue response seen in lungs, skin, and other organs; this combined response may explain the lower incidence of blastomycosis, when compared with histoplasmosis, among immunosuppressed patients.[22] After conversion to the yeast phase, the organism can spread hematogenously to many other organs.[23] Ultimately, T-cell activation is necessary for control

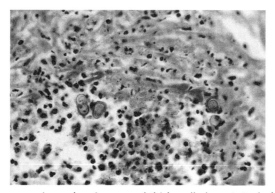

Fig. 2. A lung biopsy specimen showing several thick-walled yeasts typical of B dermatitidis (periodic acid-Schiff). Daughter buds are attached by a broad base to the mother cell.

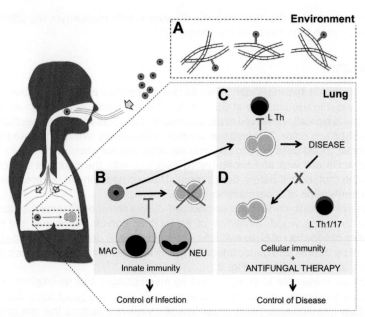

Fig. 3. Pathogenesis of blastomycosis. In the environment, *B dermatitidis* grows as branching septate hyphae that produce conidia (*A*). Infection occurs by inhalation of aerosolized conidia. After inhalation into the lungs, macrophages (MAC) and neutrophils (NEU) respond by phagocytizing and killing the conidia and preventing conversion to the yeast phase (*B*). Those conidia that escape the innate immune host defenses convert to the yeast phase (*C*). Progression of disease is facilitated by yeast-specific virulence factors that inhibit host cell cytokine production, impair T-helper lymphocyte (L Th) activation, and suppress nitric oxide production. Control of the disease typically requires Th1 and Th17 cell (L Th1/17) activation, which increases fungicidal activity of macrophages and antifungal therapy (*D*).

of this disease.[24,25] Humoral immunity seems to have little role. It is likely that in some people, a few viable organisms persist and can reactivate to cause pulmonary or extrapulmonary disease years later.[23]

CLINICAL MANIFESTATIONS

Blastomycosis causes a spectrum of illness in regard to severity and organ involvement, ranging from asymptomatic subclinical infection to widespread disseminated infection and, less commonly, fulminant pulmonary infection with ARDS. Most infected patients remain asymptomatic.[26] Blastomycosis most often involves the lungs, and symptoms appear after an incubation period of 2 to 6 weeks.[2,26] Disseminated, extrapulmonary infection can affect nearly every organ but most commonly involves the skin, bones/joints, genitourinary tract, and less often the central nervous system (CNS). Infections involving the eye, endocrine glands, larynx, breast, uterus, and peritoneum have been reported.[23]

Acute Pulmonary Blastomycosis

Approximately 50% of pulmonary infections remain subclinical, and infection seems to be limited to the lungs in 53% to 75% of patients.[8,12,27,28] Symptomatic patients with acute pulmonary blastomycosis present with cough with or without sputum, fever, chills, malaise, and pleuritic pain, similar to bacterial or viral pneumonias. These patients are often treated with antibacterial medications and may experience clinical improvement within 2 to 3 weeks of symptom onset that is falsely attributed to the antibiotic treatment rather than the self-limited nature of the infection. Even in endemic areas, blastomycosis is often only considered when symptoms persist despite multiple courses of antibacterial therapy.

The typical radiographic picture in symptomatic patients is an infiltrate in one or several lobes (**Fig. 4**). Reticulonodular and miliary patterns are seen less commonly. Hilar and mediastinal lymphadenopathy are uncommon in blastomycosis and suggest an alternative diagnosis, such as histoplasmosis. Occasionally, a chest radiograph or computed tomography (CT) scan performed for another indication reveals a nodular lesion that on biopsy is found to be *B dermatitidis* (**Fig. 5**). In order to prevent progression to chronic disease and dissemination, treatment is advised even if symptoms of the acute illness have resolved or an asymptomatic nodule is incidentally found.

Patients with acute pulmonary blastomycosis may present in extremis secondary to ARDS. ARDS can develop within a week of presentation despite appropriate antifungal treatment (**Fig. 6**). Many patients who develop ARDS are not immunocompromised and presumably had exposure to a large burden of conidia or their vigorous host response to the infection resulted in ARDS. In a recent case series, 15% of patients diagnosed with acute pulmonary blastomycosis developed ARDS, 23% required intensive care unit–level care, and mortality in those with ARDS was 47%.[29] Even though this recent experience reports improved mortality rates from those as high as 80% to 90% several decades ago, ARDS remains a very serious complication of blastomycosis.

Chronic Pulmonary Blastomycosis

Patients with chronic pulmonary blastomycosis may have fevers, weight loss, and night sweats. Persistent cough with sputum production and hemoptysis may or may not be present. The clinical syndrome is indistinguishable from that of pulmonary tuberculosis or chronic pulmonary histoplasmosis, and the radiographic findings can be similar to these diseases with upper-lobe thick-walled cavitary lesions. In other patients, sputum production is minimal and the chest radiographs show a masslike infiltrate that mimics lung cancer (**Fig. 7**). Chronic pulmonary blastomycosis is

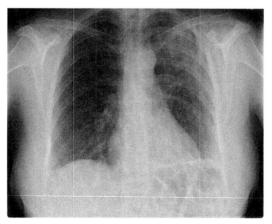

Fig. 4. Acute pulmonary blastomycosis in a 50-year-old woman whose infection subsequently progressed to involve the entire left lung.

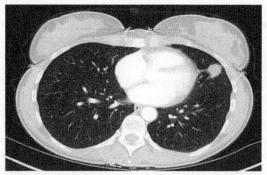

Fig. 5. CT scan of the thorax showing a solitary nodule in an asymptomatic woman in whom the CT scan was performed for another reason. Biopsy revealed typical yeast forms of *B dermatitidis*.

progressive if left untreated. Extrapulmonary manifestations are common, and finding cutaneous lesions is a clue to the diagnosis of blastomycosis.

Extrapulmonary Blastomycosis

B dermatitidis can disseminate to virtually any organ system. Approximately 25% to 40% of symptomatic blastomycosis is extrapulmonary, and manifestations often occur after the pulmonary manifestations have cleared. Unless patients give a convincing history of cutaneous inoculation, extrapulmonary involvement represents dissemination from a primary pulmonary infection.[30,31]

Skin manifestations

Cutaneous lesions occur in up to 60% of patients with extrapulmonary blastomycosis.[3] Lesions can appear at any site but are more commonly found on exposed areas. Lesions tend to be verrucous with raised, irregular borders and crusted

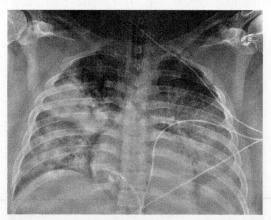

Fig. 6. ARDS in a 30-year-old healthy man who presented with progressive dyspnea and productive cough. He developed acute respiratory failure requiring intubation and ultimately extracorporeal membrane oxygenation. The diagnosis of blastomycosis was confirmed by growth of *B dermatitidis* on culture of bronchoalveolar lavage fluid.

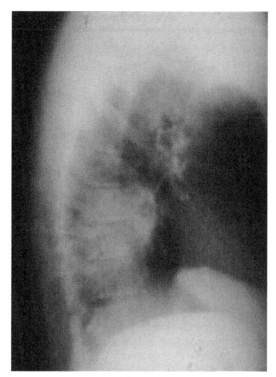

Fig. 7. Masslike lesion in the right lower lobe that was thought to be cancer but yielded *B dermatitidis* on culture of the biopsy specimen.

appearance or ulcerative with sharp borders and exudate at the base of the ulcer (**Fig. 8**). Skin lesions can also manifest as violaceous nodules or pustules or be keloid-like (**Fig. 9**). Facial lesions are common (**Fig. 10**). Cutaneous blastomycosis can be confused with basal cell or squamous cell carcinomas or pyoderma gangrenosum.[23]

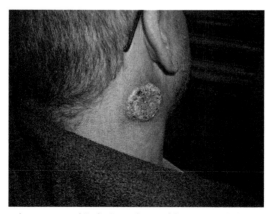

Fig. 8. One of several verrucous skin lesions due to blastomycosis in a 29-year-old man.

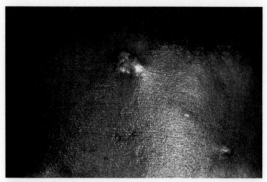

Fig. 9. Multiple pustular skin lesions that arose over several days in a patient who had disseminated blastomycosis.

Osteoarticular structures

B dermatitidis dissemination to osteoarticular structures represents about 25% of extrapulmonary infections.[23] Infection is usually indolent and most commonly involves long bones, followed by the vertebrae, although any bony structure can be involved. Patients present with localized pain, possibly a draining sinus tract, or erythema and warmth, and limitation of movement of a joint. Vertebral blastomycosis is often complicated by epidural, paravertebral, or psoas abscesses with the potential for cord compression. Radiographs show lytic lesions in the long bones, and MRI of the spine reveal discitis, vertebral body destruction, and paraspinal abscesses.[32]

Genitourinary tract

Blastomycosis involving the genitourinary tract is far more common in men than women. The prostate is most commonly affected, followed by the epididymis and testicles. Symptoms are testicular pain, dysuria, perineal discomfort, or urinary obstruction from prostate involvement.[33] In women, cases of uterine and tubo-ovarian abscesses have been reported rarely.[34] Adnexal involvement carries the potential for local extension leading to peritonitis and development of peritoneal and omental nodules.[35]

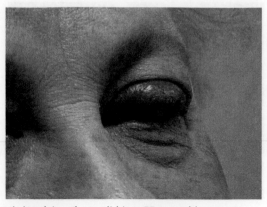

Fig. 10. Blastomycosis involving the eyelid in a 55-year-old woman.

Central nervous system

Involvement of the CNS occurs in only 5% to 10% of patients who have disseminated infection.[36] Manifestations include acute meningitis, isolated chronic meningitis, and intracranial abscesses. Patients can present with a variety of concerns, including headache, fever, altered mental status, nuchal rigidity, nausea, vomiting, visual changes, seizures, or focal neurologic deficits. In patients who have brain abscesses, contrast-enhanced CT scans or MRI show single or multiple ring-enhancing lesions in the brain and/or spinal cord.[37] In cases of chronic meningitis, examination of the cerebrospinal fluid (CSF) reveals a lymphocytic or neutrophilic predominant pleocytosis, elevated protein, and normal to low glucose.[37] Isolation of *B dermatitidis* in culture from CSF is unusual, and antigen testing is likely to be more helpful (see Diagnosis).

BLASTOMYCOSIS IN SPECIAL POPULATIONS
Immunocompromised Patients

Blastomycosis is described in patients with human immunodeficiency virus (HIV)/ AIDS, solid organ and hematopoietic cell transplant recipients, and patients who have been treated with immunosuppressive medications, including glucocorticoids, cytotoxic agents, and tumor necrosis factor (TNF)-alpha inhibitors. In one large series, only 2.7% of patients seen before 1978 were immunocompromised compared with 23.6% between 1978 and 1991.[38] Subsequent reports focused on specific populations, such as transplant recipients.[22,39,40] In general, immunocompromised patients develop more severe infection, are more likely to have symptomatic dissemination, have a greater risk of developing ARDS, and have higher mortality rates than patients who are immunocompetent.[38]

Human immunodeficiency virus/AIDS

Blastomycosis is not recognized as an AIDS-defining illness and is no more common in patients with HIV than non-HIV patients. Patients with AIDS are at risk for reactivation blastomycosis, which can occur years after initial infection.[41] Patients with AIDS with blastomycosis are more likely to manifest CNS involvement (40%) and severe pulmonary infection (20%). In early series, mortality rates were as high as 40% in the first few weeks after diagnosis.[41] Patients who received amphotericin B rather than an azole as initial therapy had better outcomes.

Transplant recipients

The overall incidence of blastomycosis among solid organ transplant recipients is low (<0.1%) and among hematopoietic cell transplant recipients is rare.[22] Transplant recipients are more likely to develop severe pulmonary disease complicated by respiratory failure.[39] There does not seem to be an increased risk of dissemination, and CNS involvement is uncommon. In one series of transplant recipients, the median time to disease onset after transplantation was 26 months (range 0.4–250.0 months).[39] To date, there are no reports of donor-derived blastomycosis.

Tumor necrosis factor–alpha inhibitor therapy

Increased use of TNF-alpha inhibitors has been accompanied by an increase in serious, often fatal, infections with the endemic mycoses.[42] In 2008, the Food and Drug Administration (FDA) issued a warning about the occurrence of fungal infections in patients receiving these agents and created a registry to monitor for endemic fungal infections.[43] A total of 7 cases of blastomycosis had been reported to the FDA by 2008. There has been no update on cases since this original release. One patient who developed CNS and disseminated blastomycosis while taking etanercept has been noted, but few clinical details were reported.[44]

Pregnancy

Blastomycosis is rare in pregnancy and is most commonly diagnosed in the second and third trimesters. Pregnant patients seem to have an increased risk of dissemination.[45] ARDS has been reported in a small number of cases.[46] The largest case series included 2 stillbirths attributed to fetal blastomycosis but also a case in which *B dermatitidis* was cultured from the placenta of a baby who remained healthy.[45] In most of the fatal cases, the mothers had not received antifungal therapy.[45,47]

Children

Children represent only 3% to 10% of all reported cases of blastomycosis.[48] Most children have pneumonia; skeletal involvement is more common than cutaneous manifestations.[49,50] CNS involvement also seems to be more common in children, with one series reporting this complication in 15% of cases, all of whom had mass lesions or abscesses.[50]

DIAGNOSIS

The diagnosis of blastomycosis is often delayed because of a low index of suspicion. In Mississippi, a state that has a high incidence of blastomycosis, pulmonary blastomycosis was correctly diagnosed at initial presentation only 5% of the time in one study.[12] If patients had both pulmonary symptoms and cutaneous lesions, the diagnosis rate increased to 64%. In nearly half of the patients, the diagnosis was made more than 30 days into their illness.[12] A thorough history that includes travel to endemic regions, recreational activities, occupation, construction in close proximity to the patients' residence, and exposure to decaying wood and compost should prompt consideration of blastomycosis in the differential diagnosis.

Culture

Definitive diagnosis is made by isolation of *B dermatitidis* in culture. In patients with pulmonary blastomycosis, diagnostic yield is high for both bronchoscopy and sputum samples.[51] Clinical samples should be plated on Sabouraud dextrose agar and typically demonstrate growth of a mold within 1 to 4 weeks.[52] A DNA probe assay is used to rapidly identify *B dermatitidis* from the culture.[1]

Histopathology

Direct visualization of *B dermatitidis* in fluid or tissues can lead to a rapid presumptive diagnosis of blastomycosis and initiation of antifungal therapy. Hematoxylin and eosin stains typically demonstrate an inflammatory, pyogranulomatous response; but fungal elements can be difficult to see.[52] The distinctive yeast form is better visualized after application of periodic acid-Schiff (see **Fig. 2**) or methenamine silver stain. A wet preparation of respiratory secretions using KOH or calcofluor white is low cost and can lead to a rapid presumptive diagnosis, as can a Papanicolaou stain on a cytology specimen of respiratory secretions.[1,23]

Antigen Detection

An enzyme immunoassay (EIA) for the detection of a polysaccharide cell wall antigen of *B dermatitidis* in urine, serum, bronchoalveolar lavage, and CSF (Mira Vista Diagnostics, Indianapolis, IN) has improved rapid diagnosis of blastomycosis.[5,53] The sensitivity of the detection of antigen in urine is reported to be 93%, but the specificity is low because of almost uniform cross reactivity in patients with histoplasmosis.[5]

Sensitivity seems to be lower for the detection of antigenemia. This test can also be used to follow the response to treatment of patients who have blastomycosis.

Serology

Serologic testing, including complement fixation, immunodiffusion, and EIA, has been used in epidemiologic studies but does not yet have a role in diagnosis because of poor sensitivity and significant cross reactivity with other dimorphic fungi, such as *Histoplasma capsulatum*. Several immunodiagnostic targets are under development for clinical use. The most promising assay seems to be an EIA using BAD-1 (formerly WI-1) antigen. Preliminary data show high sensitivity (88%) and specificity (99%) and low cross reactivity (6%) with *H capsulatum*.[54] It remains to be seen if this assay will prove useful for diagnosis.

Nucleic Acid Testing

Real time PCR assays for the rapid diagnosis of blastomycosis are currently under development. One assay demonstrated sensitivity and specificity of 100% with culture isolates and 86% in and 99% using direct clinical specimens.[55] A second assay targeting the *BAD1* gene promoter was highly specific and sensitive, detecting all haplotypes of *B dermatitidis* at low concentrations and in 5 of 6 paraffin-embedded tissues.[56] In both assays, there was no cross-reactivity with *H capsulatum* or other dimorphic fungi and time to result was 4 to 5 hours. However, neither assay is commercially available.

TREATMENT

The Infectious Diseases Society of America's guidelines for the treatment of blastomycosis emphasize that all patients with blastomycosis should receive antifungal therapy regardless of the clinical presentation because of the high likelihood of progression or recurrence of the infection if not treated.[57] The treatment of pulmonary and disseminated blastomycosis is determined by the severity of the disease, the presence of CNS involvement, and the host immune status.

Mild to Moderate Pulmonary or Disseminated Blastomycosis

Itraconazole is first-line therapy for mild to moderate blastomycosis[57,58] (**Box 1**). The usual dosage of itraconazole is 200 mg once or twice daily after an initial loading dose of 200 mg 3 times daily for 3 days.[58] Serum itraconazole levels should be obtained after steady state has been reached, typically after 2 weeks of therapy. A serum trough level greater than 1.0 mg/mL as measured by high performance liquid chromatography is recommended.[57] Patients should be treated for a minimum of 6 to 12 months.

If itraconazole is not tolerated, other azole agents can be used. Fluconazole is less active against *B dermatitidis*, and the dosage is 800 mg daily.[57,59] Voriconazole and posaconazole have excellent in vitro activity against *B dermatitidis*.[60,61] Voriconazole has been used successfully for the treatment of blastomycosis.[6,22,39] Clinical experience with posaconazole is currently limited to individual case reports.[62,63]

Moderately Severe to Severe Pulmonary or Disseminated Blastomycosis

The initial treatment of moderately severe to severe blastomycosis should be with a lipid formulation of amphotericin B, 3 to 5 mg/kg/d (**Box 2**). This treatment should be given for a few weeks until improvement is noted. If a lipid formulation of amphotericin B is not available, amphotericin B deoxycholate, 0.7 to 1.0 mg/kg/d, can be used; but this formulation is associated with more nephrotoxicity.[64]

Box 1
Treatment of pulmonary or disseminated blastomycosis, mild to moderate severity

- Preferred therapy
  - Itraconazole 200 mg TID × 3 days, then 200 mg BID

    - Measure trough levels after 2 weeks of therapy

    - Goal: 1 to 2 μg/mL combining itraconazole + hydroxyitraconazole, the active metabolite
- Alternative therapy if intolerant to itraconazole
  - Fluconazole 800 mg daily or 400 mg BID

    - Less active, monitor clinical response carefully

  - Voriconazole 400 mg BID × 1 day, then 200 mg BID

    - Measure trough serum levels after 5 days of therapy

    - Goal: 1 to 5 μg/mL

    - Highly variable serum levels requiring adjustment of the dose to achieve the safe and effective goal noted earlier
- Requires 6 to 12 months of treatment

After an initial clinical response with amphotericin B has been achieved, step-down therapy to an azole agent, usually itraconazole, is recommended for a total of at least 12 months of antifungal therapy. Voriconazole has been used in a few patients who had severe blastomycosis. The response was good in most patients[6,22]; but other reports noted mixed results,[39,40] and relapses were seen.[6]

Optimal management of blastomycosis-associated ARDS remains uncertain. Several reports suggest that intravenous methylprednisolone may be beneficial.[65,66] It is postulated that the antiinflammatory effect of corticosteroids attenuates the local

---

Box 2
Treatment of pulmonary or disseminated blastomycosis, moderately severe to severe

- Initial therapy
  - Lipid formulation amphotericin B, 3 to 5 mg/kg daily, for at least 1 to 2 weeks or until clinical response occurs
  - Amphotericin B deoxycholate, 0.7 to 1.0 mg/kg daily, can be used in children and if lipid formulation is not available
- Step-down therapy following clinical response
  - Itraconazole 200 mg TID × 3 days, then 200 mg BID

    - Measure trough levels after 2 weeks of therapy

    - Goal: 1 to 2 μg/mL combining itraconazole + hydroxyitraconazole, the active metabolite
- Alternative therapy if intolerant of itraconazole
  - Voriconazole 400 mg BID × 1 day, then 200 mg BID

    - Measure trough serum levels after 5 days of therapy

    - Goal: 1 to 5 μg/mL

    - Highly variable serum levels requiring adjustment of the dose to achieve the safe and effective goal noted earlier
- Requires 12 months of treatment

immune response and, thus, improves oxygen exchange.[66] The use of methylprednis-olone, even though not proved to be beneficial, is often used adjunctively in these very ill patients.

Extracorporeal membrane oxygenation (ECMO) has been used to support patients with severe blastomycosis-associated ARDS.[67,68] One report noted a successful outcome in 4 adult patients with blastomycosis-associated respiratory failure treated with ECMO.[69] The role of ECMO has yet to be fully elucidated.

Central Nervous System Blastomycosis

The recommended treatment of patients with CNS blastomycosis is a lipid formulation of amphotericin B, 5 mg/kg daily for 4 to 6 weeks, followed by step-down therapy with an azole for a total of at least a year of antifungal therapy (**Box 3**).

The preferred oral agent for step-down therapy in patients with CNS blastomycosis is yet to be determined. Itraconazole has excellent in vitro activity against *B dermatitidis*, but the CSF levels are very poor. Fluconazole, on the other hand, is not recommended for the treatment of blastomycosis but has excellent penetration into the CSF and has proved effective in treating CNS blastomycosis in a few patients.[70] Voriconazole achieves good CSF concentrations and also has excellent activity against the organism. Clinical experience has shown that voriconazole is effective in treating CNS blastomycosis.[5,71–73] It is likely that voriconazole will become the azole of choice for step-down therapy for CNS blastomycosis. Posaconazole does not achieve adequate levels in the CSF and should not be used. Depending on the response to therapy and the immune status of patients with CNS blastomycosis, lifelong therapy with an azole may be required to prevent relapse.[57]

Immunosuppressed Patients

Transplant recipients and other immunosuppressed patients who acquire blastomycosis should be treated initially with a lipid formulation of amphotericin B.[57] Initial azole therapy in transplant recipients has been associated with relapse and treatment

---

Box 3
Treatment of CNS blastomycosis

- Initial therapy
  - Lipid formulation amphotericin B 5 mg/kg daily for 4 to 6 weeks
- Step-down therapy
  - Voriconazole 400 mg BID × 1 day, then 200 to 300 mg BID
    - Measure trough serum levels after 5 days of therapy
    - Goal: 1 to 5 μg/mL
    - Highly variable serum levels requiring adjustment of the dose to achieve the safe and effective goal noted earlier
  - Fluconazole 800 mg daily or 400 mg BID
  - Itraconazole 200 mg TID × 3 days, then 200 mg BID
    - Measure trough levels after 2 weeks of therapy
    - Goal: 1 to 2 μg/mL combining itraconazole + hydroxyitraconazole, the active metabolite
- At least 12 months of treatment AND until resolution of CSF abnormalities
- Requires lifelong suppression with an azole in some patients

failure.[38,40] After patients show a good clinical response, therapy can be transitioned to oral itraconazole, for a total of 12 months of antifungal therapy. Voriconazole can be used for patients who cannot tolerate itraconazole.[5,6,22,39] The need for long-term secondary prophylaxis in the immunocompromised host is not well established, but persistent immunosuppression poses an increased risk for relapse and recurrence. Thus, continuation of therapy with an azole is prudent in those who remain on immunosuppressive agents.

Pregnant Women and Children

Treatment during pregnancy should prevent transplacental transmission and avoid teratogenicity. Amphotericin B remains the drug of choice in pregnant women. Azoles are teratogenic and should be avoided during pregnancy. Children tolerate amphotericin B deoxycholate better than adults and can be treated with either amphotericin B deoxycholate or a lipid formulation of amphotericin B.[57] Itraconazole is the treatment of choice for children with mild to moderate infection.

OUTCOMES

Overall mortality associated with blastomycosis is reported to be 4% to 6%.[3] Mortality rates as high as 18% have been reported in patients with CNS blastomycosis and as high as 89% in patients with ARDS.[13,37,65] Immunocompromising conditions, such as AIDS and solid organ transplantation, were associated with mortality rates as high as 25% to 41% in several earlier series.[37–41] However, more recent case series report mortality rates of 45% in patients with ARDS and no deaths from blastomycosis in organ transplant recipients.[22] There have been several large case series in the United States reporting higher mortality associated with Native American and African American race/ethnicity.[9,74] A retrospective series from Manitoba found an increased incidence of blastomycosis in Aboriginal patients but no difference in mortality.[11] The retrospective nature of all of these reports limits further analysis. Mortality rates are low in children, possibly because of fewer comorbidities and better tolerance of amphotericin B.

REFERENCES

1. Saccente M, Woods GL. Clinical and laboratory update on blastomycosis. Clin Microbiol Rev 2010;23:367–81.
2. Smith JA, Kauffman CA. Blastomycosis. Proc Am Thorac Soc 2010;7:173–80.
3. Smith JA, Gauthier G. New developments in blastomycosis. Semin Respir Crit Care Med 2015;36(5):715–28.
4. Lemos LB, Baliga M, Guo M. Acute respiratory distress syndrome and blastomycosis: presentation of nine cases and review of the literature. Ann Diagn Pathol 2001;5:1–9.
5. Bariola JR, Hage CA, Durkin M, et al. Detection of *Blastomyces dermatitidis* antigen in patients with newly diagnosed blastomycosis. Diagn Microbiol Infect Dis 2011;69:187–91.
6. Freifeld A, Proia L, Andes D, et al. Voriconazole use for endemic fungal infections. Antimicrob Agents Chemother 2009;53:1648–51.
7. Klein BS, Vergeront JM, DiSalvo AF, et al. Two outbreaks of blastomycosis along rivers in Wisconsin. Isolation of *Blastomyces dermatitidis* from riverbank soil and evidence of its transmission along waterways. Am Rev Respir Dis 1987;136: 1333–8.

8. Baumgardner DJ, Buggy BP, Mattson BJ, et al. Epidemiology of blastomycosis in a region of high endemicity in north central Wisconsin. Clin Infect Dis 1992;15: 629–35.

9. Dworkin MS, Duckro AN, Proia L, et al. The epidemiology of blastomycosis in Illinois and factors associated with death. Clin Infect Dis 2005;41:e107–11.

10. Cano MV, Ponce-de-Leon GF, Tippen S, et al. Blastomycosis in Missouri: epidemiology and risk factors for endemic disease. Epidemiol Infect 2003;131:907–14.

11. Crampton TL, Light RB, Berg GM, et al. Epidemiology and clinical spectrum of blastomycosis diagnosed at Manitoba hospitals. Clin Infect Dis 2002;34:1310–6.

12. Chapman SW, Lin AC, Hendricks KA, et al. Endemic blastomycosis in Mississippi: epidemiological and clinical studies. Semin Respir Infect 1997;12:219–28.

13. Vasquez JE, Mehta JB, Agrawal R, et al. Blastomycosis in northeast Tennessee. Chest 1998;114:436–43.

14. Carlos WG, Rose AS, Wheat LJ, et al. Blastomycosis in Indiana: digging up more cases. Chest 2010;138:1377–82.

15. De Groote MA, Bjerke R, Smith H, et al. Expanding epidemiology of blastomycosis: clinical features and investigation of 2 cases in Colorado. Clin Infect Dis 2000;30:582–4.

16. Randhawa HS, Chowdhary A, Kathuria S, et al. Blastomycosis in India: report of an imported case and current status. Med Mycol 2013;51:185–92.

17. Roy M, Benedict K, Deak E, et al. A large community outbreak of blastomycosis in Wisconsin with geographic and ethnic clustering. Clin Infect Dis 2013;57:655–62.

18. Anderson JL, Dieckman JL, Reed KD, et al. Canine blastomycosis in Wisconsin: a survey of small-animal veterinary practices. Med Mycol 2014;52:774–9.

19. Smith JA, Riddell J, Kauffman CA. Cutaneous manifestations of endemic mycoses. Curr Infect Dis Rep 2013;15:440–9.

20. Koneti A, Linke MJ, Brummer E, et al. Evasion of innate immune responses: evidence for mannose binding lectin inhibition of tumor necrosis factor alpha production by macrophages in response to *Blastomyces dermatitidis*. Infect Immun 2008;76:994–1002.

21. Girouard G, Lachance C, Pelletier R. Observations on (1-3)-beta-D-glucan detection as a diagnostic tool in endemic mycosis caused by *Histoplasma* or *Blastomyces*. J Med Microbiol 2007;56:1001–2.

22. Kauffman CA, Freifeld AG, Andes DR, et al. Endemic fungal infections in solid organ and hematopoietic cell transplant recipients enrolled in the Transplant-Associated Infection Surveillance Network (TRANSNET). Transpl Infect Dis 2014;16:213–24.

23. Bradsher RW, Bariola JR. Blastomycosis. In: Kauffman CA, Pappas PG, Sobel JD, et al, editors. Essentials of clinical mycology. 2nd edition. New York: Springer; 2011. p. 337–48.

24. Wuthrich M, Gern B, Hung CY, et al. Vaccine-induced protection against 3 systemic mycoses endemic to North America requires Th17 cells in mice. J Clin Invest 2011;121:554–68.

25. Bradsher RW, Balk RA, Jacobs RF. Growth inhibition of *Blastomyces dermatitidis* in alveolar and peripheral macrophages from patients with blastomycosis. Am Rev Respir Dis 1987;135:412–7.

26. Klein BS, Vergeront JM, Weeks RJ, et al. Isolation of *Blastomyces dermatitidis* in soil associated with a large outbreak of blastomycosis in Wisconsin. N Engl J Med 1986;314:529–34.

27. Bradsher RW. Histoplasmosis and blastomycosis. Clin Infect Dis 1996;22(Suppl 2):S102–11.

28. Pappas PG. Blastomycosis. Semin Respir Crit Care Med 2004;25:113–21.
29. Azar MM, Assi R, Relich RF, et al. Blastomycosis in Indiana: clinical and epidemiologic patterns of disease gleaned from a multicenter retrospective study. Chest 2015. http://dx.doi.org/10.1378/chest.15-0289.
30. Lemos LB, Guo M, Baliga M. Blastomycosis: organ involvement and etiologic diagnosis. A review of 123 patients from Mississippi. Ann Diagn Pathol 2000;4: 391–406.
31. Gray NA, Baddour LM. Cutaneous inoculation blastomycosis. Clin Infect Dis 2002;34:e44–9.
32. Saccente M, Abernathy RS, Pappas PG, et al. Vertebral blastomycosis with paravertebral abscess: report of eight cases and review of the literature. Clin Infect Dis 1998;26:413–8.
33. Watts B, Argekar P, Saint S, et al. Clinical problem-solving. Building a diagnosis from the ground up. N Engl J Med 2007;356:1456–62.
34. Murray JJ, Clark CA, Lands RH, et al. Reactivation blastomycosis presenting as a tubo-ovarian abscess. Obstet Gynecol 1984;64:828–30.
35. Barocas JA, Gauthier GM. Peritonitis caused by Blastomyces dermatitidis in a kidney transplant recipient: case report and literature review. Transpl Infect Dis 2014;16:634–41.
36. Bradsher RW, Chapman SW, Pappas PG. Blastomycosis. Infect Dis Clin North Am 2003;17:21–40.
37. Bariola JR, Perry P, Pappas PG, et al. Blastomycosis of the central nervous system: a multicenter review of diagnosis and treatment in the modern era. Clin Infect Dis 2010;50:797–804.
38. Pappas PG, Threlkeld MG, Bedsole GD, et al. Blastomycosis in immunocompromised patients. Medicine (Baltimore) 1993;72:311–25.
39. Gauthier GM, Safdar N, Klein BS, et al. Blastomycosis in solid organ transplant recipients. Transpl Infect Dis 2007;9:310–7.
40. Grim SA, Proia L, Miller R, et al. A multicenter study of histoplasmosis and blastomycosis after solid organ transplantation. Transpl Infect Dis 2012;14: 17–23.
41. Pappas PG, Pottage JC, Powderly WG, et al. Blastomycosis in patients with the acquired immunodeficiency syndrome. Ann Intern Med 1992;116:847–53.
42. Smith JA, Kauffman CA. Endemic fungal infections in patients receiving tumor necrosis factor-alpha inhibitor therapy. Drugs 2009;69:1403–15.
43. FDA Alert. Information for healthcare professionals: Cimzia (certolizumab pegol), Enbrel (etanercept), Humira (adalimumab), and Remicade (infliximab). Available at: http://www.fda.gov/Drugs/DrugSafety/PostmarketDrugSafetyInformationfor PatientsandProviders/ucm124185.htm. Accessed August 23, 2015.
44. Proia LA. Treatment of blastomycosis. Curr Fungal Infect Rep 2010;4:23–9.
45. Lemos LB, Soofi M, Amir E. Blastomycosis and pregnancy. Ann Diagn Pathol 2002;6:211–5.
46. MacDonald D, Alguire PC. Adult respiratory distress syndrome due to blastomycosis during pregnancy. Chest 1990;98:1527–8.
47. Maxson S, Miller SF, Tryka AF, et al. Perinatal blastomycosis: a review. Pediatr Infect Dis J 1992;11:760–3.
48. Varkey B. Blastomycosis in children. Semin Respir Infect 1997;12:235–42.
49. Schutze GE, Hickerson SL, Fortin EM, et al. Blastomycosis in children. Clin Infect Dis 1996;22:496–502.
50. Brick KE, Drolet BA, Lyon VB, et al. Cutaneous and disseminated blastomycosis: a pediatric case series. Pediatr Dermatol 2013;30:23–8.

51. Martynowicz MA, Prakash UB. Pulmonary blastomycosis: an appraisal of diagnostic techniques. Chest 2002;121:768–73.

52. Areno JP, Campbell GD Jr, George RB. Diagnosis of blastomycosis. Semin Respir Infect 1997;12:252–62.

53. Connolly P, Hage CA, Bariola JR, et al. *Blastomyces dermatitidis* antigen detection by quantitative enzyme immunoassay. Clin Vaccine Immunol 2012;19:53–6.

54. Richer SM, Smedema ML, Durkin MM, et al. Development of a highly sensitive and specific blastomycosis antibody enzyme immunoassay using *Blastomyces dermatitidis* surface protein BAD-1. Clin Vaccine Immunol 2014;21:143–6.

55. Babady NE, Buckwalter SP, Hall L, et al. Detection of *Blastomyces dermatitidis* and *Histoplasma capsulatum* from culture isolates and clinical specimens by use of real-time PCR. J Clin Microbiol 2011;49:3204–8.

56. Sidamonidze K, Peck MK, Perez M, et al. Real-time PCR assay for identification of *Blastomyces dermatitidis* in culture and in tissue. J Clin Microbiol 2012;50:1783–6.

57. Chapman SW, Dismukes WE, Proia LA, et al. Clinical practice guidelines for the management of blastomycosis: 2008 update by the Infectious Diseases Society of America. Clin Infect Dis 2008;46:1801–12.

58. Dismukes WE, Bradsher RW, Cloud GC, et al. Itraconazole therapy for blastomycosis and histoplasmosis. Am J Med 1992;93:489–97.

59. Pappas PG, Bradsher RW, Chapman SW, et al. Treatment of blastomycosis with fluconazole: a pilot study. Clin Infect Dis 1995;20:267–71.

60. Li RK, Ciblak MA, Nordoff N, et al. In vitro activities of voriconazole, itraconazole, and amphotericin B against *Blastomyces dermatitidis, Coccidioides immitis*, and *Histoplasma capsulatum*. Antimicrob Agents Chemother 2000;44:1734–6.

61. Espinel-Ingroff A. Comparison of in vitro activities of the new triazole SCH56592 and the echinocandins MK-0991 (L-743,872) and LY303366 against opportunistic filamentous and dimorphic fungi and yeasts. J Clin Microbiol 1998;36:2950–6.

62. Proia LA, Harnisch DO. Successful use of posaconazole for treatment of blastomycosis. Antimicrob Agents Chemother 2012;56:4029.

63. Day SR, Weiss DB, Hazen KC, et al. Successful treatment of osseous blastomycosis without pulmonary or disseminated disease and review of the literature. Diagn Microbiol Infect Dis 2014;79:242–4.

64. Miceli MH, Chandrasekar P. Safety and efficacy of liposomal amphotericin B for the empirical therapy of invasive fungal infections in immunocompromised patients. Infect Drug Resist 2012;5:9–16.

65. Lahm T, Neese S, Thornburg AT, et al. Corticosteroids for blastomycosis-induced ARDS: a report of two patients and review of the literature. Chest 2008;133:1478–80.

66. Plamondon M, Lamontagne F, Allard C, et al. Corticosteroids as adjunctive therapy in severe blastomycosis-induced acute respiratory distress syndrome in an immunosuppressed patient. Clin Infect Dis 2010;51:e1–3.

67. Resch M, Kurz K, Schneider-Brachert W, et al. Extracorporeal membrane oxygenation (ECMO) for severe acute respiratory distress syndrome (ARDS) in fulminant blastomycosis in Germany. BMJ Case Rep 2009;2009.

68. Dalton HJ, Hertzog JH, Hannan RL, et al. Extracorporeal membrane oxygenation for overwhelming *Blastomyces dermatitidis* pneumonia. Crit Care 1999;3:91–4.

69. Bednarczyk JM, Kethireddy S, White CW, et al. Extracorporeal membrane oxygenation for blastomycosis-related acute respiratory distress syndrome: a case series. Can J Anaesth 2015;62:807–15.

70. Pearson GJ, Chin TW, Fong IW. Case report: treatment of blastomycosis with fluconazole. Am J Med Sci 1992;303:313–5.
71. Borgia SM, Fuller JD, Sarabia A, et al. Cerebral blastomycosis: a case series incorporating voriconazole in the treatment regimen. Med Mycol 2006;44:659–64.
72. Bakleh M, Aksamit AJ, Tleyjeh IM, et al. Successful treatment of cerebral blastomycosis with voriconazole. Clin Infect Dis 2005;40:e69–71.
73. Panicker J, Walsh T, Kamani N. Recurrent central nervous system blastomycosis in an immunocompetent child treated successfully with sequential liposomal amphotericin B and voriconazole. Pediatr Infect Dis J 2006;25:377–9.
74. Khuu D, Shafir S, Bristow B, et al. Blastomycosis mortality rates, United States, 1990-2010. Emerg Infect Dis 2014;20:1789–94.

Contemporary Strategies in the Prevention and Management of Fungal Infections

Philipp Koehler, MD[a,b], Oliver A. Cornely, MD[a,b,c,d],*

KEYWORDS

- Invasive candidiasis • Invasive aspergillosis • Mucormycosis • Prophylaxis
- Empiric therapy • Targeted therapy

KEY POINTS

- The nonendemic invasive fungal infections with the highest prevalence are invasive aspergillosis, invasive candidiasis, and invasive mucormycosis.
- Lack of reliable diagnostics and high mortality lead to complex treatment strategies by means of prophylaxis, fever-driven, diagnosis-driven, and targeted treatment approaches, and combinations of these.
- Pharmacologic prophylaxis or treatment depends on clinical setting, individual risk profile, pathogen, safety profile, and concomitant medication.

INTRODUCTION

Current strategies in the prevention and management of invasive fungal infections are characterized by lack of reliable diagnostic tests and by heterogeneity of patient populations at risk. In these populations, a variety of risk factors predispose for different fungal pathogens. The major diseases are invasive candidiasis, invasive aspergillosis, and mucormycosis.[1–4] Invasive aspergillosis and mucormycosis are

Disclosure Statement: P. Koehler has received travel grants from Merck/MSD and received lecture honoraria from Astellas. O.A. Cornely has received research grants from Astellas, Basilea, Gilead, Merck/MSD, Miltenyi, Pfizer, is a consultant to Astellas, Basilea, Cidara, F2G, Gilead, Merck/MSD, Pfizer, Vical, and received lecture honoraria from Astellas, Basilea, Gilead, and Merck/MSD.

[a] Department I of Internal Medicine, University Hospital of Cologne, Kerpener Str. 62, Cologne 50937, Germany; [b] Cologne Excellence Cluster on Cellular Stress Responses in Aging-Associated Diseases (CECAD), University of Cologne, Joseph-Stelzmann-Str. 26, Cologne 50931, Germany; [c] Clinical Trials Centre Cologne, ZKS Köln, Gleueler Str. 269, Cologne 50935, Germany; [d] German Centre for Infection Research, Partner Site Bonn-Cologne, Kerpener Str. 62, Cologne 50937, Germany
* Corresponding author. Department I of Internal Medicine, University Hospital of Cologne, Kerpener Str. 62, Cologne 50937, Germany.
E-mail address: oliver.cornely@uk-koeln.de

Infect Dis Clin N Am 30 (2016) 265–275
http://dx.doi.org/10.1016/j.idc.2015.10.003
0891-5520/16/$ – see front matter © 2016 Elsevier Inc. All rights reserved.

predominantly found in patients with well-defined profound immunosuppression, whereas invasive candidiasis occurs frequently in less well-defined states of immunosuppression. Administration of systemic antifungal medication is continuously rising and antifungal stewardship programs with emphasis on diagnostic-driven approaches are needed to guide antifungal treatment, to avoid inappropriate therapies, and to save costs.[5–9]

CONTEMPORARY STRATEGIES IN THE PREVENTION AND MANAGEMENT OF INVASIVE CANDIDIASIS
Pharmacologic Prevention of Invasive Candidiasis

The non-neutropenic patient population at risk for invasive candidiasis comprises individuals on intensive care units (ICUs) and patients with gastrointestinal perforation, recent abdominal surgery, or anastomotic leakages developing intra-abdominal candidiasis.[10] In the latter cases, prophylactic use of fluconazole is recommended.[11] Trials on prophylactic antifungal medication for broader ranges of patients in the ICU did not show a reduction in mortality, but selection of less-susceptible or even resistant *Candida glabrata* strains remained a relevant problem.[12]

In terms of hematology-oncology patient populations, one should differentiate between autologous and allogeneic hematopoietic stem cell recipients (HSCT), pre or post allogeneic HSCT, and non-HSCT recipients with severe, prolonged neutropenia. For *Candida* prophylaxis during neutropenia after conditioning chemotherapy for allogeneic HSCT, azoles have been recommended,[13] in particular fluconazole[14–18] and voriconazole.[19] Micafungin and posaconazole yielded results similar to fluconazole.[20,21]

For autologous HSCT and patients with prolonged neutropenia, data are lacking. Reasons lie in the overlapping antifungal activity of prophylactic medication against *Aspergillus* as well as *Candida*. Another reason is that neutropenia during autologous HSCT is too short to impose a high risk for invasive candidiasis.[13] For patients with prolonged neutropenia, only one trial demonstrated improved survival rates with posaconazole prophylaxis, but that difference was not due to invasive candidiasis, but aspergillosis.[22]

Management of Invasive Candidiasis: Fever or Diagnostic-Driven Approach

A recent randomized, double-blind, placebo-controlled trial exploring the preemptive use of micafungin in patients undergoing emergency gastrointestinal surgery did not show significant decrease of invasive candidiasis.[23]

Risk-based strategies based on scoring systems were developed to guide clinicians regarding empirical, that is, fever-driven, antifungal therapy and to avoid treatment delays: the *Candida* score, colonization index, and different predictive rules facilitating a prediction of invasive candidiasis.[24–28]

During neutropenia, broad-spectrum antibacterial treatment is mandatory with the first fever. When fever persists for 72 to 96 hours in patients who were not on broad-spectrum antifungal prophylaxis, an antifungal will typically be added. Such empiric antifungal treatment is usually directed toward yeasts and molds. Local epidemiology informs the choice of the empiric antifungal. Broad-spectrum antifungal drugs recommended are caspofungin[29,30] and liposomal amphotericin B.[31] It is important to know that *Candida* species recovered from respiratory, urine, or stool samples proves colonization only and is not a treatment indication.[11]

Management of Invasive Candidiasis: Targeted Treatment

Microscopic evidence of yeasts in a blood culture is the easiest proof of invasive fungal infection due to *Candida* species (**Fig. 1**). On diagnosis, immediate treatment with echinocandins as the drugs of choice is recommended.[32–35] Delays to treatment

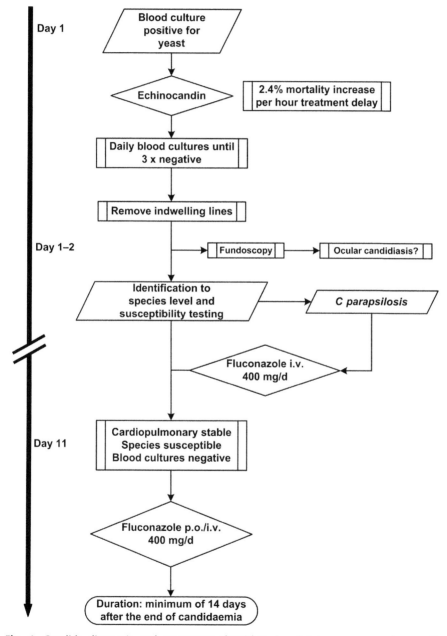

Fig. 1. *Candida* diagnosis and treatment algorithm. i.v., intravenous; p.o., by mouth. (*From* Koehler P, Tacke D, Cornely OA. Our 2014 approach to candidaemia. Mycoses 2014;57(10):582; with permission.)

start increase mortality rates so profoundly that mortality has been expressed per hour.[13,36–42] Species identification and susceptibility testing are essential to guide management.[11,36,43,44] The initial echinocandin treatment should be replaced with fluconazole if *Candida parapsilosis* is identified.[11] If a patient received previous antifungal prophylaxis, a change in drug class appears reasonable. Duration of treatment is at least 14 days after the last positive blood culture.[13] After 10 days of intravenous treatment, step down to oral fluconazole may be feasible if species is susceptible and no organ involvement has been diagnosed.[13,45–47] Prolonged intravenous treatment duration is mandatory in complicated or disseminated candidiasis.[13] To increase survival rates, the removal of indwelling catheters is recommended.[48] If removal is not possible, echinocandins and liposomal amphotericin B are preferred choices because of their biofilm activity.[49,50]

CONTEMPORARY STRATEGIES IN THE PREVENTION AND MANAGEMENT OF INVASIVE ASPERGILLOSIS
Pharmacologic Prevention of Invasive Aspergillosis

Antifungal drugs active against *Aspergillus* species are azoles (except fluconazole), echinocandins, and polyenes.[51] Patients with prolonged neutropenia or allogeneic HSCT recipients are at high risk for invasive aspergillosis. In the preengraftment phase of allogeneic HSCT, antifungal prophylaxis was successful with micafungin, posaconazole, and voriconazole.[19,20,22,51–54] Postengraftment, in particular during graft-versus-host disease (GVHD), posaconazole is protective.[21] To prevent invasive aspergillosis in patients with chemotherapy-induced neutropenia, for example, with acute myeloid leukemia, myelodysplastic syndrome, or severe aplastic anemia, posaconazole is regarded as the drug of choice.[22,51] In case of restricted bioavailability, for example, due to gastrointestinal GVHD or vomiting, posaconazole tablets are a well-tolerated alternative with more reliable pharmacokinetics.[55]

Management of Invasive Aspergillosis: Fever or Diagnostic-Driven Approach

For empiric therapy of invasive aspergillosis, caspofungin and liposomal amphotericin B are the antifungals of choice.[30,31,56] As the true incidence of invasive aspergillosis was estimated to be much lower than the number of patients receiving *Aspergillus*-directed empiric treatment, diagnostic-driven approaches were developed. With the addition of microbiological tests to radiographic imaging, the diagnostic yield increased (**Fig. 2**). Galactomannan or *Aspergillus* polymerase chain reaction assays enhance sensitivity, spare unneeded antifungal therapy, and in combination provide earlier diagnosis.[57–62]

Management of Invasive Aspergillosis: Targeted Treatment

Voriconazole is the drug of choice for invasive aspergillosis because of improved response and survival rates, and safety and tolerability when compared with amphotericin B deoxycholate[63] (**Fig. 3**A). In profoundly immunocompromised patients, liposomal amphotericin B appeared to have comparable efficacy at standard dose, although the compound has not been directly compared with voriconazole.[64] In breakthrough aspergillosis during azole prophylaxis, liposomal amphotericin B is the drug of choice. For caspofungin, data are less clear and currently it is not licensed nor recommended for first-line treatment of invasive aspergillosis.[65–67] A recent clinical trial showed similar success rates for isavuconazole and voriconazole, and better tolerability of isavuconazole, so that the new compound was approved by the US Food and Drug Administration for the treatment of invasive aspergillosis[68–71] and may be used as an alternative (see **Fig. 3**A).

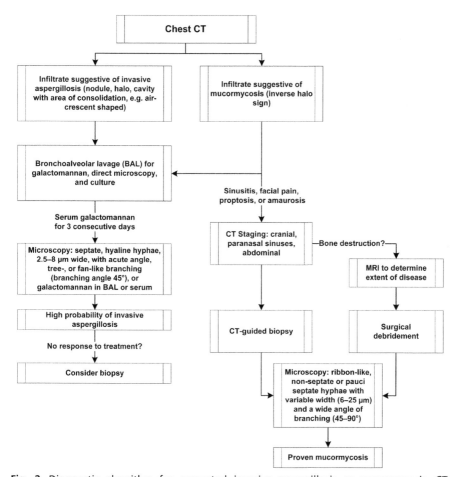

Fig. 2. Diagnostic algorithm for suspected invasive aspergillosis or mucormycosis. CT, computed tomography. (*Adapted from* Liss B, Vehreschild JJ, Bangard C, et al. Our 2015 approach to invasive pulmonary aspergillosis. Mycoses 2015;58(6):376; and Tacke D, Koehler P, Markiefka B, et al. Our 2014 approach to mucormycosis. Mycoses 2014;57(9):521.)

CONTEMPORARY STRATEGIES IN THE PREVENTION AND MANAGEMENT OF MUCORMYCOSIS

Pharmacologic Prevention of Mucormycosis

Currently, posaconazole is the drug of choice for prophylaxis, as there are only a few drugs with activity against Mucorales.[72]

Management of Mucormycosis: Targeted Treatment

Mucormycosis is an ultra-orphan disease with an estimated frequency of 0.1 per 100,000 population. Consequently no large randomized trial has been published for the treatment of mucormycosis. Surgical debridement is an integral part of the management of mucormycosis, as it has been associated with decreased mortality.[73] Additionally, immediate administration of high-dose liposomal amphotericin B is recommended. Many patients with mucormycosis have been treated with posaconazole

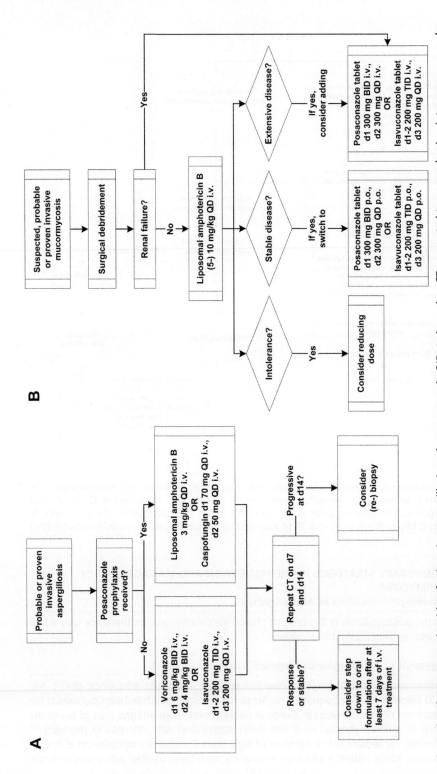

Fig. 3. (A, B) Treatment algorithm for invasive aspergillosis and mucormycosis. BID, twice a day; CT, computed tomography; i.v., intravenous; p.o., by mouth; QD, every day; TID, 3 times a day. (*Adapted from* Refs.[68,78,79].)

either first line or in salvage settings.[74–76] With the advent and approval of isavuconazole, a new treatment option is now available for mucormycosis.[69–71] A matched case-control analysis was used to compare 21 patients with primary isavuconazole treatment with 33 patients treated with amphotericin B formulations in the FungiScope registry.[68] Both groups had similar mortality so that isavuconazole is a new treatment option for mucormycosis. For extensive disease, combination treatment may be considered (see **Fig. 3**B).[68,77]

REFERENCES

1. Wisplinghoff H, Ebbers J, Geurtz L, et al. Nosocomial bloodstream infections due to *Candida* spp. in the USA: species distribution, clinical features and antifungal susceptibilities. Int J Antimicrob Agents 2014;43(1):78–81.
2. Lewis RE, Cahyame-Zuniga L, Leventakos K, et al. Epidemiology and sites of involvement of invasive fungal infections in patients with haematological malignancies: a 20-year autopsy study. Mycoses 2013;56(6):638–45.
3. Pfaller MA, Diekema DJ. Epidemiology of invasive candidiasis: a persistent public health problem. Clin Microbiol Rev 2007;20(1):133–63.
4. Maschmeyer G, Haas A, Cornely OA. Invasive aspergillosis: epidemiology, diagnosis and management in immunocompromised patients. Drugs 2007;67(11):1567–601.
5. Azoulay E, Dupont H, Tabah A, et al. Systemic antifungal therapy in critically ill patients without invasive fungal infection*. Crit Care Med 2012;40(3):813–22.
6. Valerio M, Munoz P, Rodriguez CG, et al. Antifungal stewardship in a tertiary-care institution: a bedside intervention. Clin Microbiol Infect 2015;21(5):492.e1–9.
7. Valerio M, Vena A, Bouza E, et al. How much European prescribing physicians know about invasive fungal infections management? BMC Infect Dis 2015;15:80.
8. Dellit TH, Owens RC, McGowan JE Jr, et al. Infectious Diseases Society of America and the Society for Healthcare Epidemiology of America guidelines for developing an institutional program to enhance antimicrobial stewardship. Clin Infect Dis 2007;44(2):159–77.
9. Barnes R, Earnshaw S, Herbrecht R, et al. Economic comparison of an empirical versus diagnostic-driven strategy for treating invasive fungal disease in immunocompromised patients. Clin Ther 2015;37(6):1317–28.e2.
10. Bassetti M, Righi E, Ansaldi F, et al. A multicenter multinational study of abdominal candidiasis: epidemiology, outcomes and predictors of mortality. Intensive Care Med 2015;41(9):1601–10.
11. Cornely OA, Bassetti M, Calandra T, et al. ESCMID* guideline for the diagnosis and management of Candida diseases 2012: non-neutropenic adult patients. Clin Microbiol Infect 2012;18(Suppl 7):19–37.
12. Perlin DS. Mechanisms of echinocandin antifungal drug resistance. Ann N Y Acad Sci 2015;1354:1–11.
13. Ullmann AJ, Akova M, Herbrecht R, et al. ESCMID* guideline for the diagnosis and management of Candida diseases 2012: adults with haematological malignancies and after haematopoietic stem cell transplantation (HCT). Clin Microbiol Infect 2012;18(Suppl 7):53–67.
14. Goodman JL, Winston DJ, Greenfield RA, et al. A controlled trial of fluconazole to prevent fungal infections in patients undergoing bone marrow transplantation. N Engl J Med 1992;326(13):845–51.
15. Marr KA, Seidel K, Slavin MA, et al. Prolonged fluconazole prophylaxis is associated with persistent protection against candidiasis-related death in allogeneic

marrow transplant recipients: long-term follow-up of a randomized, placebo-controlled trial. Blood 2000;96(6):2055–61.

16. Slavin MA, Osborne B, Adams R, et al. Efficacy and safety of fluconazole prophylaxis for fungal infections after marrow transplantation–a prospective, randomized, double-blind study. J Infect Dis 1995;171(6):1545–52.

17. Marr KA, Crippa F, Leisenring W, et al. Itraconazole versus fluconazole for prevention of fungal infections in patients receiving allogeneic stem cell transplants. Blood 2004;103(4):1527–33.

18. Morgenstern GR, Prentice AG, Prentice HG, et al. A randomized controlled trial of itraconazole versus fluconazole for the prevention of fungal infections in patients with haematological malignancies. U.K. Multicentre Antifungal Prophylaxis Study Group. Br J Haematol 1999;105(4):901–11.

19. Wingard JR, Carter SL, Walsh TJ, et al. Randomized, double-blind trial of fluconazole versus voriconazole for prevention of invasive fungal infection after allogeneic hematopoietic cell transplantation. Blood 2010;116(24):5111–8.

20. van Burik JA, Ratanatharathorn V, Stepan DE, et al. Micafungin versus fluconazole for prophylaxis against invasive fungal infections during neutropenia in patients undergoing hematopoietic stem cell transplantation. Clin Infect Dis 2004; 39(10):1407–16.

21. Ullmann AJ, Lipton JH, Vesole DH, et al. Posaconazole or fluconazole for prophylaxis in severe graft-versus-host disease. N Engl J Med 2007;356(4):335–47.

22. Cornely OA, Maertens J, Winston DJ, et al. Posaconazole vs. fluconazole or itraconazole prophylaxis in patients with neutropenia. N Engl J Med 2007;356(4):348–59.

23. Knitsch W, Vincent JL, Utzolino S, et al. A randomized, placebo-controlled trial of pre-emptive antifungal therapy for the prevention of invasive candidiasis following gastrointestinal surgery for intra-abdominal infections. Clin Infect Dis 2015. [Epub ahead of print].

24. Charles PE, Dalle F, Aube H, et al. *Candida* spp. colonization significance in critically ill medical patients: a prospective study. Intensive Care Med 2005;31(3): 393–400.

25. Eggimann P, Que YA, Revelly JP, et al. Preventing invasive candida infections. Where could we do better? J Hosp Infect 2015;89(4):302–8.

26. Leon C, Ruiz-Santana S, Saavedra P, et al. A bedside scoring system ("Candida score") for early antifungal treatment in nonneutropenic critically ill patients with *Candida* colonization. Crit Care Med 2006;34(3):730–7.

27. Ostrosky-Zeichner L, Sable C, Sobel J, et al. Multicenter retrospective development and validation of a clinical prediction rule for nosocomial invasive candidiasis in the intensive care setting. Eur J Clin Microbiol Infect Dis 2007;26(4):271–6.

28. Paphitou NI, Ostrosky-Zeichner L, Rex JH. Rules for identifying patients at increased risk for candidal infections in the surgical intensive care unit: approach to developing practical criteria for systematic use in antifungal prophylaxis trials. Med Mycol 2005;43(3):235–43.

29. Maertens JA, Madero L, Reilly AF, et al. A randomized, double-blind, multicenter study of caspofungin versus liposomal amphotericin B for empiric antifungal therapy in pediatric patients with persistent fever and neutropenia. Pediatr Infect Dis J 2010;29(5):415–20.

30. Walsh TJ, Teppler H, Donowitz GR, et al. Caspofungin versus liposomal amphotericin B for empirical antifungal therapy in patients with persistent fever and neutropenia. N Engl J Med 2004;351(14):1391–402.

31. Walsh TJ, Finberg RW, Arndt C, et al. Liposomal amphotericin B for empirical therapy in patients with persistent fever and neutropenia. National Institute of Allergy

and Infectious Diseases Mycoses Study Group. N Engl J Med 1999;340(10): 764–71.

32. Mora-Duarte J, Betts R, Rotstein C, et al. Comparison of caspofungin and amphotericin B for invasive candidiasis. N Engl J Med 2002;347(25):2020–9.

33. Pappas PG, Rotstein CM, Betts RF, et al. Micafungin versus caspofungin for treatment of candidemia and other forms of invasive candidiasis. Clin Infect Dis 2007; 45(7):883–93.

34. Reboli AC, Rotstein C, Pappas PG, et al. Anidulafungin versus fluconazole for invasive candidiasis. N Engl J Med 2007;356(24):2472–82.

35. Kuse ER, Chetchotisakd P, da Cunha CA, et al. Micafungin versus liposomal amphotericin B for candidaemia and invasive candidosis: a phase III randomised double-blind trial. Lancet 2007;369(9572):1519–27.

36. Cuenca-Estrella M, Verweij PE, Arendrup MC, et al. ESCMID* guideline for the diagnosis and management of Candida diseases 2012: diagnostic procedures. Clin Microbiol Infect 2012;18(Suppl 7):9–18.

37. Garey KW, Rege M, Pai MP, et al. Time to initiation of fluconazole therapy impacts mortality in patients with candidemia: a multi-institutional study. Clin Infect Dis 2006;43(1):25–31.

38. Gudlaugsson O, Gillespie S, Lee K, et al. Attributable mortality of nosocomial candidemia, revisited. Clin Infect Dis 2003;37(9):1172–7.

39. Oude Lashof AM, Donnelly JP, Meis JF, et al. Duration of antifungal treatment and development of delayed complications in patients with candidaemia. Eur J Clin Microbiol Infect Dis 2003;22(1):43–8.

40. Blot SI, Vandewoude KH, Hoste EA, et al. Effects of nosocomial candidemia on outcomes of critically ill patients. Am J Med 2002;113(6):480–5.

41. Morrell M, Fraser VJ, Kollef MH. Delaying the empiric treatment of candida bloodstream infection until positive blood culture results are obtained: a potential risk factor for hospital mortality. Antimicrob Agents Chemother 2005;49(9):3640–5.

42. Taur Y, Cohen N, Dubnow S, et al. Effect of antifungal therapy timing on mortality in cancer patients with candidemia. Antimicrob Agents Chemother 2010;54(1): 184–90.

43. Arendrup MC, Boekhout T, Akova M, et al. ESCMID and ECMM joint clinical guidelines for the diagnosis and management of rare invasive yeast infections. Clin Microbiol Infect 2014;20(Suppl 3):76–98.

44. Ullmann AJ, Cornely OA, Donnelly JP, et al. ESCMID* guideline for the diagnosis and management of Candida diseases 2012: developing European guidelines in clinical microbiology and infectious diseases. Clin Microbiol Infect 2012;18(Suppl 7):1–8.

45. Rex JH, Bennett JE, Sugar AM, et al. A randomized trial comparing fluconazole with amphotericin B for the treatment of candidemia in patients without neutropenia. Candidemia Study Group and the National Institute. N Engl J Med 1994; 331(20):1325–30.

46. Anaissie EJ, Darouiche RO, Abi-Said D, et al. Management of invasive candidal infections: results of a prospective, randomized, multicenter study of fluconazole versus amphotericin B and review of the literature. Clin Infect Dis 1996;23(5): 964–72.

47. Koehler P, Tacke D, Cornely OA. Our 2014 approach to candidaemia. Mycoses 2014;57(10):581–3.

48. Andes DR, Safdar N, Baddley JW, et al. Impact of treatment strategy on outcomes in patients with candidemia and other forms of invasive candidiasis: a patient-level quantitative review of randomized trials. Clin Infect Dis 2012;54(8): 1110–22.

49. Bernhardt H, Knoke M, Bernhardt J. Efficacy of anidulafungin against biofilms of different *Candida* species in long-term trials of continuous flow cultivation. Mycoses 2011;54(6):e821-7.
50. Kuhn DM, George T, Chandra J, et al. Antifungal susceptibility of Candida biofilms: unique efficacy of amphotericin B lipid formulations and echinocandins. Antimicrob Agents Chemother 2002;46(6):1773-80.
51. Tacke D, Buchheidt D, Karthaus M, et al. Primary prophylaxis of invasive fungal infections in patients with haematologic malignancies. 2014 update of the recommendations of the Infectious Diseases Working Party of the German Society for Haematology and Oncology. Ann Hematol 2014;93(9):1449-56.
52. Marks DI, Pagliuca A, Kibbler CC, et al. Voriconazole versus itraconazole for antifungal prophylaxis following allogeneic haematopoietic stem-cell transplantation. Br J Haematol 2011;155(3):318-27.
53. Huang X, Chen H, Han M, et al. Multicenter, randomized, open-label study comparing the efficacy and safety of micafungin versus itraconazole for prophylaxis of invasive fungal infections in patients undergoing hematopoietic stem cell transplant. Biol Blood Marrow Transplant 2012;18(10):1509-16.
54. Bow EJ, Vanness DJ, Slavin M, et al. Systematic review and mixed treatment comparison meta-analysis of randomized clinical trials of primary oral antifungal prophylaxis in allogeneic hematopoietic cell transplant recipients. BMC Infect Dis 2015;15:128.
55. Duarte RF, Lopez-Jimenez J, Cornely OA, et al. Phase 1b study of new posaconazole tablet for prevention of invasive fungal infections in high-risk patients with neutropenia. Antimicrob Agents Chemother 2014;58(10):5758-65.
56. Walsh TJ, Pappas P, Winston DJ, et al. Voriconazole compared with liposomal amphotericin B for empirical antifungal therapy in patients with neutropenia and persistent fever. N Engl J Med 2002;346(4):225-34.
57. Cordonnier C, Pautas C, Maury S, et al. Empirical versus preemptive antifungal therapy for high-risk, febrile, neutropenic patients: a randomized, controlled trial. Clin Infect Dis 2009;48(8):1042-51.
58. Girmenia C, Barosi G, Aversa F, et al. Prophylaxis and treatment of invasive fungal diseases in allogeneic stem cell transplantation: results of a consensus process by Gruppo Italiano Trapianto di Midollo Osseo (GITMO). Clin Infect Dis 2009;49(8):1226-36.
59. Maertens J, Theunissen K, Verhoef G, et al. Galactomannan and computed tomography-based preemptive antifungal therapy in neutropenic patients at high risk for invasive fungal infection: a prospective feasibility study. Clin Infect Dis 2005;41(9):1242-50.
60. Hebart H, Klingspor L, Klingebiel T, et al. A prospective randomized controlled trial comparing PCR-based and empirical treatment with liposomal amphotericin B in patients after allo-SCT. Bone Marrow Transplant 2009;43(7):553-61.
61. Pagano L, Caira M, Nosari A, et al. The use and efficacy of empirical versus preemptive therapy in the management of fungal infections: the HEMA e-Chart Project. Haematologica 2011;96(9):1366-70.
62. Aguado JM, Vazquez L, Fernandez-Ruiz M, et al. Serum galactomannan versus a combination of galactomannan and polymerase chain reaction-based Aspergillus DNA detection for early therapy of invasive aspergillosis in high-risk hematological patients: a randomized controlled trial. Clin Infect Dis 2015;60(3):405-14.
63. Herbrecht R, Denning DW, Patterson TF, et al. Voriconazole versus amphotericin B for primary therapy of invasive aspergillosis. N Engl J Med 2002;347(6):408-15.

64. Cornely OA, Maertens J, Bresnik M, et al. Liposomal amphotericin B as initial therapy for invasive mold infection: a randomized trial comparing a high-loading dose regimen with standard dosing (AmBiLoad trial). Clin Infect Dis 2007; 44(10):1289–97.
65. Viscoli C, Herbrecht R, Akan H, et al. An EORTC phase II study of caspofungin as first-line therapy of invasive aspergillosis in haematological patients. J Antimicrob Chemother 2009;64(6):1274–81.
66. Herbrecht R, Maertens J, Baila L, et al. Caspofungin first-line therapy for invasive aspergillosis in allogeneic hematopoietic stem cell transplant patients: a European Organisation for Research and Treatment of Cancer study. Bone Marrow Transplant 2010;45(7):1227–33.
67. Cornely OA, Vehreschild JJ, Vehreschild MJ, et al. Phase II dose escalation study of caspofungin for invasive Aspergillosis. Antimicrob Agents Chemother 2011; 55(12):5798–803.
68. US Food and Drug Administration. Isavuconazonium—invasive aspergillosis and invasive mucormycosis. Advisory Committee Briefing Document 2015. Available at: www.FDAgov/downloads/advisory committees/committeesmeetingmaterials/drugs/anti-infectivedrugs advisorycommittee/ucm430748pdf. Accessed August 16, 2015.
69. Ananda-Rajah MR, Kontoyiannis D. Isavuconazole: a new extended spectrum triazole for invasive mold diseases. Future Microbiol 2015;10(5):693–708.
70. McCormack PL. Isavuconazonium: first global approval. Drugs 2015;75(7): 817–22.
71. Miceli MH, Kauffman CA. Isavuconazole: a new broad-spectrum triazole antifungal agent. Clin Infect Dis 2015;61(10):1558–65.
72. Cornely OA, Arikan-Akdagli S, Dannaoui E, et al. ESCMID and ECMM joint clinical guidelines for the diagnosis and management of mucormycosis 2013. Clin Microbiol Infect 2014;20(Suppl 3):5–26.
73. Tedder M, Spratt JA, Anstadt MP, et al. Pulmonary mucormycosis: results of medical and surgical therapy. Ann Thorac Surg 1994;57(4):1044–50.
74. Greenberg RN, Mullane K, van Burik JA, et al. Posaconazole as salvage therapy for zygomycosis. Antimicrob Agents Chemother 2006;50(1):126–33.
75. van Burik JA, Hare RS, Solomon HF, et al. Posaconazole is effective as salvage therapy in zygomycosis: a retrospective summary of 91 cases. Clin Infect Dis 2006;42(7):e61–5.
76. Vehreschild JJ, Birtel A, Vehreschild MJ, et al. Mucormycosis treated with posaconazole: review of 96 case reports. Crit Rev Microbiol 2013;39(3):310–24.
77. Pagano L, Cornely OA, Busca A, et al. Combined antifungal approach for the treatment of invasive mucormycosis in patients with hematologic diseases: a report from the SEIFEM and FUNGISCOPE registries. Haematologica 2013; 98(10):e127–30.
78. Liss B, Vehreschild JJ, Bangard C, et al. Our 2015 approach to invasive pulmonary aspergillosis. Mycoses 2015;58(6):375–82.
79. Tacke D, Koehler P, Markiefka B, et al. Our 2014 approach to mucormycosis. Mycoses 2014;57(9):519–24.

Approach to the Solid Organ Transplant Patient with Suspected Fungal Infection

CrossMark

Judith A. Anesi, MD[a], John W. Baddley, MD, MSPH[b,c],*

KEYWORDS

- Solid organ transplant • Invasive fungal infection • Candida • Aspergillus
- Endemic fungi • Cryptococcus • Mold

KEY POINTS

- Identification of invasive fungal infections (IFIs) can be challenging, because the signs and symptoms are similar to other infections and diagnostic techniques are limited.
- *Aspergillus* and *Candida* species are the most frequent causes of IFIs in solid organ transplant (SOT) recipients.
- When an SOT recipient presents with pulmonary symptoms, chest imaging should be performed to evaluate for a fungal cause, which typically presents with nodular opacities.
- Because of immunosuppression, typical morphology of fungal skin lesions may be altered in SOT recipients, making skin biopsy an essential step for diagnosis.

INTRODUCTION

In solid organ transplant (SOT) recipients, invasive fungal infections (IFIs) are associated with significant morbidity and mortality. Detection of IFIs can be difficult because the signs and symptoms are similar to those of viral or bacterial infections or noninfectious illness, and diagnostic techniques have limited sensitivity and specificity. As a result, to aid in the diagnosis of IFI, clinicians often must rely on knowledge of the patient's risk factors for fungal infection.

In this article, an approach to diagnosis of IFIs is described on the basis of the SOT patient's clinical presentation and risk factors. Specifically, the spectrum of suspected

Disclosure Statement: Dr J.A. Anesi has nothing to disclose; Dr J.W. Baddley consults for Merck, Astellas, and Pfizer.
[a] Division of Infectious Diseases, University of Pennsylvania, 3400 Spruce Street, 3 Silverstein, Suite E, Philadelphia, PA 19104, USA; [b] Department of Medicine, University of Alabama at Birmingham, 1900 University Boulevard, 229 THT, Birmingham, AL 35294, USA; [c] Medical Service, Birmingham VA Medical Center, 700 South 19th street, Birmingham, AL 35233, USA
* Corresponding author. Department of Medicine, University of Alabama at Birmingham, 1900 University Boulevard, 229 THT, Birmingham, AL 35294.
E-mail address: jbaddley@uab.edu

Infect Dis Clin N Am 30 (2016) 277–296
http://dx.doi.org/10.1016/j.idc.2015.10.001
0891-5520/16/$ – see front matter © 2016 Elsevier Inc. All rights reserved.

id.theclinics.com

IFIs that may be present in patients who present with clinical syndromes is outlined, including respiratory illness, neurologic illness, cutaneous manifestations, and a sepsis syndrome. Relevant fungal pathogens associated with these clinical syndromes, an initial diagnostic approach, and considerations for empiric antifungal therapy are discussed.

EPIDEMIOLOGY OF INVASIVE FUNGAL INFECTIONS AFTER SOLID ORGAN TRANSPLANTATION

The timing and incidence of IFIs vary by the organ transplanted and the use of antifungal prophylaxis. Candidiasis and aspergillosis have historically caused—and continue to cause—most IFIs in SOT recipients, although there are increasing reports of non-*albicans Candida* and non-*Aspergillus* molds complicating SOT in recent years[1–5] (**Table 1**).

There have been 2 recent multicenter, observational studies describing the epidemiology of IFIs in SOT patients.[6,7] The first, by Pappas and colleagues,[6] analyzed data from the Transplant-Associated Infection Surveillance Network. The group described 1208 IFIs among 1063 SOT recipients (kidney, liver, pancreas, lung, heart, and small bowel) over a follow-up period of up to 5 years. The overall incidence of IFIs was 3.1%.[6] The second study, by Neofytos and colleagues,[7] used data collected from the Prospective Antifungal Therapy Alliance registry. In this study, 515 IFIs among 429 SOT recipients (liver, lung, kidney, heart, small bowel, islet cell, and pancreas) were described, with a follow-up time of up to 3 years. Both studies revealed similar IFI epidemiology: the most common IFIs were invasive candidiasis, invasive aspergillosis, and cryptococcosis. Invasive candidiasis was the most common IFI in all transplant types except in lung recipients, where aspergillosis was most common. Non-*Aspergillus* molds, endemic fungi, zygomycosis, and pneumocytosis were less commonly observed.[6,7]

Timing of Invasive Fungal Infections After Solid Organ Transplant

In general, invasive candidiasis is an early complication of SOT, and other IFIs are more likely late complications, although the timing may vary based on antifungal prophylaxis and transplant type (**Fig. 1**).[1,6–8] With current antifungal prophylaxis strategies, the time to onset of invasive candidiasis ranges between 3 and 6 months.[6,7]

Table 1
Epidemiology of invasive fungal infection in solid organ transplant recipients

Organ Transplanted	IFIs in Order of Decreasing Frequency
Kidney	Candida > Crypto > Aspergillus > Endemic mycoses > Molds > PJP
Liver	Candida > Aspergillus > Crypto > Endemic mycoses > Molds > PJP
Pancreas	Candida > Endemic mycoses > Aspergillus ≈ Crypto > Molds > PJP
Lung	Aspergillus > Candida > Molds > Crypto > PJP > Endemic mycoses
Heart	Candida > Aspergillus > Molds > Crypto > Endemic mycoses > PJP
Small bowel	Candida > Crypto > Aspergillus > Endemic mycoses > Molds > PJP

Abbreviation: Crypto, *Cryptococcus.*

Adapted from Pappas PG, Alexander BD, Andes DR, et al. Invasive fungal infections among organ transplant recipients: results of the Transplant-Associated Infection Surveillance Network (TRANSNET). Clin Infect Dis 2010;50:1101–11; and Neofytos D, Fishman JA, Horn D, et al. Epidemiology and outcome of invasive fungal infections in solid organ transplant recipients. Transpl Infect Dis 2010;12:220–9.

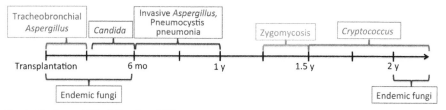

Fig. 1. Timing of IFIs following SOT.

The timing of aspergillosis is dependent on the site of infection: tracheobronchial or anastomotic *Aspergillus* infections typically occur within 90 days, whereas other forms of invasive aspergillosis occur later (6–12 months).[6,7,9,10]

Zygomycosis and other non-*Aspergillus* mold infections tend to present later after SOT, with average time to onset of 312 to 467 days (10–14 months).[6,7] Of note, a study reported time to mold infection of 81 days (2.7 months) in liver recipients, but 533 days (1.5 years) for nonliver SOT recipients, suggesting that liver recipients are an outlier with much earlier onset of both *Aspergillus* and non-*Aspergillus* mold infections.[11] This phenomenon of early mold infections after liver transplantation has been described in other studies as well.[12]

Endemic fungi also tend to be a late complication following SOT, with a median time to onset of 343 days (11.4 months), although one study found that the timing may be bimodal with 40% of infections occurring within the first 6 months after transplant and 34% occurring between 2 and 11 years after transplant.[6,13]

Pneumocystosis is now predominantly a late complication of SOT. Before the advent of prophylaxis, it generally occurred between 3 and 6 months after transplant. Studies in the era of widespread prophylaxis, however, have shown that it now occurs typically more than 180 days (6 months) after transplant, after prophylaxis has been discontinued. Most cases occur within 1 year of transplant.[14]

Cryptococcosis is one of the latest infectious complications after SOT, with a median time to onset between 1.5 and 5 years after SOT.[6,7]

Risk Factors for Invasive Fungal Infections Following Solid Organ Transplant

Knowledge and recognition of risk factors for IFI play an important role in evaluation of the patient with suspected IFI. Risk factors for IFI vary by the organ transplanted (**Table 2**). In liver recipients, the major risk factors associated with IFIs are predominantly surgical factors, as increased technical complexity, prolonged operation time, greater transfusion requirements, Roux-en-Y biliary anastomosis, retransplantation, and bleeding complications requiring reoperation have been associated with increased risk of IFIs.[15–18] Nonsurgical factors that are associated with increased risk for IFIs in liver recipients include hepatic and renal dysfunction, particularly when requiring hemodialysis,[19,20] and immunomodulatory viral infections, including cytomegalovirus (CMV) and human herpesvirus-6 (HHV-6).[15,21–23]

In lung recipients, airway colonization with *Aspergillus* has been associated with increased risk for subsequent invasive aspergillosis.[24] Other risk factors for invasive aspergillosis include CMV infection, ischemia of the anastomosis, receipt of a single lung transplant, hypogammaglobulinemia, and augmented immunosuppression; it remains controversial whether allograft rejection is a significant risk factor.[19,25–28]

In kidney recipients, the major risk factors for IFIs include diabetes, prolonged pretransplant dialysis, allograft rejection, the use of tacrolimus, and graft failure requiring reinitiation of hemodialysis.[29] An increased risk for invasive aspergillosis specifically

Table 2
Risk factors for invasive fungal infections by organ type

Organ Transplanted	Risk Factors
Liver[15–23]	Increased technical complexity of surgery Prolonged operation time Greater transfusion requirements Roux-en-Y biliary anastomosis Retransplantation Bleeding complications requiring reoperation Hepatic dysfunction Renal dysfunction, especially requiring HD CMV infection HHV6 infection
Lung[19,24–28]	Airway colonization with *Aspergillus* CMV infection Ischemia of the anastomosis Receipt of a single lung transplant Hypogammaglobulinemia Augmented immunosuppression
Kidney[29–31]	Diabetes mellitus Prolonged pretransplant dialysis Allograft rejection Tacrolimus Graft failure requiring reinitiation of HD Corticosteroids
Heart[1,8,32–34]	Broad-spectrum antibiotics Prolonged duration of antibiotics Central venous catheters ECMO Hemodialysis *Aspergillus* on BAL Reoperation CMV infection
Pancreas[36]	Increased donor age Enteric drainage (rather than bladder drainage) Transplantation after kidney transplantation Preoperative peritoneal dialysis Retransplantation
Small bowel[37]	Graft rejection or dysfunction Enhanced immunosuppression Anastomotic disruption Abdominal reoperation Multivisceral transplant

Abbreviation: HD, hemodialysis.

has been associated with high dose and prolonged duration of corticosteroids, and graft failure requiring hemodialysis and enhanced immunosuppression.[19,30,31]

In heart transplant recipients, invasive candidiasis has been associated with use of broad-spectrum antibiotics, prolonged duration of antibiotic use, presence of central-venous catheters, and need for hemodialysis.[1,8] Invasive aspergillosis has been associated with isolation of *Aspergillus* on bronchoalveolar lavage (BAL), reoperation, CMV disease, and posttransplant hemodialysis.[32–34] The use of extracorporeal membrane oxygenation (ECMO) is also associated with increased risk for IFIs.[35]

Risk factors for IFIs in pancreas recipients include increased donor age, enteric drainage (rather than bladder drainage), pancreas transplantation after kidney transplantation, preoperative peritoneal dialysis, and pancreatic retransplantation.[36]

With small bowel transplantation, patients are thought to be particularly high risk for IFIs, especially candidiasis, when there is graft rejection or dysfunction, enhanced immunosuppression, anastomotic disruption, abdominal reoperation, and multivisceral transplantation.[37] Infections with non-*albicans* *Candida* species have been associated with the use of fluconazole prophylaxis.[3]

RECOGNITION OF INVASIVE FUNGAL INFECTIONS BY CLINICAL SYNDROME

Given the lack of diagnostic tests with high sensitivity and specificity for detecting IFIs, the diagnosis of an IFI in an SOT recipient is often made based on the patient's clinical presentation, knowledge of fungal infections by site, and patient risk factors. In this section, suspected IFI by clinical syndrome is approached. Specifically discussed are patients who present with pulmonary symptoms, neurologic symptoms, cutaneous eruptions, and sepsis syndrome without localizing symptoms.

Pulmonary Fungal Infections

When a transplant recipient presents with respiratory symptoms, pulmonary fungal infections should be considered, particularly if the patient is more than 6 months after transplantation. Patients with pulmonary mycosis often present with nonspecific symptoms such as cough (either dry or productive) and fever. They may also endorse hemoptysis, dyspnea, and systemic symptoms of weight loss and fatigue.

Among transplant recipients, fungi are much less common causes of pneumonia than are bacteria or viruses—fungi account for approximately 6% of all pneumonias.[38] Molds, especially *Aspergillus* species, cause the greatest number of pulmonary fungal infections in SOT recipients.[38,39] Less commonly, *Fusarium*, *Scedosporium*, agents of mucormycosis, and dematiaceous fungi may be causative. *Cryptococcus*, and the dimorphic endemic fungi, such as *Histoplasma*, *Blastomyces*, and *Coccidioides*, should be considered on the basis of clinical presentation and geography. In studies conducted before the widespread use of prophylaxis, the incidence of *Pneumocystis jiroveci* pneumonia (PJP) varied between 5% and 15% depending on the organ type and immunosuppressive regimen; in the era of prophylaxis, the incidence of PJP within the first year after SOT is estimated to be less than 1%, although higher rates (up to 15%) have been reported after 1 year.[40–43]

Initial evaluation of the transplant patient with suspected pulmonary mycosis typically involves chest imaging. Radiographic findings, especially subcentimeter lesions, may be difficult to appreciate on chest radiograph alone, so chest computed tomographic scan is the best imaging modality.[44] Imaging may reveal nodular or masslike opacities (with or without the halo sign), which may progress to cavitary lesions. Ground-glass opacities (GGOs) and lobar infiltrates can also be seen with some types of fungal infections.[45–47] It is not uncommon to have concurrent bacterial or viral pulmonary infection in patients with a pulmonary fungal infection, sometimes complicating radiographic interpretation. The following sections highlight suspected fungal infections on the basis of imaging findings (**Table 3**).

Pulmonary nodules or masses

Nodules are the most common radiographic findings of pulmonary fungal infections.[48,49] In SOT recipients, aspergillosis should be considered strongly when nodular opacities are seen, because it is the most common cause of nodular

Table 3
Pulmonary invasive fungal infections based on radiographic findings

Radiographic Findings	Causative Fungi
Pulmonary nodules or masses	*Aspergillus*
	Histoplasma
	Blastomyces
	Coccidioides
	Cryptococcus
	Agents of mucormycosis
	Fusarium
	Phaeohyphomycosis
Pulmonary GGOs	PJP
	Histoplasma

Data from Refs.[44–47]

pneumonia.[38,50,51] The halo sign is much less sensitive for aspergillosis in SOT patients than for neutropenic patients with hematologic malignancy.[52] Specific risk factors that should increase suspicion for pulmonary aspergillosis include retransplantation, reoperation, renal failure, and transplantation for fulminant liver failure in liver recipients[53–57]; single lung transplants, early airway ischemia, CMV infection, *Aspergillus* colonization, acquired hypogammaglobulinemia, and rejection in lung recipients[25–28,58–60]; colonization of the respiratory tract with *Aspergillus*, reoperation, CMV disease, and posttransplant hemodialysis in heart recipients[32–34]; and graft failure requiring hemodialysis, and prolonged duration of corticosteroid exposure in renal recipients.[19,30,31]

Endemic fungi can also cause nodular pneumonias in SOT recipients. Although endemic fungi may rarely occur outside of the typical geographic regions, donor-derived infection can be another cause of endemic fungal infections outside of the endemic regions and should always be considered. Histoplasmosis is endemic to the Ohio and Mississippi River Valleys. Patients with exposures to bats, caves, and construction sites are at increased risk. In the southwest United States and parts of Mexico, *Coccidioides* infection may result in nodular pneumonia in SOT patients.[61,62] Risk factors for coccidioidomycosis among SOT recipients include treatment of acute rejection and African American race.[62,63]

Nodular pneumonia is the most common presentation of cryptococcosis in SOT patients.[49,64] Patients receiving calcineurin-inhibitor immunosuppression are at increased risk of pulmonary cryptococcosis.[65] Other risk factors include corticosteroids, alemtuzumab, and antithymocyte use.[66–70] Concomitant meningitis may also be a clue to cryptococcal infection.

The agents of mucormycosis, *Fusarium*, and phaeohyphomycoses may cause pneumonia that manifests with nodular opacities. These emerging fungi are most common among liver and lung transplant recipients.[6] Other risk factors include breaks in skin integrity, chronic respiratory disease, and prior exposure to azoles (that may select for less common fungi).[71–77]

Pulmonary ground-glass opacities

PJP often presents with diffuse interstitial infiltrates and GGOs on chest imaging. Lung and combined heart-lung recipients are at higher risk for PJP than other organ types.[43] Other risk factors for PJP include prolonged corticosteroid courses, antilymphocyte

therapy, alemtuzumab therapy, CMV disease, allograft rejection, and lack of PJP prophylaxis.[78–81] Other fungal infections that may present with GGOs include aspergillosis, histoplasmosis, and coccidioidomycosis.[46,61,82]

Diagnostic evaluation for pulmonary fungal infections

Diagnosis of pulmonary IFI in SOT patients is difficult, because clinical signs and radiographic changes may be nonspecific. Historically, microscopy of clinical specimens
from sputum or bronchoscopy has been useful, specifically for diagnosis of PJP.[83]
Culture of clinical specimens remains an important method of diagnosis, but many
fungi are difficult to grow in culture, and thus, the utility in establishing a diagnosis
is limited.[84,85] Even when there is growth on culture, there may be difficulties in identification on the basis of macroscopic and microscopic morphologic characteristics.

Serologic testing has become a useful adjunct for diagnosing pulmonary IFI in SOT
recipients. Serologic testing is used frequently for cryptococcosis, histoplasmosis,
aspergillosis, and coccidioidomycosis.[83] Serum cryptococcal antigen testing can
detect both *Cryptococcus neoformans* and *Cryptococcus gattii*; the serum test has
a relatively high sensitivity for detecting cryptococcal meningitis but has a lower diagnostic yield for isolated pulmonary cryptococcosis in SOT patients (approximately
50%).[86] *Histoplasma* urine antigen testing has a sensitivity of 92% for patients with
disseminated disease, 80% with diffuse pulmonary disease, 34% with subacute pulmonary disease, and 14% with chronic pulmonary disease.[87–89] The antibody test for
Coccidioides may be positive in 50% to 70% of patients with pneumonia and can also
be falsely positive in the setting of histoplasmosis.[90,91]

Serum or BAL galactomannan testing may aid in the diagnosis of aspergillosis, but
the sensitivity and specificity have not been reliable in SOT patients. For example, a
recent meta-analysis showed a sensitivity of 22% and specificity of 84% in SOT recipients.[92] β-D-Glucan, a nonspecific marker of fungal infection, was found to have a mar-
ginal positive predictive value when used in lung transplant patients, although the
negative predictive value was high.[93]

Thus, despite laboratory advances, the clinical presentation, chest imaging, and
clinical suspicion on the basis of risk factors and epidemiology are essential to the
diagnosis of pulmonary IFI. If an SOT recipient presents with fever, cough, and chest
imaging concerning for fungal pneumonia, relevant serologic studies should be obtained early in the process. In addition, bronchoscopy should be considered early in
the process.

Central Nervous System Fungal Infections

Fungal infections of the central nervous system (CNS) in SOT patients are associated
with significant mortality, necessitating careful evaluation of the patient with suspected CNS infection. IFIs may cause meningitis, brain abscesses, and frontal lobe
destruction associated with sinus disease (**Table 4**). Patients may present with headache, neck stiffness, focal neurologic deficits, altered mental status, somnolence, cranial nerve palsy, or seizures; they may not have fever. The most common fungal
infection of the CNS in SOT patients is cryptococcal meningitis, occurring in 0.2%
to 5% of SOT patients.[64] Less commonly, *Candida* species, molds, and endemic fungi
can infect the CNS and may result in a variety of lesions on brain imaging.

Meningitis

Cryptococcal meningitis may present with minimal abnormalities on brain imaging
particularly in early disease, although later in the disease process meningeal enhancement is expected, along with gelatinous pseudocyst formation in the basal ganglia and

Table 4
Cental nervous system invasive fungal infections based on presenting signs and symptoms

Presenting Symptoms	Differential of IFIs
Meningitis	*Cryptococcus*
	Histoplasma
	Coccidioides
CNS abscess	*Candida*
	Aspergillus
	Agents of mucormycosis
	Dematiaceous fungi
	Coccidioides
	Blastomyces
	Histoplasma
Frontal lobe lesions ± sinus disease	*Aspergillus*
	Agents of mucormycosis
	Fusarium
	Scedosporium

Data from Refs.[94,98,100]

findings of hydrocephalus.[94] In advanced disease, cryptococcomas may be seen, particularly with *C gattii* infection.[94,95] Lumbar puncture (LP) should be performed when symptoms of meningitis are present. It is of critical importance that an opening pressure be measured when performing the LP, because elevated intracranial pressure is associated with poor outcomes.[64] Cerebrospinal fluid (CSF) testing should include measurement of cell counts, protein, glucose, as well as aerobic/anaerobic cultures, mycobacterial culture, fungal culture, and cryptococcal antigen testing. The CSF cryptococcal antigen assay is more sensitive and specific than fungal culture or India ink staining.[65,96,97] A serum cryptococcal antigen assay has a sensitivity approaching 90% for detection of CNS disease and can be sent as an adjunct.[97]

Rarely, endemic fungi including *Coccidioides* and *Histoplasma* cause meningitis, with headache, altered mental status, and minimal changes on brain imaging.[94,98–100] Serologic testing is often required to diagnose *Coccidioides* meningitis. The detection of *Coccidioides* antibodies in the CSF is nearly as specific as recovery of the organism on culture; alternatively, this diagnosis can be inferred from CSF with a lymphocytic pleocytosis in the setting of known coccidioidomycosis.[100] Urine antigen or serum antibody testing is often required for diagnosing *Histoplasma*. The *Histoplasma* antigen and antibody tests can be tested on CSF, although the sensitivity of the antigen test is estimated to be around 38%, and the specificity around 96%.[101–103] The serum antibody test for *Histoplasma* has been shown to detect the organism in about 80% of cases (not specifically with CNS disease), although it may be less accurate in the SOT population.[87,101,104]

Brain abscess

Candidiasis may cause fungal brain abscesses. Typically, there are multiple small abscesses (often <3 mm) at the gray-white junction or perforating arterial zones.[94] As it is generally from hematogenous spread, risk factors for candidemia should be considered, and blood cultures should be performed. Candidal infections with dissemination to the CNS usually occur within the first 3 months after transplant, in contrast to other IFIs, which tend to occur later after transplant.[1,8,105,106]

When there is a single large brain abscess, molds including *Aspergillus*, agents of mucormycosis, and dematiaceous fungi should be considered as causes, particularly in the more profoundly immunocompromised SOT recipients.[107–111] *Aspergillus* can also cause multifocal hemorrhagic lesions with associated infarcts, in addition to nodules.[94] Endemic fungi, in particular *Coccidioides*, *Blastomyces*, and *Histoplasma*, can also cause abscesses, although it is an uncommon presentation for each of these causes. Aspiration of the abscess is often necessary in order to establish these diagnoses.

Frontal lobe lesions with sinus disease

Frontal lobe lesions should prompt an evaluation of the sinuses as a possible source of fungal infection due to direct extension. Typically, there is evidence of bony erosion on imaging, and the orbits and optic nerves may also be affected. Molds, in particular *Aspergillus* and the agents of mucormycosis, should be considered in these cases.[112,113] Other molds that may cause rhino-orbital cerebral infection include *Fusarium* and *Scedosporium*. Invasive mucormycosis among SOT patients has been reported to be particularly prevalent in patients who also have diabetes mellitus, renal failure, and prior voriconazole or caspofungin use.[113] Diagnosis is usually made via endoscopic sinus evaluation with histopathologic evaluation and culture of biopsies.

Cutaneous Manifestations of Invasive Fungal Infections

Dermatologic diseases are common in SOT patients. Because of immune suppression and lack of inflammatory response in tissues, the typical morphology of skin lesions may be altered, making diagnosis difficult. Unusual pathogens should always be considered, even when skin lesions appear typical. For example, cryptococcal cellulitis may be indistinguishable from cellulitis caused by pathogens such as *Staphylococcus* or *Streptococcus*. Definitive diagnosis of fungal skin lesions is often made by skin biopsy with routine examination, special staining, and tissue cultures.

Fungal infections are among the most common skin infections in SOT patients and may be present in up to 50% of patients.[114,115] However, most are superficial infections and are not described herein. There are several scenarios wherein cutaneous fungal infections may occur: (1) primary skin infections such as tinea infections; (2) primary skin infections caused by opportunistic pathogens, which may remain localized or invade; and (3) secondary skin infections caused by dissemination from other sites. This section reviews skin manifestations of selected invasive mycoses in SOT recipients (**Table 5**).

Aspergillosis

Cutaneous aspergillosis may present as primary or secondary skin lesions. A recent review of a prospective multicenter aspergillosis database in France identified approximately 1% (15/1410) of patients having cutaneous infections: 5 with primary infection and 10 with secondary infection (cutaneous plus disseminated aspergillosis).[116] Of these, 3 were SOT recipients. Primary skin infection with aspergilli may occur as a result of burns, trauma, or infected catheters.[116–118] Typical skin lesions appear as erythematous papules and plaques. Lesions may become necrotic or develop hemorrhagic eschar.[116–118] In primary disease, extensive surgical debridement is often required.

Secondary infections usually result from hematogenous spread or direct spread from other foci of infection, both of which are associated with high mortality. Lesions may present as cellulitis, pustules, nodules, subcutaneous abscesses, ulcerations, or hemorrhagic blisters.[116] Skin biopsy may show blood vessel involvement and branching, septate hyphae.

Table 5	
Cutaneous presentations of invasive fungal infections in solid organ transplant recipients	
IFI Cause	**Cutaneous Presentations**
Aspergillosis	Erythematous papules and plaques
	Necrotic or hemorrhagic eschar
	Cellulitis
	Pustules and subcutaneous abscesses
	Nodules
	Ulcers
	Hemorrhagic bullae
Cryptococcosis	Abscesses
	Pustules
	Papules
	Plaques
	Purpura
	Ulcers
	Cellulitis
	Sinus tracts
Mucormycosis	Necrotic eschar with surrounding erythema
	Cellulitis with necrosis
	Erythematous macules, nodules, or plaques
Phaeohyphomycosis	Nodules
	Cysts
	Cellulitis
	Plaques
	Eschars
	Ulcerations

Adapted from Virgili A, Zampino MR, Mantovani L. Fungal skin infections in organ transplant recipients. Am J Clin Dermatol 2002;3:19–35, with permission; and Lima AM, Rocha SP, Reis Filho EG, et al. Study of dermatoses in kidney transplant patients. An Bras Dermatol 2013;88:361–7.

Cryptococcosis

Skin involvement occurs in up to 20% of SOT patients with cryptococcosis and may manifest as primary or secondary infection.[119–122] There may be a variety of lesions, including pustules, papules, purpura, ulcers, cellulitis, superficial granulomas or plaques, abscesses, and sinus tracts.[119,120,123] Cases of necrotizing cellulitis have also been described in SOT recipients.[124,125] Cellulitis not responding to routine antibacterial agents should prompt evaluation for cryptococcal infection or other unusual pathogens. Cryptococcal cellulitis is often present in patients receiving systemic corticosteroids or other immunosuppressive therapy and is characterized by prominent erythema and induration; development of blisters or ulcerations may also occur.[126,127] Skin biopsy for routine examination and culture is the most sensitive test for the diagnosis of cryptococcal skin disease.

Mucormycosis

SOT patients comprise fewer than 10% of patients with mucormycosis.[128,129] Cutaneous disease is seen in approximately 20% of cases.[130] Primary cutaneous mucormycosis results from inoculation of the fungus into the skin and often occurs at the site of external catheters.[131] Secondary cutaneous mucormycosis is seen after dissemination from pulmonary sites of infection but is very rare among patients with pulmonary mucormycosis.[132] Cutaneous mucormycosis typically presents with a necrotic eschar and surrounding erythema.[131] Other less common lesions include cellulitis with necrosis, erythematous macules or nodules, and plaques.[133,134]

Phaeohyphomycosis

There are more than one hundred species of dematiaceous, or pigmented, fungi that cause human disease. Common causative species in SOT patients include *Alternaria*, *Exophiala*, *Cladophialophora*, and *Ochroconis*.[5,135] Among transplant patients with phaeohyphomycosis, skin and soft tissue infections are present in most cases.[5,135] Lesions are frequently on the extremities and result from traumatic inoculation, but lesions as a result of dissemination are also common. Manifestations are quite variable and may include nodules, cysts, cellulitis, plaques, eschars, and ulcerations.[5,136] Skin biopsy for routine examination and culture, with special staining (Gomori-Methenamine silver or Fontana-Masson), will identify pigmented fungal forms.

Invasive Fungal Infections Causing a Sepsis Syndrome

SOT recipients often present with a sepsis syndrome but without any localizing symptoms. In these cases, it is important to consider IFIs, particularly candidemia/candidiasis. Candidiasis is more common among small bowel, pancreas, and liver transplant recipients than among kidney, heart, or lung recipients.[6] The risk for disseminated candidiasis is also increased in patients who have received prolonged courses of antimicrobials, parenteral nutrition, those who have had a prolonged ICU stay, recent CMV disease, primary graft failure, or early surgical re-exploration, and those with diabetes or on renal replacement therapy.[137,138] When assessing for candidiasis, at least 2 sets of blood cultures should be obtained, because *Candida* species can be grown on routine blood cultures, although the sensitivity remains around 70% even with newer techniques.[139] Another diagnostic tool to consider is the β-D-glucan assay, which has a sensitivity of 70% and specificity of 87% among patients with invasive candidiasis.[140–142]

In addition to candidiasis, another IFI to consider in the setting of a sepsis syndrome is progressive disseminated histoplasmosis (PDH), which may include extrapulmonary infection with gastrointestinal disease, hepatitis, mucosal/skin abnormalities, and hepatosplenomegaly.[143] The diagnosis of PDH is made frequently with blood or tissue cultures or with urine *Histoplasma* antigen testing, which has a sensitivity of 92% in patients with disseminated disease.[87–89]

EMPIRIC ANTIFUNGAL THERAPY FOR SUSPECTED INVASIVE FUNGAL INFECTIONS

For suspected IFI in the SOT recipient, empiric antifungal therapy should be considered, especially in patients who have potentially life-threatening conditions (pneumonia, meningitis, or a sepsis syndrome). It is important to evaluate risk factors for IFI and the likelihood of the specific fungal pathogen based on clinical signs and symptoms, radiography, and site of infection. Important considerations when deciding to administer antifungal therapy include current antifungal prophylaxis, institutional resistance patterns, and potential drug interactions and adverse effects.

In the SOT recipient who presents with respiratory symptoms and nodular opacities on chest imaging, it is reasonable to empirically start antifungal therapy after bronchoscopy and cultures have been performed. A third-generation triazole such as voriconazole is reasonable, because *Aspergillus* is the most common fungal cause. An amphotericin B preparation may also be considered, based on the patient's history and risk factors, especially if agents of mucormycosis or endemic fungi are likely. For the SOT patient with respiratory symptoms and GGOs on chest imaging, empiric therapy for PJP with trimethoprim-sulfamethoxazole should be considered if the patient is severely ill. Supportive risk factors would include chronic high-dose corticosteroids, lack of PJP prophylaxis, and recent rejection.

For patients presenting with meningitis but without mass lesions on brain imaging, empiric therapy for cryptococcosis is not often warranted, as CSF cryptococcal antigen testing can be rapidly performed and definitive diagnosis made quickly. However, if empiric therapy is needed, current treatment guidelines recommend amphotericin B preparations plus flucytosine.[64] If there are numerous microabscesses suggestive of a disseminated *Candida* infection, then an azole or amphotericin B preparation could be used empirically.[144] Of note, echinocandins do not have adequate CNS penetration and should be avoided when there is CNS IFI.[145–148] If there is a single large abscess or solid nodules, then amphotericin B would be a reasonable choice until the specific cause is identified.

For patients who present with a sepsis syndrome and no localizing symptoms, candidiasis is the most common IFI, so therapy recommended for candidiasis, such as an echinocandin, may be administered, especially in the critically ill.[144] For suspected PDH, empiric therapy with a lipid amphotericin B preparation may be necessary.[144]

SUMMARY

In SOT recipients, IFIs are associated with significant morbidity and mortality, and consequently, are important to identify and treat as early as possible to minimize poor outcomes. Detection of IFIs can be difficult, because presenting symptoms are similar to those of other infections, and available fungal diagnostic techniques are limited. Clinicians often must rely on the patient's risk factors and clinical presentation to aid in diagnosis and management of infection. Knowledge of the epidemiology of IFIs in SOT recipients and clinical presentation patterns may enable clinicians to suspect fungal infections earlier and lead to more rapid diagnosis and appropriate therapy.

REFERENCES

1. Patterson JE. Epidemiology of fungal infections in solid organ transplant patients. Transpl Infect Dis 1999;1:229–36.
2. Fortun J, Lopez-San Roman A, Velasco JJ, et al. Selection of Candida glabrata strains with reduced susceptibility to azoles in four liver transplant patients with invasive candidiasis. Eur J Clin Microbiol Infect Dis 1997;16:314–8.
3. Primeggia J, Matsumoto CS, Fishbein TM, et al. Infection among adult small bowel and multivisceral transplant recipients in the 30-day postoperative period. Transpl Infect Dis 2013;15:441–8.
4. Johnson LS, Shields RK, Clancy CJ. Epidemiology, clinical manifestations, and outcomes of Scedosporium infections among solid organ transplant recipients. Transpl Infect Dis 2014;16:578–87.
5. Schieffelin JS, Garcia-Diaz JB, Loss GE Jr, et al. Phaeohyphomycosis fungal infections in solid organ transplant recipients: clinical presentation, pathology, and treatment. Transpl Infect Dis 2014;16:270–8.
6. Pappas PG, Alexander BD, Andes DR, et al. Invasive fungal infections among organ transplant recipients: results of the Transplant-Associated Infection Surveillance Network (TRANSNET). Clin Infect Dis 2010;50:1101–11.
7. Neofytos D, Fishman JA, Horn D, et al. Epidemiology and outcome of invasive fungal infections in solid organ transplant recipients. Transpl Infect Dis 2010; 12:220–9.
8. Silveira FP, Husain S. Fungal infections in solid organ transplantation. Med Mycol 2007;45:305–20.

9. Singh N, Husain S. Aspergillus infections after lung transplantation: clinical differences in type of transplant and implications for management. J Heart Lung Transplant 2003;22:258–66.
10. Sole A, Morant P, Salavert M, et al. Aspergillus infections in lung transplant recipients: risk factors and outcome. Clin Microbiol Infect 2005;11:359–65.
11. Park BJ, Pappas PG, Wannemuehler KA, et al. Invasive non-Aspergillus mold infections in transplant recipients, United States, 2001-2006. Emerg Infect Dis 2011;17:1855–64.
12. Neofytos D, Treadway S, Ostrander D, et al. Epidemiology, outcomes, and mortality predictors of invasive mold infections among transplant recipients: a 10-year, single-center experience. Transpl Infect Dis 2013;15:233–42.
13. Kauffman CA, Freifeld AG, Andes DR, et al. Endemic fungal infections in solid organ and hematopoietic cell transplant recipients enrolled in the Transplant-Associated Infection Surveillance Network (TRANSNET). Transpl Infect Dis 2014;16:213–24.
14. Neff RT, Jindal RM, Yoo DY, et al. Analysis of USRDS: incidence and risk factors for Pneumocystis jiroveci pneumonia. Transplantation 2009;88:135–41.
15. Collins LA, Samore MH, Roberts MS, et al. Risk factors for invasive fungal infections complicating orthotopic liver transplantation. J Infect Dis 1994;170:644–52.
16. Kusne S, Dummer JS, Singh N, et al. Infections after liver transplantation. An analysis of 101 consecutive cases. Medicine (Baltimore) 1988;67:132–43.
17. Tollemar J, Ericzon BG, Barkholt L, et al. Risk factors for deep candida infections in liver transplant recipients. Transplant Proc 1990;22:1826–7.
18. Paya CV, Hermans PE, Washington JA 2nd, et al. Incidence, distribution, and outcome of episodes of infection in 100 orthotopic liver transplantations. Mayo Clin Proc 1989;64:555–64.
19. Paterson DL, Singh N. Invasive aspergillosis in transplant recipients. Medicine (Baltimore) 1999;78:123–38.
20. Singh N, Arnow PM, Bonham A, et al. Invasive aspergillosis in liver transplant recipients in the 1990s. Transplantation 1997;64:716–20.
21. Kusne S, Torre-Cisneros J, Manez R, et al. Factors associated with invasive lung aspergillosis and the significance of positive Aspergillus culture after liver transplantation. J Infect Dis 1992;166:1379–83.
22. Dockrell DH, Mendez JC, Jones M, et al. Human herpesvirus 6 seronegativity before transplantation predicts the occurrence of fungal infection in liver transplant recipients. Transplantation 1999;67:399–403.
23. Rogers J, Rohal S, Carrigan DR, et al. Human herpesvirus-6 in liver transplant recipients: role in pathogenesis of fungal infections, neurologic complications, and outcome. Transplantation 2000;69:2566–73.
24. Paradowski LJ. Saprophytic fungal infections and lung transplantation–revisited. J Heart Lung Transplant 1997;16:524–31.
25. Husni RN, Gordon SM, Longworth DL, et al. Cytomegalovirus infection is a risk factor for invasive aspergillosis in lung transplant recipients. Clin Infect Dis 1998;26:753–5.
26. Higgins R, McNeil K, Dennis C, et al. Airway stenoses after lung transplantation: management with expanding metal stents. J Heart Lung Transplant 1994;13:774–8.
27. Westney GE, Kesten S, De Hoyos A, et al. Aspergillus infection in single and double lung transplant recipients. Transplantation 1996;61:915–9.
28. Goldfarb NS, Avery RK, Goormastic M, et al. Hypogammaglobulinemia in lung transplant recipients. Transplantation 2001;71:242–6.

29. Abbott KC, Hypolite I, Poropatich RK, et al. Hospitalizations for fungal infections after renal transplantation in the United States. Transpl Infect Dis 2001;3:203–11.
30. Gustafson TL, Schaffner W, Lavely GB, et al. Invasive aspergillosis in renal transplant recipients: correlation with corticosteroid therapy. J Infect Dis 1983; 148:230–8.
31. Panackal AA, Dahlman A, Keil KT, et al. Outbreak of invasive aspergillosis among renal transplant recipients. Transplantation 2003;75:1050–3.
32. Berenguer J, Munoz P, Parras F, et al. Treatment of deep mycoses with liposomal amphotericin B. Eur J Clin Microbiol Infect Dis 1994;13:504–7.
33. Munoz P, Rodriguez C, Bouza E, et al. Risk factors of invasive aspergillosis after heart transplantation: protective role of oral itraconazole prophylaxis. Am J Transplant 2004;4:636–43.
34. Munoz P, Alcala L, Sanchez Conde M, et al. The isolation of Aspergillus fumigatus from respiratory tract specimens in heart transplant recipients is highly predictive of invasive aspergillosis. Transplantation 2003;75:326–9.
35. Tissot F, Pascual M, Hullin R, et al. Impact of targeted antifungal prophylaxis in heart transplant recipients at high risk for early invasive fungal infection. Transplantation 2014;97:1192–7.
36. Singh N. Antifungal prophylaxis for solid organ transplant recipients: seeking clarity amidst controversy. Clin Infect Dis 2000;31:545–53.
37. Silveira FP, Kusne S, AST Infectious Diseases Community of Practice. Candida infections in solid organ transplantation. Am J Transplant 2013;13(Suppl 4): 220–7.
38. Giannella M, Munoz P, Alarcon JM, et al. Pneumonia in solid organ transplant recipients: a prospective multicenter study. Transpl Infect Dis 2014;16:232–41.
39. Eyuboglu FO, Kupeli E, Bozbas SS, et al. Evaluation of pulmonary infections in solid organ transplant patients: 12 years of experience. Transplant Proc 2013; 45:3458–61.
40. Choi YI, Hwang S, Park GC, et al. Clinical outcomes of Pneumocystis carinii pneumonia in adult liver transplant recipients. Transplant Proc 2013;45: 3057–60.
41. Gerrard JG. Pneumocystis carinii pneumonia in HIV-negative immunocompromised adults. Med J Aust 1995;162:233–5.
42. Hoyo I, Sanclemente G, Cervera C, et al. Opportunistic pulmonary infections in solid organ transplant recipients. Transplant Proc 2012;44:2673–5.
43. Fishman JA. Prevention of infection due to Pneumocystis carinii. Antimicrob Agents Chemother 1998;42:995–1004.
44. De Pauw B, Walsh TJ, Donnelly JP, et al. Revised definitions of invasive fungal disease from the European Organization for Research and Treatment of Cancer/ Invasive Fungal Infections Cooperative Group and the National Institute of Allergy and Infectious Diseases Mycoses Study Group (EORTC/MSG) Consensus Group. Clin Infect Dis 2008;46:1813–21.
45. Connolly JE Jr, McAdams HP, Erasmus JJ, et al. Opportunistic fungal pneumonia. J Thorac Imaging 1999;14:51–62.
46. Park YS, Seo JB, Lee YK, et al. Radiological and clinical findings of pulmonary aspergillosis following solid organ transplant. Clin Radiol 2008;63:673–80.
47. Copp DH, Godwin JD, Kirby KA, et al. Clinical and radiologic factors associated with pulmonary nodule etiology in organ transplant recipients. Am J Transplant 2006;6:2759–64.
48. Klein DL, Gamsu G. Thoracic manifestations of aspergillosis. AJR Am J Roentgenol 1980;134:543–52.

49. Patz EF Jr, Goodman PC. Pulmonary cryptococcosis. J Thorac Imaging 1992;7: 51–5.

50. Gazzoni FF, Hochhegger B, Severo LC, et al. High-resolution computed tomographic findings of Aspergillus infection in lung transplant patients. Eur J Radiol 2014;83:79–83.

51. Lee P, Minai OA, Mehta AC, et al. Pulmonary nodules in lung transplant recipients: etiology and outcome. Chest 2004;125:165–72.

52. Park SY, Kim SH, Choi SH, et al. Clinical and radiological features of invasive pulmonary aspergillosis in transplant recipients and neutropenic patients. Transpl Infect Dis 2010;12:309–15.

53. Gavalda J, Len O, San Juan R, et al. Risk factors for invasive aspergillosis in solid-organ transplant recipients: a case-control study. Clin Infect Dis 2005; 41:52–9.

54. Singh N, Paterson DL. Aspergillus infections in transplant recipients. Clin Microbiol Rev 2005;18:44–69.

55. Singh N, Paterson DL, Gayowski T, et al. Preemptive prophylaxis with a lipid preparation of amphotericin B for invasive fungal infections in liver transplant recipients requiring renal replacement therapy. Transplantation 2001;71:910–3.

56. Fortun J, Martin-Davila P, Moreno S, et al. Risk factors for invasive aspergillosis in liver transplant recipients. Liver Transpl 2002;8:1065–70.

57. Singh N, Avery RK, Munoz P, et al. Trends in risk profiles for and mortality associated with invasive aspergillosis among liver transplant recipients. Clin Infect Dis 2003;36:46–52.

58. Cahill BC, Hibbs JR, Savik K, et al. Aspergillus airway colonization and invasive disease after lung transplantation. Chest 1997;112:1160–4.

59. Nunley DR, Ohori P, Grgurich WF, et al. Pulmonary aspergillosis in cystic fibrosis lung transplant recipients. Chest 1998;114:1321–9.

60. Helmi M, Love RB, Welter D, et al. Aspergillus infection in lung transplant recipients with cystic fibrosis: risk factors and outcomes comparison to other types of transplant recipients. Chest 2003;123:800–8.

61. Blair JE. Coccidioidomycosis in patients who have undergone transplantation. Ann N Y Acad Sci 2007;1111:365–76.

62. Blair JE, Logan JL. Coccidioidomycosis in solid organ transplantation. Clin Infect Dis 2001;33:1536–44.

63. Keckich DW, Blair JE, Vikram HR, et al. Reactivation of coccidioidomycosis despite antifungal prophylaxis in solid organ transplant recipients. Transplantation 2011;92:88–93.

64. Baddley JW, Forrest GN, AST Infectious Diseases Community of Practice. Cryptococcosis in solid organ transplantation. Am J Transplant 2013;13(Suppl 4): 242–9.

65. Singh N, Alexander BD, Lortholary O, et al. Cryptococcus neoformans in organ transplant recipients: impact of calcineurin-inhibitor agents on mortality. J Infect Dis 2007;195:756–64.

66. Baddley JW, Perfect JR, Oster RA, et al. Pulmonary cryptococcosis in patients without HIV infection: factors associated with disseminated disease. Eur J Clin Microbiol Infect Dis 2008;27:937–43.

67. Diamond RD, Bennett JE. Prognostic factors in cryptococcal meningitis. A study in 111 cases. Ann Intern Med 1974;80:176–81.

68. Dromer F, Mathoulin S, Dupont B, et al. Individual and environmental factors associated with infection due to Cryptococcus neoformans serotype D. French Cryptococcosis Study Group. Clin Infect Dis 1996;23:91–6.

69. Pappas PG, Perfect JR, Cloud GA, et al. Cryptococcosis in human immunodeficiency virus-negative patients in the era of effective azole therapy. Clin Infect Dis 2001;33:690–9.
70. Silveira FP, Husain S, Kwak EJ, et al. Cryptococcosis in liver and kidney transplant recipients receiving anti-thymocyte globulin or alemtuzumab. Transpl Infect Dis 2007;9:22–7.
71. Wingard JR. The changing face of invasive fungal infections in hematopoietic cell transplant recipients. Curr Opin Oncol 2005;17:89–92.
72. Richardson M, Lass-Florl C. Changing epidemiology of systemic fungal infections. Clin Microbiol Infect 2008;14(Suppl 4):5–24.
73. Barnes PD, Marr KA. Risks, diagnosis and outcomes of invasive fungal infections in haematopoietic stem cell transplant recipients. Br J Haematol 2007; 139:519–31.
74. Fleming RV, Walsh TJ, Anaissie EJ. Emerging and less common fungal pathogens. Infect Dis Clin North Am 2002;16:915–33.
75. Kontoyiannis DP, Lewis RE. Invasive zygomycosis: update on pathogenesis, clinical manifestations, and management. Infect Dis Clin North Am 2006;20:581–607.
76. Siwek GT, Dodgson KJ, de Magalhaes-Silverman M, et al. Invasive zygomycosis in hematopoietic stem cell transplant recipients receiving voriconazole prophylaxis. Clin Infect Dis 2004;39:584–7.
77. Marty FM, Cosimi LA, Baden LR. Breakthrough zygomycosis after voriconazole treatment in recipients of hematopoietic stem-cell transplants. N Engl J Med 2004;350:950–2.
78. Martin SI, Marty FM, Fiumara K, et al. Infectious complications associated with alemtuzumab use for lymphoproliferative disorders. Clin Infect Dis 2006;43:16–24.
79. Fishman JA. Prevention of infection caused by Pneumocystis carinii in transplant recipients. Clin Infect Dis 2001;33:1397–405.
80. Lufft V, Kliem V, Behrend M, et al. Incidence of Pneumocystis carinii pneumonia after renal transplantation. Impact of immunosuppression. Transplantation 1996; 62:421–3.
81. Arend SM, Westendorp RG, Kroon FP, et al. Rejection treatment and cytomegalovirus infection as risk factors for Pneumocystis carinii pneumonia in renal transplant recipients. Clin Infect Dis 1996;22:920–5.
82. Conces DJ Jr. Endemic fungal pneumonia in immunocompromised patients. J Thorac Imaging 1999;14:1–8.
83. Lease ED, Alexander BD. Fungal diagnostics in pneumonia. Semin Respir Crit Care Med 2011;32:663–72.
84. Tarrand JJ, Lichterfeld M, Warraich I, et al. Diagnosis of invasive septate mold infections. A correlation of microbiological culture and histologic or cytologic examination. Am J Clin Pathol 2003;119:854–8.
85. Kontoyiannis DP, Wessel VC, Bodey GP, et al. Zygomycosis in the 1990s in a tertiary-care cancer center. Clin Infect Dis 2000;30:851–6.
86. Singh N, Alexander BD, Lortholary O, et al. Pulmonary cryptococcosis in solid organ transplant recipients: clinical relevance of serum cryptococcal antigen. Clin Infect Dis 2008;46:e12–8.
87. Williams B, Fojtasek M, Connolly-Stringfield P, et al. Diagnosis of histoplasmosis by antigen detection during an outbreak in Indianapolis, Ind. Arch Pathol Lab Med 1994;118:1205–8.
88. Wheat LJ, Conces D, Allen SD, et al. Pulmonary histoplasmosis syndromes: recognition, diagnosis, and management. Semin Respir Crit Care Med 2004; 25:129–44.

89. Hage CA, Ribes JA, Wengenack NL, et al. A multicenter evaluation of tests for diagnosis of histoplasmosis. Clin Infect Dis 2011;53:448–54.
90. Blair JE, Coakley B, Santelli AC, et al. Serologic testing for symptomatic coccidioidomycosis in immunocompetent and immunosuppressed hosts. Mycopathologia 2006;162:317–24.
91. DiTomasso JP, Ampel NM, Sobonya RE, et al. Bronchoscopic diagnosis of pulmonary coccidioidomycosis. Comparison of cytology, culture, and transbronchial biopsy. Diagn Microbiol Infect Dis 1994;18:83–7.
92. Pfeiffer CD, Fine JP, Safdar N. Diagnosis of invasive aspergillosis using a galactomannan assay: a meta-analysis. Clin Infect Dis 2006;42:1417–27.
93. Alexander BD, Smith PB, Davis RD, et al. The (1,3){beta}-D-glucan test as an aid to early diagnosis of invasive fungal infections following lung transplantation. J Clin Microbiol 2010;48:4083–8.
94. Starkey J, Moritani T, Kirby P. MRI of CNS fungal infections: review of aspergillosis to histoplasmosis and everything in between. Clin Neuroradiol 2014;24: 217–30.
95. McMullan BJ, Sorrell TC, Chen SC. Cryptococcus gattii infections: contemporary aspects of epidemiology, clinical manifestations and management of infection. Future Microbiol 2013;8:1613–31.
96. Husain S, Wagener MM, Singh N. Cryptococcus neoformans infection in organ transplant recipients: variables influencing clinical characteristics and outcome. Emerg Infect Dis 2001;7:375–81.
97. Wu G, Vilchez RA, Eidelman B, et al. Cryptococcal meningitis: an analysis among 5,521 consecutive organ transplant recipients. Transpl Infect Dis 2002; 4:183–8.
98. Grim SA, Proia L, Miller R, et al. A multicenter study of histoplasmosis and blastomycosis after solid organ transplantation. Transpl Infect Dis 2012;14:17–23.
99. Holt CD, Winston DJ, Kubak B, et al. Coccidioidomycosis in liver transplant patients. Clin Infect Dis 1997;24:216–21.
100. Johnson RH, Einstein HE. Coccidioidal meningitis. Clin Infect Dis 2006;42: 103–7.
101. Wheat LJ, Batteiger BE, Sathapatayavongs B. Histoplasma capsulatum infections of the central nervous system. A clinical review. Medicine (Baltimore) 1990;69:244–60.
102. Wheat LJ, Kohler RB, Tewari RP, et al. Significance of Histoplasma antigen in the cerebrospinal fluid of patients with meningitis. Arch Intern Med 1989;149:302–4.
103. Wheat LJ, Connolly-Stringfield PA, Baker RL, et al. Disseminated histoplasmosis in the acquired immune deficiency syndrome: clinical findings, diagnosis and treatment, and review of the literature. Medicine (Baltimore) 1990;69:361–74.
104. Ordonez N, Arango M, Gomez B, et al. The value of immunological assays in the diagnosis of meningeal histoplasmosis. Rev Neurol 1997;25:1376–80 [in Spanish].
105. Zaoutis TE, Webber S, Naftel DC, et al. Invasive fungal infections in pediatric heart transplant recipients: incidence, risk factors, and outcomes. Pediatr Transplant 2011;15:465–9.
106. Zicker M, Colombo AL, Ferraz-Neto BH, et al. Epidemiology of fungal infections in liver transplant recipients: a six-year study of a large Brazilian liver transplantation centre. Mem Inst Oswaldo Cruz 2011;106:339–45.
107. Aldape KD, Fox HS, Roberts JP, et al. Cladosporium trichoides cerebral phaeohyphomycosis in a liver transplant recipient. Report of a case. Am J Clin Pathol 1991;95:499–502.

108. Vukmir RB, Kusne S, Linden P, et al. Successful therapy for cerebral phaeohyphomycosis due to Dactylaria gallopava in a liver transplant recipient. Clin Infect Dis 1994;19:714–9.
109. Revankar SG, Sutton DA, Rinaldi MG. Primary central nervous system phaeohyphomycosis: a review of 101 cases. Clin Infect Dis 2004;38:206–16.
110. Levin TP, Baty DE, Fekete T, et al. Cladophialophora bantiana brain abscess in a solid-organ transplant recipient: case report and review of the literature. J Clin Microbiol 2004;42:4374–8.
111. Erdogan E, Beyzadeoglu M, Arpaci F, et al. Cerebellar aspergillosis: case report and literature review. Neurosurgery 2002;50:874–6 [discussion: 876–7].
112. Almyroudis NG, Sutton DA, Linden P, et al. Zygomycosis in solid organ transplant recipients in a tertiary transplant center and review of the literature. Am J Transplant 2006;6:2365–74.
113. Singh N, Aguado JM, Bonatti H, et al. Zygomycosis in solid organ transplant recipients: a prospective, matched case-control study to assess risks for disease and outcome. J Infect Dis 2009;200:1002–11.
114. Virgili A, Zampino MR, Mantovani L. Fungal skin infections in organ transplant recipients. Am J Clin Dermatol 2002;3:19–35.
115. Lima AM, Rocha SP, Reis Filho EG, et al. Study of dermatoses in kidney transplant patients. An Bras Dermatol 2013;88:361–7.
116. Bernardeschi C, Foulet F, Ingen-Housz-Oro S, et al. Cutaneous invasive aspergillosis: retrospective multicenter study of the French invasive-aspergillosis registry and literature review. Medicine (Baltimore) 2015;94:e1018.
117. Chakrabarti A, Gupta V, Biswas G, et al. Primary cutaneous aspergillosis: our experience in 10 years. J Infect 1998;37:24–7.
118. Galimberti R, Kowalczuk A, Hidalgo Parra I, et al. Cutaneous aspergillosis: a report of six cases. Br J Dermatol 1998;139:522–6.
119. Sun HY, Alexander BD, Lortholary O, et al. Cutaneous cryptococcosis in solid organ transplant recipients. Med Mycol 2010;48:785–91.
120. Biancheri D, Kanitakis J, Bienvenu AL, et al. Cutaneous cryptococcosis in solid organ transplant recipients: epidemiological, clinical, diagnostic and therapeutic features. Eur J Dermatol 2012;22:651–7.
121. Zorman JV, Zupanc TL, Parac Z, et al. Primary cutaneous cryptococcosis in a renal transplant recipient: case report. Mycoses 2010;53:535–7.
122. Neuville S, Dromer F, Morin O, et al. Primary cutaneous cryptococcosis: a distinct clinical entity. Clin Infect Dis 2003;36:337–47.
123. Mitchell TG, Perfect JR. Cryptococcosis in the era of AIDS–100 years after the discovery of Cryptococcus neoformans. Clin Microbiol Rev 1995;8:515–48.
124. Baer S, Baddley JW, Gnann JW, et al. Cryptococcal disease presenting as necrotizing cellulitis in transplant recipients. Transpl Infect Dis 2009;11:353–8.
125. Yoneda T, Itami Y, Hirayama A, et al. Cryptococcal necrotizing fasciitis in a patient after renal transplantation–a case report. Transplant Proc 2014;46:620–2.
126. Anderson DJ, Schmidt C, Goodman J, et al. Cryptococcal disease presenting as cellulitis. Clin Infect Dis 1992;14:666–72.
127. Dall Bello AG, Severo CB, Schio S, et al. First reported case of cellulitis due to Cryptococcus gattii in lung transplantation recipient: a case report. Dermatol Online J 2013;19:20395.
128. Pagano L, Valentini CG, Posteraro B, et al. Zygomycosis in Italy: a survey of FIMUA-ECMM (Federazione Italiana di Micopatologia Umana ed Animale and European Confederation of Medical Mycology). J Chemother 2009;21:322–9.

129. Bitar D, Van Cauteren D, Lanternier F, et al. Increasing incidence of zygomycosis (mucormycosis), France, 1997-2006. Emerg Infect Dis 2009;15:1395–401.
130. Torres-Narbona M, Guinea J, Martinez-Alarcon J, et al. Impact of zygomycosis on microbiology workload: a survey study in Spain. J Clin Microbiol 2007;45:2051–3.
131. Petrikkos G, Skiada A, Lortholary O, et al. Epidemiology and clinical manifestations of mucormycosis. Clin Infect Dis 2012;54(Suppl 1):S23–34.
132. Roden MM, Zaoutis TE, Buchanan WL, et al. Epidemiology and outcome of zygomycosis: a review of 929 reported cases. Clin Infect Dis 2005;41:634–53.
133. Garcia-Pajares F, Sanchez-Antolin G, Almohalla Alvarez C, et al. Cutaneous mucormycosis infection by Absidia in two consecutive liver transplant patients. Transplant Proc 2012;44:1562–4.
134. Ashkenazi-Hoffnung L, Bilavsky E, Avitzur Y, et al. Successful treatment of cutaneous zygomycosis with intravenous amphotericin B followed by oral posaconazole in a multivisceral transplant recipient. Transplantation 2010;90:1133–5.
135. McCarty TP, Baddley JW, Walsh TJ, et al. Phaeohyphomycosis in transplant recipients: results from the Transplant Associated Infection Surveillance Network (TRANSNET). Med Mycol 2015;53:440–6.
136. Patel U, Chu J, Patel R, et al. Subcutaneous dematiaceous fungal infection. Dermatol Online J 2011;17:19.
137. Hadley S, Samore MH, Lewis WD, et al. Major infectious complications after orthotopic liver transplantation and comparison of outcomes in patients receiving cyclosporine or FK506 as primary immunosuppression. Transplantation 1995;59:851–9.
138. Marik PE. Fungal infections in solid organ transplantation. Expert Opin Pharmacother 2006;7:297–305.
139. Berenguer J, Buck M, Witebsky F, et al. Lysis-centrifugation blood cultures in the detection of tissue-proven invasive candidiasis. Disseminated versus single-organ infection. Diagn Microbiol Infect Dis 1993;17:103–9.
140. Obayashi T, Negishi K, Suzuki T, et al. Reappraisal of the serum (1–>3)-beta-D-glucan assay for the diagnosis of invasive fungal infections–a study based on autopsy cases from 6 years. Clin Infect Dis 2008;46:1864–70.
141. Odabasi Z, Mattiuzzi G, Estey E, et al. Beta-D-glucan as a diagnostic adjunct for invasive fungal infections: validation, cutoff development, and performance in patients with acute myelogenous leukemia and myelodysplastic syndrome. Clin Infect Dis 2004;39:199–205.
142. Ostrosky-Zeichner L, Alexander BD, Kett DH, et al. Multicenter clinical evaluation of the (1–>3) beta-D-glucan assay as an aid to diagnosis of fungal infections in humans. Clin Infect Dis 2005;41:654–9.
143. Miller R, Assi M, AST Infectious Diseases Community of Practice. Endemic fungal infections in solid organ transplantation. Am J Transplant 2013;13(Suppl 4):250–61.
144. Pappas PG, Kauffman CA, Andes D, et al. Clinical practice guidelines for the management of candidiasis: 2009 update by the Infectious Diseases Society of America. Clin Infect Dis 2009;48:503–35.
145. Riddell Jt, Comer GM, Kauffman CA. Treatment of endogenous fungal endophthalmitis: focus on new antifungal agents. Clin Infect Dis 2011;52:648–53.
146. Groll AH, Mickiene D, Petraitis V, et al. Compartmental pharmacokinetics and tissue distribution of the antifungal echinocandin lipopeptide micafungin (FK463) in rabbits. Antimicrob Agents Chemother 2001;45:3322–7.

147. Groll AH, Gullick BM, Petraitiene R, et al. Compartmental pharmacokinetics of the antifungal echinocandin caspofungin (MK-0991) in rabbits. Antimicrob Agents Chemother 2001;45:596–600.

148. Groll AH, Mickiene D, Petraitiene R, et al. Pharmacokinetic and pharmacodynamic modeling of anidulafungin (LY303366): reappraisal of its efficacy in neutropenic animal models of opportunistic mycoses using optimal plasma sampling. Antimicrob Agents Chemother 2001;45:2845–55.

Index

Note: Page numbers of article titles are in **boldface** type.

A

ABPA. *See* Allergic bronchopulmonary aspergillosis (ABPA)
Abscess(es)
  brain
    dematiaceous molds and, 172–173
    in SOT recipients, 284–285
Acute disseminated candidiasis
  IC and, 109
Acute pulmonary blastomycosis, 250–251
Acute pulmonary histoplasmosis, 210
  treatment of, 220
Adenitis
  mediastinal
    histoplasmosis presenting as, 212, 214
      nontreatment for, 221
AIDS/HIV patients
  blastomycosis effects in, 255
Allergic bronchopulmonary aspergillosis (ABPA), 129–130
  dematiaceous molds and, 172
Allergic disease
  dematiaceous molds and, 171–172
AmB. *See* Amphotericin B (AmB)
Amphotericin B (AmB)
  in coccidioidomycosis management, 237–238
  in IC management, 115
  in invasive aspergillosis management, 135–136
Antibody testing
  in fungal disease, 39
  in histoplasmosis, 219
Antifungal agents, **51–83**. *See also* Polyene(s); *specific types and agents, e.g.,* Azole(s)
  azoles, 60–68
  in coccidioidomycosis management, 237–241
  echinocandins, 68–70
  empiric
    in SOT recipients, 287–288
  evolution of, 51–52
  flucytosine, 59–60
  introduction, 51–52
  in mucormycoses management, 151–152
  pharmacologic considerations, 53
  polyenes, 53–59

Infect Dis Clin N Am 30 (2016) 297–312
http://dx.doi.org/10.1016/S0891-5520(16)00009-X
0891-5520/16/$ – see front matter © 2016 Elsevier Inc. All rights reserved.

id.theclinics.com

Antifungal resistance
  to invasive aspergillosis, 136–137
  trends in
    in fungal identification, 23–25
Antifungal susceptibility testing
  in fungal identification, 18–23
  in IC, 106–108
Antigen(s)
  in fungal disease
    detection of, 39–43 (See also specific types)
      Aspergillus GM, 39, 42
      BDG, 39
      cryptococcal antigen, 42
      for dimorphic fungi, 42
      histology and special stains, 43
Antigen testing
  in blastomycosis, 256–257
  in histoplasmosis, 217–219
Arthritis
  IC and, 109–110
Aspergilloma, 129
Aspergillosis. See also Invasive aspergillosis
  allergic bronchopulmonary, 129–130
  clinical manifestations of, 129
  CNS, 132
  epidemiology of, 126–128
  host susceptibility to, 128–129
  invasive, 125–142 (See also Invasive aspergillosis)
  mycology of, 126–128
  noninvasive disease, 129–130
  ocular, 131–132
  pulmonary
    chronic forms of, 130
    invasive, 130–131
  in SOT recipients, 285
  spectrum of, 125–126
  tracheobronchial, 131
Aspergillosis rhinosinusitis, 131
Aspergillus galactomannan (GM)
  detection of, 39, 42
Aspergillus spp.
  A. fumigatus
    azole resistance to, 24–25
  A. osteomyelitis, 132
  fungal diseases due to
    global burden of, 4
Azole(s), 60–68
  clinical indications for, 65–67
  in coccidioidomycosis management, 238–239
  described, 60–61
  drug–drug interactions with, 67–68

pharmacology of, 62–65
resistance of, 61–62
    to *Aspergillus fumigatus,* 24–25
spectrum of activity and resistance, 61–62
toxicities of, 67

B

BDG. *See* (1,3)-β-D-Glucan (BDG)
Blastomyces dermatitidis
    fungal diseases due to
        global burden of, 6
Blastomycosis, **247–264**
    in children, 256
        treatment of, 260
    clinical manifestations of, 250–255
        acute pulmonary blastomycosis, 250–251
        chronic pulmonary blastomycosis, 251–252
        extrapulmonary blastomycosis, 252–255
    CNS
        treatment of, 259
    diagnosis of, 256–257
    disseminated
        treatment of, 257–259
    epidemiology of, 248–249
    extrapulmonary, 252–255
    in immunosuppressed patients
        treatment of, 259–260
    introduction, 247–248
    mortality data, 260
    outcomes of, 260
    pathogenesis of, 249–250
    in pregnancy, 256
        treatment of, 260
    pulmonary
        acute, 250–251
        chronic, 251–252
        treatment of, 257–259
    in special populations, 255–256
    treatment of, 257–260
Brain abscess
    dematiaceous molds and, 172–173
    in SOT recipients, 284–285
Breakthrough infections
    invasive aspergillosis–related, 137
Broncholithiasis
    histoplasmosis presenting as, 215

C

Candida glabrata
    echinocandin resistance in, 23–24

Candida infections, **85–102**
  global burden of, 2–3
  introduction, 85–86
  monogenic inheritance of, 86–93
    CMC associated with primary immunodeficiencies, 92
    HIES, 87–92
    invasive infections, 92–93
    isolated CMC, 86–87
    syndromic CMC, 87–92
  polygenic inheritance of, 93–96
Candidemia
  IC and, 108
Candidiasis
  acute disseminated
    IC and, 109
  chronic disseminated
    IC and, 110
  chronic mucocutaneous (*See* Chronic mucocutaneous candidiasis (CMC))
  hepatosplenic
    IC and, 110
  invasive, **103–124** (*See also* Invasive candidiasis (IC))
  neonatal
    IC and, 108–109
Central nervous system (CNS)
  aspergillosis effects on, 132
  blastomycosis effects on, 255
    treatment of, 259
  cryptococcosis effects on, 185–186
Central nervous system (CNS) infections
  in SOT recipients, 283–285
Children
  blastomycosis effects in, 256
    treatment of, 260
Chronic disseminated candidiasis
  IC and, 110
Chronic mucocutaneous candidiasis (CMC)
  isolated, 86–87
  primary immunodeficiencies and, 92
  syndromic, 87–92
Chronic pulmonary blastomycosis, 251–252
Chronic pulmonary histoplasmosis, 210
  treatment of, 220
CMC. *See* Chronic mucocutaneous candidiasis (CMC)
CNS. *See* Central nervous system (CNS)
Coccidioidal meningitis, 235–236
Coccidioides spp.
  C. immitis
    fungal diseases due to
      global burden of, 5–6
  C. posadasii
    fungal diseases due to

      global burden of, 5–6
Coccidioidomycosis, **229–246**
   clinical manifestations of, 232–237
      diffuse pneumonia, 233–234
      extrapulmonary disease, 235
      meningitis, 235–236
      primary pulmonary infection, 232–233
      residual nodule, cavity, and chronic infiltrates, 234–235
   described, 232
   diagnosis of, 230–232
   epidemiology of, 230
   in immunocompromised patients, 236–237
   introduction, 229–230
   treatment of, 237–241
      AmB in, 237–238
      antifungal agents in, 237–241
      azoles in, 238–239
      echinocandins in, 240
      future therapies in, 240–241
      IFN-γ in, 240
      isavuconazole in, 240
      posaconazole in, 239–240
      voriconazole in, 239–240
CRAG. *See* Cryptococcal antigen (CRAG)
Cryptococcal antigen (CRAG)
   detection of, 42
Cryptococcal antigen (CRAG) lateral flow assay
   in fungal identification, 17–18
Cryptococcosis, **179–206**
   causes of, 180–182
   clinical manifestations of, 184–188
      CNS infection, 185–186
      eye infection, 186
      IRIS, 187–188
      prostate infection, 186
      pulmonary infection, 184–185
      skin infection, 186
   epidemiology of, 182–184
   host immunity to, 182–184
   introduction, 179–180
   laboratory diagnosis of, 188–190
   pathogenesis of, 182–184
   risk factors for, 182–184
   in SOT recipients, 286
   treatment of, 190–196
      antiretroviral therapy in
         timing of, 192–193
      basic principles in, 190–192
      ICP management in, 193–194
      in non–HIV-infected, nontransplant patients, 193
      in nonmeningeal disease, 194–195

Cryptococcosis (*continued*)
    in organ transplant recipients, 193
    for persistent and relapsed infection, 194
    prevention-related, 195–196
    screening in, 195–196
Cryptococcus spp.
    C. gattii
        cryptococcosis due to, 180–182
    C. neoformans
        cryptococcosis due to, 180–182
    infections due to
        global burden of, 3–4

D

Dematiaceous
    defined, 165
Dematiaceous molds, **165–178**
    clinical syndromes, 168–174 (*See also specific syndromes, e.g.,* Onychomycosis)
        ABPA, 172
        allergic disease, 171–172
        brain abscess, 172–173
        disseminated infection, 173
        keratitis, 170
        onychomycosis, 169
        pneumonia, 172
        subcutaneous lesions, 170
        superficial infections, 169–171
    diagnosis of, 167
    introduction, 165–166
    mycology of, 166
    pathogenesis of, 167
    treatment of, 168–174
    in vitro susceptibility to, 167–168
Diffuse pneumonia
    coccidioidomycosis presenting as, 233–234
Disseminated blastomycosis
    treatment of, 257–259
Disseminated candidiasis
    acute
        IC and, 109
Disseminated histoplasmosis, 215
    progressive
        treatment of, 220–221
Disseminated infection
    dematiaceous molds and, 173
DNA sequence analysis
    in fungal identification, 14–15

E

Echinocandin(s), 68–70
　clinical indications for, 69
　in coccidioidomycosis management, 240
　described, 68
　drug–drug interactions with, 69–70
　in IC management, 111, 114
　in invasive aspergillosis management, 135
　pharmacology of, 68–69
　resistance of
　　to *Candida glabrata,* 23–24
　spectrum of activity and resistance, 68
　toxicities of, 69
Endemic molds
　fungal diseases due to
　　global burden of, 5–6
　　　Blastomyces dermatitidis, 6
　　　Coccidioides immitis and *Coccidioides posadasii,* 5–6
　　　Histoplasma capsulatum, 5
　　　Paracoccidioides brasiliensis, 6
　　　Talatomyces marneffei, 6
Endophthalmitis
　IC and, 110
Endovascular infection
　IC and, 109
Eumycetoma
　organisms causing, 6
Extrapulmonary blastomycosis, 252–255
Extrapulmonary coccidioidomycosis, 235
Eye infections. *See entries under* Ocular

F

Fibrosis
　mediastinal
　　histoplasmosis presenting as, 214
　　　nontreatment for, 222
Fluconazole
　clinical indications for, 65
　pharmacology of, 62
　spectrum of activity and resistance, 61
Flucytosine, 59–60
Frontal lobe lesions with sinus disease
　in SOT recipients, 285
Fungal diseases. *See also* Fungal infections
　global burden of, **1–11** (*See also specific diseases and causes*)
　　emerging pathogens, 7
　　eumycetoma, 6
　　introduction, 1–2

Fungal (*continued*)
    molds, 4–6
    PCP, 4
    yeasts, 2–4
  nonculture diagnostics in, **37–49**
    antibody detection, 39–43
    introduction, 37
    nucleic acid techniques, 43–46
Fungal identification
  in clinical setting, 14–16
    MALDI-TOF MS in, 15–16
    morphologic/phenotypic characteristics and DNA sequence analysis in, 14–15
  CRAG lateral flow assay in, 17–18
  direct specimens in, 16–18
  introduction, 13–14
  susceptibility testing in, 18–23
  trends in antifungal resistance in, 23–25
  T2-weighted MRI in, 17
  update on, **13–25**
Fungal infections. *See also specific types and* Fungal diseases
  prevention and management of
    contemporary strategies in, **265–275** (*See also specific infections, e.g.,* Invasive
      candidiasis (IC))
    IC, 266–268
    introduction, 265–266
    invasive aspergillosis, 268
    mucormycoses, 269–271
  suspected
    in SOT recipients, **277–296**
      aspergillosis, 285
      brain abscess, 284–285
      CNS infections, 283–285
      cryptococcosis, 286
      cutaneous manifestations of, 285–287
      empiric anti fungal agents for, 287–288
      epidemiology of, 278
      frontal lobe lesions with sinus disease, 285
      introduction, 277–278
      meningitis, 283–284
      mucormycoses, 286
      phaeohyphomycosis, 287
      pulmonary fungal infections, 281–283
      pulmonary GGOs, 282–283
      recognition of, 281–287
      risk factors for, 279–281
      sepsis syndrome, 287
      timing of, 278–279
Fungal sinusitis, 171–172
Fungus(i)
  dimorphic
    antigen detection for, 42

identification of, **13–25** (*See also* Fungal identification)
Fusarium spp.
    fungal diseases due to
        global burden of, 5

G

Galactomannan (GM)
    Aspergillus
        detection of, 39, 42
Genitourinary tract
    blastomycosis effects on, 254
Genus/species–specific approaches
    in fungal disease detection, 44–45
GGOs. *See* Ground-glass opacities (GGOs)
(1,3)-β-D-Glucan (BDG)
    detection of, 39
GM. *See* Galactomannan (GM)
Granuloma(s)
    mediastinal
        histoplasmosis presenting as, 214
            nontreatment for, 222
Ground-glass opacities (GGOs)
    pulmonary
        in SOT recipients, 282–283

H

Hepatosplenic candidiasis
    IC and, 110
HIES. *See* Hyper–immunoglobulin (Ig) E syndrome (HIES)
Histoplasma capsulatum
    fungal diseases due to
        global burden of, 5
Histoplasmoma, 214
Histoplasmosis, **207–227**
    clinical presentations of, 210–215
        acute pulmonary histoplasmosis, 210
            treatment of, 220
        broncholithiasis, 215
        chronic pulmonary histoplasmosis, 210
            treatment of, 220
        disseminated histoplasmosis, 215
            treatment of, 220–221
        histoplasmoma, 214
        mediastinal adenitis, 212, 214
        mediastinal fibrosis, 214
            nontreatment for, 222
        mediastinal granuloma, 214
            nontreatment for, 222
        mediastinal lymphadenopathy, 212, 214

Histoplasmosis (*continued*)
    nontreatment for, 221
    presumed ocular histoplasmosis, 215
      nontreatment for, 222
    pulmonary nodules, 210, 212
      nontreatment for, 221
    subacute pulmonary histoplasmosis, 210
      nontreatment for, 221
    untreated, 221–222
  diagnosis of, 215–219
    antibody testing in, 219
    antigen testing in, 217–219
    culture in, 217
    molecular, 219
    pathology in, 215–217
  disseminated, 215
  epidemiology of, 208
  introduction, 207
  ocular
    presumed, 215
      nontreatment for, 222
  pathogenesis of, 208–210
  pulmonary (*See* Pulmonary histoplasmosis)
  treatment of, 219–222
    manifestations usually treated, 220–221
HIV/AIDS patients
  blastomycosis effects in, 255
Hyper–immunoglobulin (Ig) E syndrome (HIES), 87–92

I

IC. *See* Invasive candidiasis (IC)
ICP. *See* Intracranial pressure (ICP)
IFN-γ. *See* Interferon gamma (IFN-γ) therapy
Immune reconstitution inflammatory syndrome (IRIS)
  cryptococcosis and, 187–188
Immunocompromised patients
  blastomycosis in, 255
  coccidioidomycosis in, 236–237
Immunodeficiency(ies)
  primary
    CMC associated with, 92
Immunosuppressed patients
  blastomycosis in
    treatment of, 259–260
Infection(s). *See specific types, e.g., Candida* infections
Interferon gamma (IFN-γ) therapy
  in coccidioidomycosis management, 240
Intracranial pressure (ICP)
  management of
    in cryptococcosis treatment, 193–194

Invasive aspergillosis, **125–142**. *See also* Aspergillosis
    antifungal resistance to, 136–137
    aspergillosis rhinosinusitis, 131
    Aspergillus osteomyelitis, 132
    breakthrough infections, 137
    clinical manifestations of, 129
    CNS aspergillosis, 132
    diagnosis of, 132–133
    epidemiology of, 126–128
    extrapulmonary involvement in, 131
    host susceptibility to, 128–129
    introduction, 125–126
    invasive pulmonary aspergillosis, 130–131
    mycology of, 126–128
    ocular aspergillosis, 131–132
    prevention and management of
        contemporary strategies in, 268
    TA, 131
    treatment of, 133–136
        AmB in, 135–136
        combination therapy in, 136
        echinocandins in, 135
        isavuconazole in, 135
        itraconazole in, 135
        posoconazole in, 134–135
        triazoles in, 133–134
        voriconazole in, 134
Invasive candidiasis (IC), **103–124**
    antifungal susceptibility testing in, 106–108
    clinical manifestations of, 108–110
    diagnosis of, 105–106
    epidemiology of, 103–104
    introduction, 103
    pathogenesis of, 105
    prevention and management of, 111–116
        AmB in, 115
        contemporary strategies in, 266–268
            fever or diagnostic-driven approaches, 266
            pharmacologic prevention, 266
            targeted treatment, 267–268
        echinocandins in, 111, 114
        empiric therapy in, 115
        general principles of, 111
        triazoles in, 114–115
Invasive pulmonary aspergillosis, 130–131
IRIS. *See* Immune reconstitution inflammatory syndrome (IRIS)
Isavuconazole
    clinical indications for, 67
    in coccidioidomycosis management, 240
    in invasive aspergillosis management, 135
    pharmacology of, 64–65

Isavuconazole (*continued*)
    spectrum of activity and resistance, 62
Isolated chronic mucocutaneous candidiasis (CMC), 86–87
Itraconazole
    clinical indications for, 65–66
    in invasive aspergillosis management, 135
    pharmacology of, 62–63
    spectrum of activity and resistance, 61

K

Keratitis, 170

L

Lymphadenopathy
    mediastinal
        histoplasmosis presenting as, 212, 214
            nontreatment for, 221

M

Magnetic resonance imaging (MRI)
    T2-weighted
        in fungal identification, 17
MALDI-TOF MS. *See* Matrix-assisted laser desorption/ionization time-of-flight mass
    spectrometry (MALDI-TOF MS)
Matrix-assisted laser desorption/ionization time-of-flight mass spectrometry
    (MALDI-TOF MS)
    in fungal identification, 15–16
Mediastinal adenitis
    histoplasmosis presenting as, 212, 214
        nontreatment for, 221
Mediastinal fibrosis
    histoplasmosis presenting as, 214
        nontreatment for, 222
Mediastinal granuloma
    histoplasmosis presenting as, 214
        nontreatment for, 222
Mediastinal lymphadenopathy
    histoplasmosis presenting as, 212, 214
        nontreatment for, 221
Meningitis
    coccidioidal, 235–236
    in SOT recipients, 283–284
Mold(s)
    dematiaceous, **165–178** (*See also* Dematiaceous molds)
    fungal diseases due to
        global burden of, 4–6
            Aspergillus, 4
            endemic molds, 5–6 (*See also* Endemic molds)

Fusarium, 5
Mucormycetes, 5
Scedosporium, 5
Molecular markers of resistance
  detection of
    in fungal disease detection, 45–46
MRI. *See* Magnetic resonance imaging (MRI)
Mucormycetes spp.
  fungal diseases due to
    global burden of, 5
Mucormycosis(es), **143–163**
  clinical manifestations of, 147–148
  diagnosis of, 148–151
  epidemiology of, 144–145
  future directions related to, 153
  introduction, 143–144
  pathogenesis of, 145–147
  prevention and management of
    contemporary strategies in, 269–271
  in SOT recipients, 286
  treatment of
    adjunctive therapy in, 152–153
    antifungal agents in, 151–152

N

Neonatal candidiasis
  IC and, 108–109
Nodule(s)
  pulmonary
    histoplasmosis presenting as, 210, 212
      nontreatment for, 221
    in SOT recipients, 281–282
Nucleic acid detection techniques
  in blastomycosis, 257
  in fungal disease, 43–46
    genus/species–specific approaches, 44–45
    molecular markers of resistance, 45–46
    pan-fungal approaches, 44

O

Ocular aspergillosis, 131–132
Ocular cryptococcosis, 186
Ocular histoplasmosis
  presumed, 215
    nontreatment for, 222
Onychomycosis, 169
Organ transplant recipients
  cryptococcosis in
    management of, 193

Osteoarticular structures
    blastomycosis effects on, 254
Osteomyelitis
    IC and, 109–110

P

Pan-fungal approaches
    in fungal disease detection, 44
Paracoccidioides brasiliensis
    fungal diseases due to
        global burden of, 6
PCP. *See Pneumocystis* pneumonia (PCP)
Phaeohyphomycosis
    in SOT recipients, 287
Pneumocystis pneumonia (PCP)
    global burden of, 4
Pneumonia(s)
    dematiaceous molds and, 172
    diffuse
        coccidioidomycosis presenting as, 233–234
    Pneumocystis
        global burden of, 4
Polyene(s), 53–59
    clinical indications for, 58
    described, 53
    drug–drug interactions with, 59
    pharmacology of, 53–55
    spectrum of activity and resistance, 53
    toxicities of, 58–59
Posaconazole
    clinical indications for, 67
    in coccidioidomycosis management, 239–240
    in invasive aspergillosis management, 134–135
    pharmacology of, 64
    spectrum of activity and resistance, 61
Pregnancy
    blastomycosis effects in, 256
        treatment of, 260
Presumed ocular histoplasmosis, 215
    nontreatment for, 222
Primary pulmonary infection
    coccidioidomycosis presenting as, 232–233
Progressive disseminated histoplasmosis
    treatment of, 220–221
Prostate infection
    cryptococcosis and, 186
Pulmonary aspergillosis
    chronic forms of, 130
    invasive, 130–131
Pulmonary blastomycosis

acute, 250–251
chronic, 251–252
treatment of, 257–259
Pulmonary fungal infections
    in SOT recipients, 281–283
Pulmonary ground-glass opacities (GGOs)
    in SOT recipients, 282–283
Pulmonary histoplasmosis
    acute, 210
        treatment of, 220
    chronic, 210
        treatment of, 220
    subacute, 210
        nontreatment for, 221
Pulmonary infection
    cryptococcosis and, 184–185
    primary
        coccidioidomycosis presenting as, 232–233
Pulmonary nodules
    histoplasmosis presenting as, 210, 212
        nontreatment for, 221
    in SOT recipients, 281–282

R

Rhinosinusitis
    aspergillosis, 131

S

Scedosporium spp.
    fungal diseases due to
        global burden of, 5
Sepsis syndrome
    invasive fungal infections causing
        in SOT recipients, 287
Sinus disease
    frontal lobe lesions with
        in SOT recipients, 285
Sinusitis
    fungal, 171–172
Skin
    blastomycosis effects on, 252–253
    invasive fungal infections effects on
        in SOT recipients, 285–287
Skin infection
    cryptococcosis and, 186
Solid organ transplant (SOT) recipients
    with suspected fungal infection
        approach to, **277–296** (*See also* Fungal infections, suspected, in SOT recipients)
SOT recipients. *See* Solid organ transplant (SOT) recipients

Subacute pulmonary histoplasmosis, 210
   nontreatment for, 221
Subcutaneous lesions
   dermatiaceous, 170
Susceptibility testing
   antifungal
      in fungal identification, 18–23
      in IC, 106–108
Syndromic chronic mucocutaneous candidiasis (CMC), 87–92

T

TA. *See* Tracheobronchial aspergillosis (TA)
Talatomyces marneffei
   fungal diseases due to
      global burden of, 6
Tracheobronchial aspergillosis (TA), 131
Transplant recipients
   blastomycosis in, 255
Triazole(s)
   in IC management, 114–115
   in invasive aspergillosis management, 133–134
Tumor necrosis factor–alpha (TNF–α) inhibitor therapy
   blastomycosis effects on, 255

V

Voriconazole
   clinical indications for, 66–67
   in coccidioidomycosis management, 239–240
   in invasive aspergillosis management, 134
   pharmacology of, 63–64
   spectrum of activity and resistance, 61

Y

Yeast(s)
   fungal diseases due to
      global burden of, 2–4
         Candida spp., 2–3
         Cryptococcus spp., 3–4

Moving?

Make sure your subscription moves with you!

To notify us of your new address, find your **Clinics Account Number** (located on your mailing label above your name), and contact customer service at:

Email: journalscustomerservice-usa@elsevier.com

800-654-2452 (subscribers in the U.S. & Canada)
314-447-8871 (subscribers outside of the U.S. & Canada)

Fax number: 314-447-8029

Elsevier Health Sciences Division
Subscription Customer Service
3251 Riverport Lane
Maryland Heights, MO 63043

*To ensure uninterrupted delivery of your subscription, please notify us at least 4 weeks in advance of move.

Printed and bound by CPI Group (UK) Ltd, Croydon, CR0 4YY

14/05/2025

01870847-0003